THE
FOODBIBLE

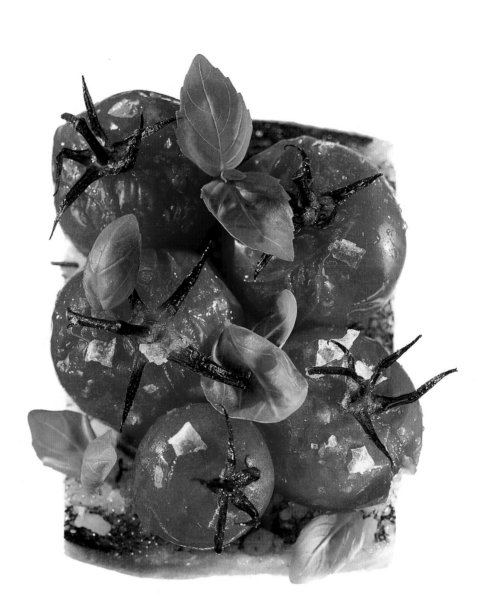

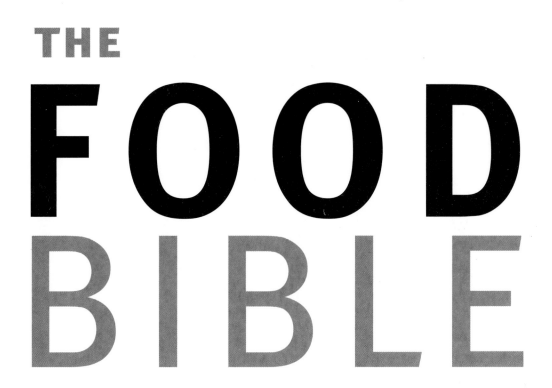

THE FOOD BIBLE

JUDITH WILLS

A Fireside Book
Published by Simon & Schuster

To Gail Pollard with thanks for her invaluable assistance, knowledge and advice.

The recipes in the book are for 2 people unless otherwise stated.

Throughout this book, the exact nutritional analysis of foods has been based on their weight in grams, but wherever possible we have also given the nearest approximate equivalent in everyday cup or spoon measures for ease of use.

The publishers recommend that you seek professional medical advice before following any of the dietary plans or remedies suggested in the book.

Art Director Mary Evans
Publishing Director Anne Furniss
Editor and Project Manager Lewis Esson
Art Editor Vanessa Courtier
Nutritionist Gail Pollard BSc, SRD
Photography Martin Brigdale, Gus Filgate, Patrick McLeavey
Home Economists Maxine Clarke, Zoe Sharp, Jane Stevenson, Nicole Szabason
Stylists Penny Markham, Luckie Smith, Helen Trent
Artwork Lynne Robinson
Production Candida Jackson, Vincent Smith
Typesetting Gina Hochstein, Peter Howard
American Editor Norma Macmillan
American Nutritionist Rita Zemaitis

F FIRESIDE
Rockefeller Center
1230 Avenue of the Americas
New York, NY 10020

Text copyright © 1998 by Judith Wills
Design and layout copyright © 1998 by Quadrille Publishing Ltd.
All rights reserved, including the right of reproduction in whole or in part in any form.

Published by arrangement with Quadrille Publishing Limited
First published in Great Britain in 1998 by Quadrille Publishing Limited

FIRESIDE and colophon are registered trademarks of Simon & Schuster Inc.

10 9 8 7 6 5 4 3 2 1

Library of Congress Cataloging-in-Publication Data
Wills. Judith.
     The food bible / Judith Wills.
     p.   cm.
     "A Fireside Book."
     Includes index.
     1. Food—Health aspects—Popular works.
     2. Nutrition—Popular works. 3. Diet—Popular works. 4. Consumer education. I. Title
     RA784.W645   1999   98-48065
     613.2—dc21   CIP

ISBN 0-684-85692-1
Printed and bound by Mohndruck Graphische Betriebe GmbH, Germany

Contents

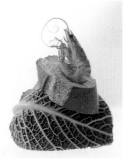
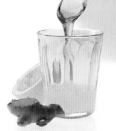

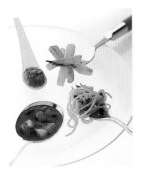
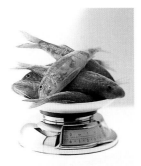
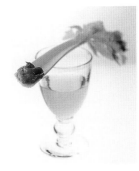
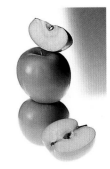

Introduction

What you eat and what you drink really are vital parts of what you are—and what you will become.

From before you are born all the way into old age, sustenance isn't just survival, it is your strength, your size, your short-term health, your long-term health, and—all other factors being equal—the length and quality of your life.

Every time you choose a meal, a snack, a food, a drink, you are making a decision that affects you and your body in a positive or a negative way.

You may feel that this is exaggerating the power of food. However, thanks to the efforts of people like Professor Philip James—regarded by many as the UK's leading expert on food and health, who is playing a leading role in setting the parameters of the British government's new Food Standards Agency—the role of diet in health and well-being is becoming more recognized.

Professor James believes that moderating diet can sometimes have a greater impact on public health than drugs. In a lecture given at the end of 1997, he said that nutrition will be at the center of health in the new millennium, and he states that "half the middle-aged people in Britain have overt nutritional disease."

We now know that heart disease, high blood pressure, diabetes, and many other major and minor ailments and diseases, including cancers, are often, at least in part, linked to poor nutrition.

The US has one of the highest rates of heart disease in the world. Over one half (97 million) of the adults in the US are overweight. The majority of adults with diabetes have the type that is often triggered by weight-gain and, therefore, diet. More than 1.2 million new cases of cancer are diagnosed each year, and it is estimated that 35 percent of them are related to diet.

Moreover, these diseases cost the US many billions of dollars each year. The cost of obesity alone in the US is over $99 billion. More than $10 billion is spent on cancer. Heart disease is the leading cause of death in the US, and heart disease mortality is about 23 percent for women and 30 percent for men. Much of all this could be prevented with greater attention to diet.

The fact is that food is not only vital fuel but also vital medicine, and it is time that we began to pay as much attention to the quality of the fuel that we feed our bodies as we do to the quality of fuel we put into our automobiles. I have compiled *The Food Bible* to help you make the right choices. Here is all the information you need for positive nutrition—food to keep you fit and well, strong and vital, all through your life.

We also examine, in detail, the negative aspects of food and help you to make choices about what to avoid, or cut back on, to maintain that health.

The book also provides all the latest thinking and research on what foods you should eat, or avoid, when you have special needs or problems.

I feel qualified to write this book because, over the past few years, I have changed from caring little about food other than for its taste and ease of preparation, into someone who believes, passionately, that everybody deserves good food and good nutrition. If I can change, I believe everybody can. I believe that good, healthy food is also delicious appealing food, and I hope to make everyone realize that eating for health doesn't mean compromise in those areas.

I hope that, with the help of *The Food Bible*, you will decide to take responsibility for your own diet—as far as is currently possible. Long term, if we vote for good food through what we buy, then good food is what we will get.

Keep thinking "five-star fuel" and remember, everybody deserves good food.

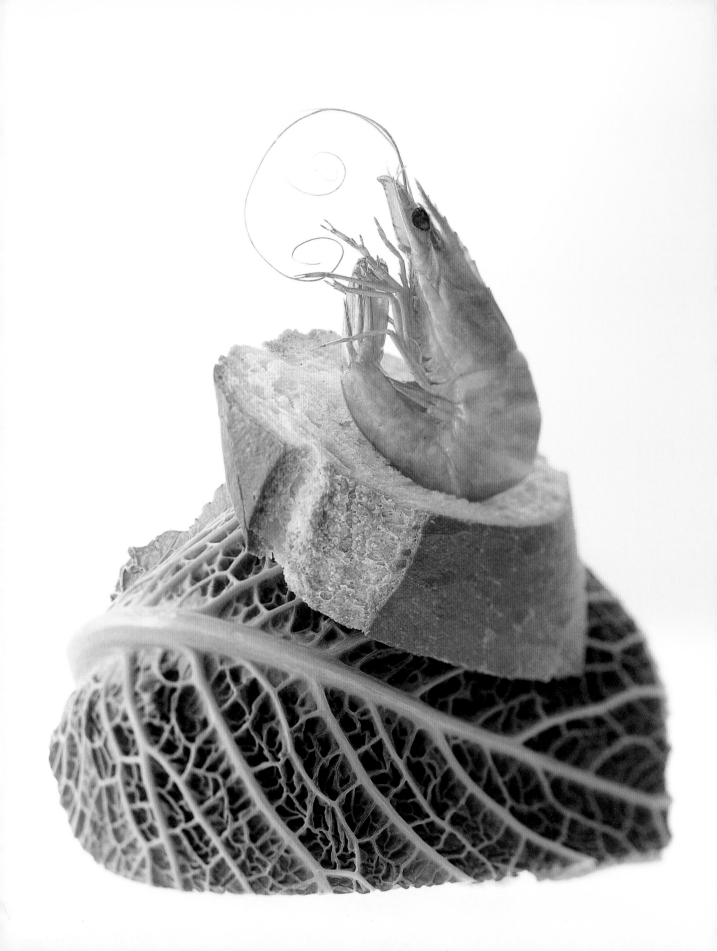

Food for a balanced diet

The experts are always telling you that you ought to eat a balanced diet. In fact, you've heard the message so often you probably know it by heart—eat less fat and more fruit and veggies and fiber. But what exactly does that mean, and how do you know you're achieving the correct balance? Most of us, for example, still fall well short of eating enough healthy carbohydrates; and many of us who try to follow a diet very low in fat may be doing just as much harm to our health as those who eat a high-fat diet. Then there's the advice to eat at least "five a day" of fruit and vegetables. What is a portion? And which fruits and vegetables can be included? Most people haven't got a clue—because no one has ever told them.

And what about the other nutrients you hardly ever hear about? For instance, did you know that many of us eat far more protein than we really need, and that too much can be bad for you? That some fats are vital to our well-being and aren't all that easy to find in a typical diet? And that many of us in the US fall short of at least some of the vitamins and minerals our bodies need? Here you will find out all you need to know about the things the experts don't usually bother to tell you, in a way you can understand.

The following two pages show a perfect day's eating for an average woman, containing all the carbohydrates, fat, protein, vitamins, minerals, fiber, etc. that are needed, in all the right quantities. Using this as our blueprint, we go on to show how you can achieve your own perfect diet. Your diet won't necessarily look the same (an average man needs about 30% more calories, for instance), or indeed contain more than a couple of the same foods, because your needs, lifestyle, and preferences may be different. That's the beauty of food—there is so much available in so much variety that you can eat "a balanced diet" without compromising your own needs. Section One sets out the foundation of your own diet for health and well-being, and shows how to give your body the fuel it needs for life.

THE BUILDING BLOCKS OF A HEALTHY DIET

To form our blueprint, the photographs on these pages show a perfect day's eating for an average woman, according to official FDA nutritional guidelines, containing all the carbohydrates, fat, protein, vitamins, minerals, fiber, etc. that are needed, in all the right quantities.

Taken together, the breakfast, lunch, main meal, and snack (together with 7 fl oz (200 ml) low-fat 2% milk and unlimited water to drink) give a total of 2,225 calories; 69 g total fat (28% of daily energy intake); 17 g saturated fat (6.8% of daily total energy intake); 18.6 g polyunsaturated fat (7.5% of daily energy intake); 28.2 g monounsaturated fat (11.4% of daily energy intake); 67 g protein (12% of daily energy intake); 334 g carbohydrate (60% of daily energy intake); 38 g fiber; contains only 1,251 mg sodium and gives 100% or more of the Reference Daily Intake for all the other major vitamins and minerals.

Breakfast
1 cup (240 ml) orange juice, 2 oz (50 g) 100%-natural cereal with raisins and dates, ⅔ cup (85 g) fresh raspberries, 5 tablespoons low-fat 2% milk, 2 slices whole-wheat bread, 2 teaspoons low-fat spread, 1½ teaspoons honey.

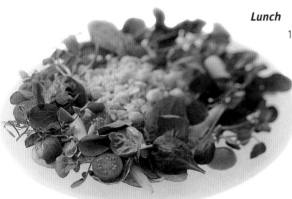

Lunch

1¼ cups (175 g) cooked weight brown rice combined into a salad with: ¾ cup (50 g) cooked chickpeas, 1½ teaspoons (7 g) pine nuts, 2 tablespoons (25 g) cooked baby corn, ¼ cup (80 g) tomato, ⅓ cup (25 g) watercress, ⅓ cup (25 g) raw baby spinach, all tossed in 1 tablespoon olive oil and balsamic vinegar or lemon juice or wine vinegar.

Snacks

1 large banana (approx. 6 oz/175 g weighed with skin, 5 oz/120 g without skin)
2 tablespoons (15 g) shelled almonds

½ cup (50 g) ready-to-eat dried apricots
1 oz (30 g) unsalted crackers

Evening meal

3 oz (85 g) salmon fillet, lightly broiled, ½ cup (50 g) sliced red bell pepper, ⅓ cup (50 g) broccoli florets, ¼ cup (25 g) scallion, sliced, ¼ cup (25 g) snow peas stir-fried in 2 teaspoons (8 g) sesame oil, tossed in lime juice and black pepper, served with ¾ cup (100 g) cooked weight whole-wheat noodles, 1 cup (125 g) cantaloupe (orange-fleshed) melon, 1 (30 g) dinner roll, 2 teaspoons (5 g) low-fat spread.

Energy-giving carbohydrates

Your body's most constant and basic requirement—apart, perhaps, from water—is energy. Energy to breathe, to move, to function, to power itself, for repair and growth. Like machines, we need an outside source of energy, but our fuel has to come from what we eat and drink.

That energy is measured in kilocalories (popularly just called calories). When you expend energy you "burn up" calories, and when you eat you consume calories. The amount of energy or calories your body needs in a day depends on your size, age, proportion of muscle to fat, activity levels, and many other factors.

However, the Food and Drug Administration and the US Department of Agriculture have laid down guidelines—called Reference Daily Intake (RDI) and Daily Reference Values (DRV)—which help meet most individuals nutritional needs. RDIs replace the term "RDAs" (Recommended Daily Allowances), which were introduced in 1973 as a reference value for vitamins, minerals, and protein, while DRVs are for the energy-producing nutrients (fat, carbohydrate, protein, and fiber) and are based on the number of calories consumed per day. The table below lists reference values, which should cover the energy needs for most healthy people in the US. Energy needs for children, teenagers, pregnancy, lactation, and the elderly differ and are discussed in Section Three. (In these days of metrication, energy is also sometimes measured in kilojoules, and 1 kilocalorie = 4.18 kilojoules.)

In order to maintain a reasonable and stable body weight, energy (food) intake and energy expenditure need to be balanced. Too little intake and too much expenditure can result in weight loss and being too thin; too much intake and too little expenditure can result in weight gain (from the surplus calories converting themselves into body fat) and eventual obesity. More about maintaining the correct energy balance appears later in Section Four, Food for Weight Control.

All food and drink containing calories can supply you with energy, in the form of carbohydrate, fat, protein, or alcohol. Hardly any foods contain only one of these elements—the main exceptions being oils, which contain nothing but fat, and sugar, which contains nothing but carbohydrate. Most foods are a mixture of more than one element (along with combinations of the vitamins and minerals).

For example, bread is high in carbohydrate, but also contains protein and fat; whole milk contains carbohydrate, fat, and protein, each in reasonable quantity; meat is a mixture of protein and fat; and so on.

The Food Charts at the end of the book give the protein, fat, and carbohydrate content of about 400 items, along with the other elements important for good health. Reading the next few pages will help you interpret these charts.

Although all types of calorie—be they from carbohydrate, fat, protein, or alcohol—supply you with energy, the majority of your energy supplies should come from carbohydrate. The wheel chart opposite shows you the proportions of each of the energy-giving nutrients that a healthy diet should contain, based on DRVs.

In the US, the new DRV for carbohydrates is 60% of total caloric intake; this has changed from the old RDA of 55%. Yet some international authorities recommend even lower levels for carbohydrates (e.g. UK 47–50%) which may seem quite low, however; the UK does have a 5% allowance for alcohol that we do not have in the US. If the World Health Organization (WHO) says 55–75% of our total caloric intake should be from carbohydrates, then certainly an increase up to 60% (this is done by reducing fat and protein intake and is further discussed on pages 15–21) of intake is likely to be both good for your health and achievable.

There are two main sorts of carbohydrate—starches and sugars. At the moment, around 60% of the carbohydrates that we eat are starches and about 40% are sugars. Starchy foods are plant-based foods, such as breakfast cereals, bread, potatoes, legumes, pasta, and rice. Vegetables also contain starch in varying amounts; most fruits contain none, the main exception being bananas. The carbohydrates in these foods are called polysaccharides and are known as complex carbohydrates.

RECOMMENDED ENERGY INTAKE FOR ADULTS*

Sex	Age	Light activity Cals/day	Moderate activity Cals/day	Heavy activity Cals/day
Female	19–24	2,000	2,100	2,600
	25–50	2,000	2,300	2,800
Male	19–24	2,700	3,000	3,600
	25–50	3,000	3,200	4,000

* These are only reference values for healthy adults and may vary according to weight, height, activity level, body size, and metabolism. This information is from the National Academy of Sciences' 1989 Recommended Dietary Allowances.

Sugars are either intrinsic, such as those found in fruits (the carbohydrates in almost all fruits are sugars) and vegetables (usually a mixture of both sugars and starches), which are part of the cellular structure of the food, or extrinsic (sometimes called "free"), such as those found in table sugar, honey, fruit drinks, cakes, cookies, confectionery, and so on, and which are not bound into the cellular structure of the food but are "refined", depleted of fiber, or added during manufacture. Milk contains an extrinsic sugar, lactose, which is not normally grouped with the other extrinsic sugars for nutrition purposes.

It is the complex carbohydrates and intrinsic sugars that should form the bulk of your healthy diet. The WHO suggests that at least 50% of the calories in your diet should come from complex carbohydrates. These are the plant foods that not only supply your body with an easily converted form of energy, but that also contain a whole range of other vital nutrients. They also have few health drawbacks and can therefore happily fill the energy gap left when we cut down on fats (see pages 15–19).

Carbohydrates also "spare" protein from being converted into energy, which can be important if protein needs are high or intakes poor.

The more unrefined the carbohydrate that you eat, the better for your health. Low-carbohydrate diets high in fats are linked with increased risk of many diseases, including heart disease, some cancers, especially bowel cancer, constipation, and obesity.

Unrefined foods or marginally refined foods, such as brown rice, whole-grain bread, fresh vegetables and fruits, legumes, nuts, and seeds, contain all or most of the original nutrients, including fiber, vitamins, minerals, and those recently-discovered, exciting compounds called phytochemicals (see page 34).

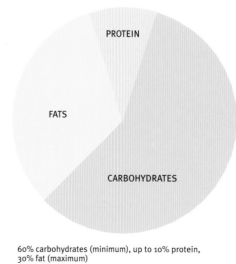

Refined carbohydrates, such as white rice, white pasta, and white flour, contain less of these elements, although they are still worth eating.

Many common manufactured starchy products, such as mass-produced cakes, packaged desserts and cookies, have lost much of their natural fibers, vitamins and minerals, and phytochemicals, and may also contain high levels of the less healthy types of fat and extrinsic sugars, and are therefore worth cutting right down on.

The USDA's "Dietary Guidelines for Americans" recommends using sugars in moderation—sparingly if your calorie needs are low. This conforms to the WHO's recommendations that extrinsic sugars can be eaten in moderation as part of a healthy diet. Another reason for limiting sugar intake is that high consumption, with inadequate oral hygiene, is a major cause of tooth decay.

Another important issue is that a diet high in sugary, fatty foods, such as snack foods, candies, and cakes, may also be low in essential nutrients (as seen above), while contributing high amounts of calories. Many experts agree that the US's ever-rising consumption of these types of foods is linked to our steadily rising levels of overweight and obesity (see Food for Weight Control).

It is all too easy to consume more extrinsic sugars than you would think. Generally speaking the major health hazard from eating too much sugar is tooth decay and most Americans do consume relatively large amounts of sugar (over 100 pounds a year). Considering the fact that extrinsic sugars may provide a high proportion of calories with low nutrient content, which in turn may lead to obesity and promote tooth decay, then moderation is advisable.

A GOOD BALANCE OF NUTRIENTS FOR ADULTS

PROTEIN

FATS

CARBOHYDRATES

60% carbohydrates (minimum), up to 10% protein, 30% fat (maximum)

Foods for fiber

One of the major reasons that the unrefined or low-refined complex carbohydrates are so important in our diet is that—along with vegetables and fruits—they are the best sources of dietary fiber.

Fiber is now more correctly called NSP, or non-starch polysaccharides. NSP, such as cellulose and pectin, comes mainly from plant cell walls. It passes undigested through the small intestine into the bowel, where it is fermented by bacteria.

There are two kinds of NSP—insoluble and soluble. Most plant foods contain both types, but proportions vary. *Insoluble fiber* is mainly cellulose and is found in all plants. Good sources are grains, especially wheat, corn, and rice, vegetables, and legumes. Insoluble fiber is important for avoiding constipation and hemorrhoids. Taken with sufficient fluids, a high-fiber diet increases stool bulk, speeds the passage of stools through the bowel, and may help to prevent bowel cancer, diverticulitis, and irritable bowel syndrome. It is also important in helping stave off hunger, as (with extra fluids) it helps us to feel full.

There are various types of *soluble fiber*, such as *pectin* (good sources are citrus fruits and apples), *beta-glucans*, (oats, barley, and rye), and *arabinose* (legumes). Several studies conclude that soluble fiber can help reduce LDL blood cholesterol levels (see Heart Disease, page 118 and overleaf). It also helps control blood sugar levels by slowing sugar absorption (see Section Four, Food for Weight Control), which may also help in diabetes. It can also play a role in stopping the absorption of a small amount of fat in the digestive system.

Resistant starch (present, for example, in cooked and cooled starchy foods, especially potatoes and cereals) is similar to fiber in that it passes undigested through the intestines until it reaches the bowel, where it may help to bulk out the stools. Lignin is another fibrous compound also found in plant cell walls, although not a NSP. It may be important for health (see Cancer, page 96) and is found mainly in flax seed, whole grains, berry fruits, and some vegetables.

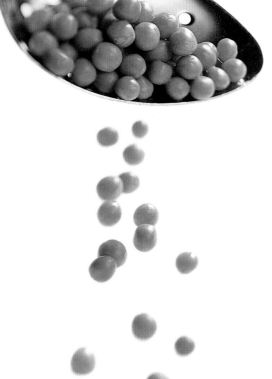

SELECTED GOOD SOURCES OF FIBER (NSP)

Food and average portion size	Total NSP (g)	Soluble (g)
Navy beans, ¼ cup (50 g) dry weight	8.5	4.0
Lima beans, ¼ cup (50 g) dry weight	8.0	3.2
Red kidney beans, ¼ cup (50 g) dry weight	7.8	3.5
Soybeans, ¼ cup (50 g) dry weight	7.8	3.4
Whole-grain barley, ¼ cup (50 g) dry weight	7.4	2.0
All Bran, ½ cup (30 g) serving	7.3	1.2
Whole-wheat bread, 3 slices (100 g)	5.8	1.6
Peas, frozen, ⅔ cup (100 g)	5.1	1.6
Mango, 1 average	4.9	3.0
Papaya, 1 average	4.7	2.8
Parsnips, ⅔ cup (100 g)	4.6	2.6
Shredded Wheat, 2	4.4	0.9
Whole-wheat pasta, ¼ cup (50 g) dry weight	4.2	1.0
Brussels sprouts, ⅔ cup (100 g)	4.1	2.2
Dried apricots, ½ cup (50 g)	3.8	2.3
Dried figs, ½ cup (50 g)	3.8	2.0
Almonds, shelled, ⅓ cup (50 g)	3.7	0.6
Black currants, ⅔ cup (100 g)	3.6	1.6
Pear, 1 dessert	3.5	1.1
Collard greens, ⅔ cup (100 g)	3.4	1.7
Hazelnuts, shelled, ⅓ cup (50 g)	3.3	1.3
Prunes, pitted, ¼ cup (50 g)	2.8	2.0
Orange, 1	2.7	1.8

■ How much fiber is enough?

In Western countries, most of us still don't get enough fiber in our diets, the average intake in the US of total fiber being approximately 13 g a day. The FDA recommends 11.5 g per 1,000 calories, with 20–30 g as a good average, although for people prone to chronic constipation up to 35 g a day (with extra fluids) may be a good idea. Beyond 35 g a day there are no proven benefits and indeed there may be drawbacks, such as a possible malabsorption of minerals.

In any case, it is always best to get your fiber naturally, from high-fiber wholefoods, rather than from a bran supplement—the phytates (see page 29) in raw bran may prevent the absorption of vital minerals, including calcium and iron, and this may be of some significance, especially for women and the elderly.

The chart opposite lists selected good sources of total NSP and soluble fiber. The Food Charts (pages 260–317) list fiber content for a wide range of foods.

The facts about fats

In dietary terms, fat has been the wicked witch of the late twentieth century. Every time we grab a fatty snack, we feel guilty. Yet we're still eating too much of the wrong kinds of fat—and probably too little of some of the healthy types. Here's what you need to know.

Fat is made up mainly of fatty acids and glycerol, along with some other compounds—fatty acids being by far the largest component (glycerol comprises roughly 3% of total fat energy intake: glycerol is naturally present as a building block of fats and you do not need to be concerned about intake). The fatty acids can be divided into three main groups— saturated fatty acids, polyunsaturated fatty acids, and monounsaturated fatty acids.

HOW MUCH FAT SHOULD YOU EAT?
(to total 30% energy intake)

	Total fat	% Sat	% Poly	% Mono
% of total energy intake	30 max	10 max	6 min	12 min
Grams/day for women (2,200 Cals/day)	73 g	24 g	15 g	29 g
Grams/day for men (2,700 Cals/day)	90 g	30 g	18 g	36 g

All fat-containing foods contain all three types of fatty acid, but in varying proportions. When people say, for example, that "butter is a saturated fat," that is not really true. Certainly the majority of the fat in butter is saturated (67%), but it also contains 25% monounsaturated fat and even a little polyunsaturated. Beef, another food that people typically think of as containing saturated fat, contains virtually as much monounsaturated fat as saturated, at 43%.

The Food Charts at the back of the book give percentages of all the fatty acids in about 400 foods. To help you balance the fats in your diet, the wheel chart on the right gives ideal (average in the case of glycerols) percentages for each type of fat.

Currently, about 42% of our total daily calorie intake is in the form of fats. Fat is mainly used by the body as energy—it provides more than twice as many calories per gram as either carbohydrate or protein (9 calories a gram). If fat surplus to energy needs is eaten, however, it stores itself in the body as adipose tissue (fat!). This can later be converted into energy if needed— i.e., if food intake doesn't match energy output (the basis of weight-loss diets). A small amount of fat is also needed because it "carries" the fat-soluble vitamins A, D, and E (see pages 22–4).

Polyunsaturated fats are also needed to supply the body with essential fatty acids (see overleaf).

Because a high-fat diet has been strongly linked with heart disease as well as some forms of cancer, obesity, and other ills, however, the FDA advises us to cut our fat intake down to 30% or less, and no more than 10% from saturated fat. It is no good just saying, "cut down on fat," because in terms of health all fats are not equal.

IDEAL DISTRIBUTION OF FATS IN THE DIET

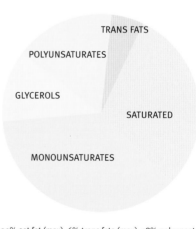

30% sat fat (max), 6% trans fats (max), 18% polyunsat fat (min), 36% monounsat fat (min), 9% glycerols (ave)

SELECTED FOODS HIGH IN SATURATED FATTY ACIDS
(all per 3½ oz/100 g weight)

	Saturated fatty acids (g)	Total fat (g)
Cocoa butter	59.7	100
Suet, animal	56.0	100
Butter	53.5	80
Lard	41.0	100
Hard margarine	35.0	80
Shortening	30.6	100
Mascarpone cheese	30.5	46
Cream cheese	30.0	48
Heavy cream	30.0	48
Crème fraîche	26.5	40
American cheese	20	31
Blue cheese	19	30
Chocolate	18.5	31
Fried bacon, lean and fat	16.0	41
Pork sausage	11.3	31
Basic piecrust	10.0	28
Potato chips	9.0	37
Ground beef	7.0	16
Lamb shoulder, roast	6.5	14

■ Saturated fat
This is the kind of fat that is usually solid at room temperature and is often found in largest quantities in animal produce such as meat, cheese, cream, milk, eggs, butter and lard, and in milk chocolate and many manufactured goods, such as pies, pastries, cakes, and cookies.

It has been proved that a diet high in saturated fats can raise levels of the "bad" blood cholesterol, LDL, which is a major risk factor in heart disease, our biggest killer. A diet high in saturated fat may also be linked with other ailments and problems, including cancer and obesity. It may also predispose to nutritional imbalances—people who eat a diet high in saturates (particularly with between-meal snacking on high-fat, high-sugar items) may find their appetite satisfied without eating enough of the other foods that provide a range of nutrients. Currently our saturated fat intake is more than 15% of our total

calorie intake (42% of fat intake) and the FDA estimates that if we reduced our intake to 10% then risk of CHD (coronary heart disease, see page 118) would be "reduced substantially."

■ Polyunsaturated fat
The largest amounts of this type of fat are usually contained in the kinds of fat that are liquid at room temperature or cooler—vegetable oils, such as corn oil, safflower oil, sunflower oil, and walnut oil are high in polyunsaturates, as are most nuts. Polyunsaturated fats have the opposite effects of saturates by lowering LDL blood cholesterol, but experts believe that high levels of polyunsaturated fat intake may nevertheless not be a good idea, especially used in cooking, because they may be easily oxidized in the body, producing free radicals which can damage body cells and may actually help cancers and other diseases to form. (A diet high in antioxidants will help

counteract his effect). For that reason a reduction in overall fat intake and a varied diet is recommended by the USDA.

However, a certain amount of polyunsaturated fats ARE needed in our diets because they contain what are termed the *essential fatty acids* (EFAs) that our bodies need for normal health—*linoleic acid* (one of the n-6 group of PUFAs, often called omega-6s) and *alpha-linolenic acid*, one of the n-3 group of PUFAs, often called omega-3s. These are called essential because they are the only fats that our bodies actually need from food, as other fats can be manufactured in the body. Good sources of EFAs are shown in the boxes on page 19.

The essential fats are needed in very small but nutritionally important amounts—a minimum 1% of total energy intake for linoleic acid (about 2 g) and 0.2% for alpha-linolenic acid (about 0.5 gram)—according to some European experts. Evidence is, however, amassing that an adequate intake of EFAs may help in prevention or control of all kinds of ailments and conditions, such as heart disease, cancers, immune system deficiencies, arthritis, skin complaints, PMS, menopausal symptoms, and more.

One special type of n-6 PUFA is *gamma-linolenic acid* (GLA), which can be manufactured in the body from linoleic acid (but this process may occasionally be hindered) and is found in greatest quantities in evening primrose and starflower oils. This may be of particular help to women with PMS and

OMEGA-3 FATTY ACID OF FISH

(g per 3½ oz/100 g fish)	
Mackerel	1.8
Herring	1.8
Salmon	1.8
Tuna, fresh	1.4
Trout	1.0

menopausal symptoms. Two other fatty acids of importance are the n-3 *eicosapentaenoic acid* (EPA) and *docosahexaenoic acid* (DHA), which are found in greatest quantities in oily fish and fish oils. These omega-3 oils have been shown to be particularly beneficial in reducing the "stickiness" of the blood and its tendency to clot, and therefore in helping to prevent coronary heart disease and stroke. A list of good sources of omega-3 fish oils appears below left. Two to three portions a week of oily fish have been shown to have a beneficial effect. EPA and DHA can also be made in the body from alpha-linolenic acid. Linseed (flax seed) oil contains high levels of alpha-linolenic acid.

Polyunsaturated fats are also one of few rich sources of natural vitamin E, an important antioxidant vitamin.

■ Trans Fats

There is another type of related fat called the trans fats. Most of the trans fats in the diet are unsaturated fats which have been altered—hydrogenated—usually in food processing, and become hard at room temperature, such as when some margarines (which are a blend of oils) are manufactured. These hydrogenated fats then become

SELECTED RICH SOURCES OF POLYUNSATURATED FATTY ACIDS (PUFAS) (all per 3½ oz/100 g weight)

	Polyunsaturated fatty acids (g)	Total fat (g)
Safflower oil	74	100
Walnut oil	70	100
Sunflower oil	63	100
Corn oil	51	100
Blended vegetable oil	48	100
Walnuts	47	68.0
Sesame oil	44	100
Mayonnaise, commercial	44	75.5
Sunflower margarine	37	84.0
Brazil nuts	23	68.0
Low-fat margarine, typical	10	40.0
Sardines, canned in oil, drained	5	13.5
Tuna, canned in oil, drained	5	9.0

more like saturated fats in the manner in which they act in the body.

It has been suspected for some years that trans fats may be no better for us than saturated fats, but more evidence is emerging and it now seems that perhaps trans fats can actually be more damaging, for instance in the case of heart disease. It now appears, according to a very large American trial, that trans fats not only raise levels of LDL blood cholesterol (the "baddie") but also lower levels of the "good" cholesterol, HDL.

Trans fats are the only types of fat to do this—natural saturated fats, such as butter or cheese, may raise LDL levels but also raise HDL levels. Currently there is no recommendation for trans fats, but in view of the latest evidence it may be wise to consider trying to reduce them in our diets.

The amount of trans fats within manufactured foods is not usually listed on the nutrition label, but in general most hard margarines and cooking fats contain the highest concentrations. They will also generally be found

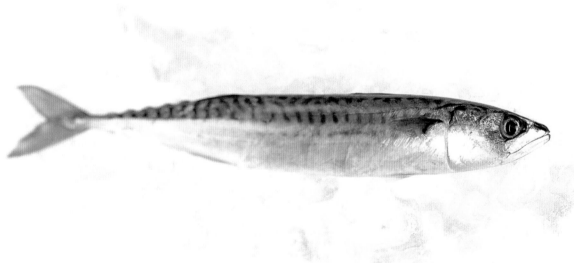

SELECTED RICH SOURCES OF MONOUNSATURATED FATTY ACIDS (MFAS)

(all per 3½ oz/100 g weight)

	Monounsaturated fatty acids (g)	Total fat (g)
Olive oil	73	100
Macadamia nuts (shelled)	61	78
Canola oil	59	100
Hazelnuts (shelled)	50.5	64
Lard	44	100
Peanut oil	44	100
Sesame oil	38	100
Blended vegetable oil	36	100
Almonds, shelled	35	56
Olive oil margarine (60% fat)	32.5	60
Corn oil	30	100
Brazil nuts (shelled)	26	68
Duck, roasted, with skin	19	38
Hummus	18	29
Low-fat margarine, typical	17.5	40
Beef, ground	11	24
Avocado	8	17
Mackerel fillet	8	16
Sour cream	7	22
Canadian bacon, broiled	7	18

in quite significant quantities in many mass-produced baked goods, such as cookies and cakes, in many soft margarines, and in take-out foods such as hamburger and fries.

In the Food Charts at the back of the book, trans fats are included in the Total Fat column.

■ Monounsaturated fat

This, the last of the types of fat, is also usually liquid at room temperature but may solidify when cooled (say, in the refrigerator), and is found in greatest quantities in olive oil, canola oil, and peanut oil, as well as in olives them-selves and many nuts and in avocados, but it is also present in fairly reasonable quantities in all fats, most dairy prod-ucts, eggs, fish, meat, and many other types of foods.

BEST SOURCES OF EFA LINOLEIC ACID

(g per 3½ oz/100 g)

Safflower oil	73.9
Evening primrose oil	68.4
Grapeseed oil	67.8
Sunflower oil	63.2
Walnut oil	58.4
Soybean oil	51.5
Corn oil	50.4
Sesame oil	43.1
Margarine	33.8
Sunflower seeds	32.8
Peanut oil	31
Walnuts	29.5
Sesame seeds	25.3
Pine nuts	24.9
Brazil nuts	22.9
Canola oil	19.7
Pumpkin seeds	19.3
Linseed oil	15
Almonds	9.8
Cashew nuts	8.1
Olive oil	7.5
Pistachio nuts	7.1
Linseeds	5.7
Oat crackers	4.7
Hazelnuts	3.7
Soy flour, full-fat	3.6

BEST SOURCES OF EFA ALPHA-LINOLENIC ACID

(g per 3½ oz/100 g)

Linseed oil	53.1
Linseeds	14
Walnut oil	11.5
Canola oil	9.6
Evening primrose oil	8.2
Soybean oil	7.3
Walnuts	5.6
Quail, raw, meat and skin	2.3
Margarine, soft polyunsaturated	2.1
Soy flour, full-fat	1.7
Butter, unsalted	1.2
Rabbit, raw	1.0
Corn oil	0.9
Butter, slightly salted	0.9
Tuna, canned in oil, drained	0.9
Pine nuts	0.8
Peanut oil	0.8
Olive oil	0.7
Cream, heavy	0.7
Lard	0.6
Sardines, canned in oil, drained	0.4
Grapeseed oil	0.4
Ghee, vegetable	0.3
Sardines	0.3
Sesame oil	0.3
Salmon	0.2

Monounsaturated fats were, at first, thought to have no effect on blood cholesterol levels, but it is now known that they actually have a better overall effect than polyunsaturated fats—by not only lowering the "bad" LDL cholesterol but by maintaining or even slightly raising the levels of the "good" HDL cholesterol.

There is also evidence that a diet rich in monounsaturates is linked with good health in other ways—the typical "Mediterranean" diet is rich in these oils and is linked not only with less heart disease but also with increased longevity, lower levels of obesity, and less cancers than the American diet. Oils high in monounsaturates are also often rich sources of the antioxidant vitamin E.

The FDA recommends that the remainder of the fatty acids in our diet not eaten as saturated or polyunsaturated or trans fats should be eaten as monounsaturated. However, for the sake of your heart, your circulation, and your general health it would probably be wise to replace more of the saturated and trans fats in the diet with monounsaturates, i.e. aim to eat less than 10% of total energy as saturates and more than 12% as monounsaturates. To do this would mean eating more plant-based foods and less animal-based and commercially produced foods (the advice given on pages 118–119 will help you to do this with ease).

■ Cholesterol

Cholesterol is present in many foods of animal origin, including meat and dairy products, eggs, fish (especially shellfish), and many fatty manufactured products. There are two types of cholesterol—low-density lipoprotein (LDL) and high-density lipoprotein (HDL). A surplus of LDL in the blood is a major factor in the "furring" of the arteries and formation of the plaques that lead to atherosclerosis, heart disease, and stroke; whereas HDL—often called "good" cholesterol—actually helps to remove cholesterol from the tissues and delivers it to the liver for excretion.

Although high levels of LDL blood cholesterol are not good news, a certain amount of cholesterol is necessary for cell functioning, and about three-quarters of what we need is manufactured in the body, while one-quarter comes from the diet. Dietary cholesterol has a diverse effect on blood cholesterol levels, but for people with CHD or risk factors (see Heart Disease, page 118), or raised blood LDL cholesterol levels, it is wise to avoid too many cholesterol-rich foods.

The WHO sets an upper limit for daily cholesterol intake from foods at 300 mg a day. This is roughly equivalent to, for example, one large egg and 3½ oz (100 g) of beef steak, or 3½ oz (100 g) shelled shrimp and 1 cup (250 ml) low-fat 2% milk. The Food Charts at the back of the book list the cholesterol content of over 300 foods. See also the Healthy Heart Diet on page 142.

Protein

Any child will tell you that protein is what we need to eat to build us up and keep us strong—and it is true. Adequate protein is essential. How much is enough, though, and can you get too much?

For a start, enough protein is definitely essential. It is essential for growth and development in children, for cell maintenance and repair (especially those muscles), for the regulation of all body functions, and for various other jobs that fat and carbohydrate just can't do. It is the "clever" nutrient. While it is likely that many people get more than enough, some people are going short.

■ What is protein?

Protein is a component of very many foods, but it doesn't always take the same form. It is made up of *amino acids*, like building blocks. Proteins from different food sources contain different amino acids. Twenty-two of these amino acids are used in the body in different combinations to make the body's own proteins, such as muscle, and for all the other activities outlined above.

The amino acids can be divided into two broad types—non-essential amino acids and essential amino acids. *Non-*

ESTIMATED PROTEIN NEEDS (kg body weight x 0.75)	
Body weight	g/protein per day
113 lb (51 kg)	38
125 lb (57 kg)	43
140 lb (63.5 kg)	48
154 lb (70 kg)	52
169 lb (76.5 kg)	57
183 lb (83 kg)	62
196 lb (89 kg)	67
210 lb (95.5 kg)	72
225 lb (102 kg)	77

essential amino acids can be made from an excess of other amino acids in the diet. *Essential amino acids* cannot be made like this and so must be provided in the diet. There are eight essential amino acids for adults—isoleucine, leucine, lysine, methionine, phenylalanine, threonine, tryptophan, and valine.

■ How much should we be eating?

As we saw on the wheel chart on page 13, as a rough guide the FDA allows for about 10% of the calories in our diet to be from protein. The WHO also suggests 10–15%, a figure that is recognized by most nutrition professionals. A more accurate guide for individuals is to reckon 0.75 g of protein per day for every kg of your body weight, which does work out at nearer the 10% level for most people. This is also less than the amount we are currently eating on average (15.6% according to the USDA's Continuing Survey of Food Intakes by Individuals), which means that many of us are actually getting more protein than we need. Cutting down a little will allow more calories to come from the complex carbohydrates, which are so important for health. The chart above shows suggested protein intake based on the 0.75 formula.

■ What happens if we eat too much?

Each gram of protein contains 4 calories. Any protein that we eat, which isn't needed for the tasks described above, can be converted into glucose and used for energy. Bearing in mind that the traditional animal sources of protein are more expensive to buy than the cheaper carbohydrate sources of energy, your budget may also prefer that you don't waste money on protein you don't need!

Of course, if 15.6% is our current average protein intake, it follows that some people will be eating much more than that. A high-protein diet (especially one high in animal protein) has been linked with bone demineralization—more calcium is excreted in the urine (see Osteoporosis, page 130), so it may be particularly important for women to keep their protein intake to less than 15%. There is strong evidence that a high-protein diet—particularly one high in animal protein—has a detrimental long-term effect on kidney function. There is a small amount of evidence that high protein intakes may also be linked to higher blood pressure levels.

For these reasons, the it is recommended that daily protein intakes over 1.5 g per kilo of body weight be avoided. To give an example, for a woman of 63.5 kg (140 pounds) this works out at 95 g protein per day or just under 20% of total daily calories—showing that, while enough protein is essential, it doesn't need much extra on a regular basis to pose possible problems.

■ Which are good sources of protein?

Animal sources of protein, such as all animal meats, dairy products, fish, and eggs, contain all eight essential amino acids within themselves, which is why they have been called "first-class" proteins. All vegetable sources of protein—with the exception of soybeans—don't, which is why they have been called "second-class" proteins.

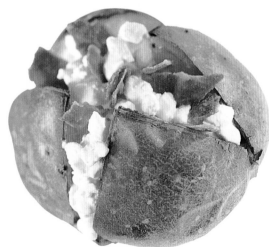

SELECTED GOOD SOURCES OF ANIMAL PROTEIN

Food	(g/average portion)	
	Protein	Total fat
Chicken breast portion without skin	42	2.9
Ostrich, 3½ oz (100 g)	39	3.4
Beef, roast, lean, 3½ oz (100 g)	32	5
Cod, 6 oz (175 g)	31.5	1.2
Venison, 3½ oz (100 g)	22	1.6
Hamburger, quarter-pounder	21	19
Salmon fillet, 3½ oz (100 g)	20	11*
Shrimp, peeled, 2¾ oz (75 g)	17	0.6
Cheddar, half-fat, 2 oz (50 g)	16	7.5
Eggs, 2 large	14.2	12.2
Cottage cheese, ½ cup (100 g)	14	4
Beef taco, 3½ oz (100 g)	13	13
Cheddar, full-fat, 2 oz (50 g)	13	17
Blue cheese, 2 oz (50 g)	11	15
Bacon, Canadian broiled, 2 slices, 2 oz (50 g)	11	4
Quark, 0% fat, ½ cup (100 g)	7.7	0.2
Milk, skim or nonfat, ¾ cup (200 ml)	6.6	0.2
Plain low-fat yogurt, ½ cup (100 g)	5	0.8

* Low in saturates

SELECTED GOOD SOURCES OF PLANT PROTEIN

Food	(g/average portion)	
	Protein	Total fat
Soybeans, ¼ cup (50 g) dry weight	18	9.3*
Peanuts, fresh, ½ cup (50 g)	13	23*
Almonds, ⅓ cup (50 g)	12	28*
Black-eyed peas, ¼ cup (50 g) dry weight	12	0.8
Lentils, ¼ cup (50 g) dry weight	12	0.9
Red kidney beans, ¼ cup (50 g) dry weight	11	0.7
Cashews, ⅓ cup (50 g)	8.9	24*
Baked potato, 8 oz (225 g) cooked weight	8.7	0.5
Vegetable burger, one 1¾ oz (50 g)	8.3	5.6
Tofu, 3½ oz (100 g)	8	4.2
Pasta, whole-wheat, ¼ cup (50 g) dry weight	6.7	1.3
Pasta, white, ¼ cup (50 g) dry weight	6	1.0
Soy milk, ¾ cup (200 ml)	6	3.8
Peas, frozen, ⅔ cup (50 g)	5.6	0.7
Whole-wheat bread, 2 slices (60 g)	5.5	1.5
Whole-grain barley, ¼ cup (50 g) dry weight	5.3	1.0
Couscous, ⅓ cup (50 g) dry weight	5.3	1.0

* Low in saturates

Some vegetable sources have certain amino acids but not others, and they need to be combined with the correct "missing" amino acids in other forms of protein in order to be utilized in the body. For example, the protein from legumes forms a complete protein when mixed with grains or with nuts and seeds, e.g. rice with beans, or hummus with pita bread, or bean taco. For more on protein in the diet of vegetarians and vegans, see pages 60–63.

As we've seen, a diet too high in saturated fats and trans fats is best avoided, and so protein sources containing too much of these types of fat are also best limited. Ironically, some of the more traditional sources ARE high in saturated fats—Cheddar cheese, for instance, is 24% protein but a whopping 75% fat, of which 64% is saturated. So, if choosing protein from animal sources, it is important to choose plenty of the lower-fat varieties. In general, fish is the best low-fat source of animal protein and standard dairy products the highest in fat.

As we've also seen, we should be eating MORE complex carbohydrates for good health, and so eating more protein from plant sources is a good idea for most of us. However, many people don't realize that all kinds of plant foods do contain protein. All legumes are a particularly good source. Many of the high-starch foods, like potatoes, bread, rice, and pasta—because they are eaten in bulk—are quite good sources. They are also, naturally combined with other protein foods and so provide "complete protein." For example, one average baked potato (7¾ oz/220 g cooked weight) will provide about 4.7 g of protein, which is 10% of the calories in the potato and approximately one-tenth an average woman's daily needs, while giving less than 0.3% fat, of which only a trace is saturated.

Unlike animal proteins, plant proteins are not totally digested in the body and nutritionists usually allow a conversion factor of 85%, i.e. 85 g of animal protein is equal to 100 g of plant protein. A person who relies mostly on plant protein, therefore, may want to eat slightly more than the minimum levels.

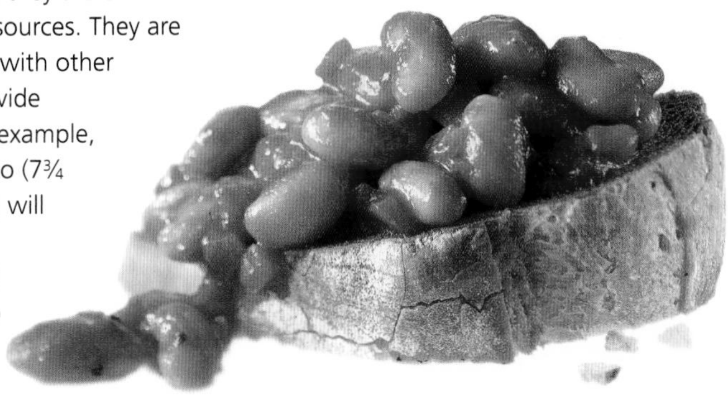

Vital vitamins

Vitamins are the "unseen" components of a healthy diet—the tiny particles without which we wouldn't survive. We are discovering more information about their importance in the diet all the time...

Vitamins are organic substances that are indispensable for the everyday functioning of our bodies, for our good health and proper development. Each has a different role to play and most have to be provided in what we eat and drink. We need only very small amounts of the vitamins—normally just a few milligrams (1,000 mg = 1 gram) or even micrograms (1,000 μg [micrograms] = 1 milligram) a day. Vitamins A, D, E, and K are fat-soluble vitamins and can thus be stored in the body. Vitamins C and the B group are water-soluble vitamins and can't be stored—excess is excreted in the urine—and so they need to be consumed on a regular basis. Each of the eleven vitamins is discussed separately in the pages ahead.

* Recommended amounts are given for each vitamin for adults. The FDA offers Reference Daily Intakes (RDIs) which were set in 1996 and which they say will be enough for the majority of the healthy US population. Some nutritionists believe that some of these levels have been set too high and so, for comparison, we include the EC's RDAs (recommended daily amounts) which are used in EC countries for the purposes of food labeling, and the UK RNIs. (Recommended amounts for children, pregnancy, and the elderly appear in Section Three.)

* A short explanation of the role of each vitamin is given, followed by general sources, and symptoms of deficiency and excess.

* "Best sources" charts list selected top sources for each per 100 g (approx. 3½ oz) of

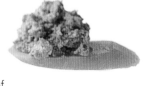

food item. Other items may provide more of the vitamins per 100 g, but may have been omitted because they are not normally eaten in large enough quantities to make a real contribution—e.g. parsley contains a creditable 673 μg vitamin A retinol equivalent per 100 g, but a normal portion is about 2 g.

* If you want to know whether a particular food, which isn't listed here, contains a certain vitamin, the Food Charts at the back of the book list the significant vitamin content of about 400 foods.

* Many people use vitamin pill supplements—often in the belief that if enough is good, more is even better. Although this may sometimes be true for some people and of some of the vitamins and minerals, it is by no means always a good idea to take more than the RDI. Indeed, most vitamins and minerals can be toxic in excess. The use of supplements is discussed in more detail in Section Two on page 146.

■ Vitamin A

RETINOL AND RETINOL EQUIVALENTS
USA RDI 1,500 μg **UK** RNI 600 μg (female), 700 μg (male) **EC** RDA 800μg

Vitamin A (retinol) is essential for healthy vision, eyes, skin, and growth. Symptoms of deficiency include poor night vision, gradual loss of sight, and reduced resistance to infection. Excess vitamin A is stored in the liver and can be

SELECTED BEST SOURCES OF VITAMIN A (μg per 100 g)	
Lambs' liver	17,300
Chicken liver	9,700
Liver pâté	7,400
Cod liver oil	1,800
Butter	887
Heavy cream	654
Blue cheese	386
Cheddar cheese, average	363
Brie	320
Eggs	190

poisonous, causing liver and bone damage, headache, double vision, and other side-effects. Excess retinol consumption is linked with certain birth defects and foods high in retinol, such as liver, should be avoided by pregnant women (see Pregnancy section on pages 172–5). It is advised that regular intakes should not exceed 7,500 μg in women and 9,000 μg in men.

Retinol is found only in foods from animal sources, such as liver, milk, butter, cheese, eggs, and oily fish, but the body can convert carotenes—particularly beta-carotene, the pigment found in greatest quantities in orange-fleshed and dark green vegetables and fruits—into retinol. Beta-carotene is also an important nutrient in its own right. Adequate intake of beta-carotene has been linked with low risk of certain cancers and it is an

SELECTED BEST SOURCES OF BETA-CAROTENE (µg per 100 g)

	Beta-carotene Equivalents	Retinol
Carrots, old	8,118	1,353
Sweet potato (orange-fleshed), baked	5,130	855
Swiss chard	4,596	766
Chili peppers	4,110	685
Red bell peppers	3,840	640
Spinach	3,840	640
Butternut squash	3,270	545
Curly kale	3,144	524
Collard greens	2,628	438
Frozen mixed vegetables	2,520	420
Cantaloupe melon	1,998	333
Mango	1,800	300
Tomato paste	1,300	217
Savoy cabbage	990	165
Dark-leaf lettuce	910	151
Tomatoes	640	107
Broccoli	575	96

SELECTED BEST SOURCES OF VITAMIN D (µg per 100 g)

Cod liver oil	210
Kipper fillet, baked	25
Red salmon, canned in brine, drained	23.1
Herring fillet, broiled	16.1
Pilchards, canned in tomato sauce	14
Sardines, broiled	12.3
Rainbow trout, broiled	11
Salmon, broiled	9.6
Smoked mackerel fillet	8
Margarine, fortified	7.9
Tuna, fresh	7.2
Sardines canned in oil, drained	5
Tuna canned in water, drained	4
Tuna canned in oil, drained	3
Milk, fortified (1 cup)	2.5
Bran Flakes, Fruit 'n Fibre, Cornflakes	2.1
Eggs	1.8

antioxidant (see page 24). For this reason, beta-carotene sources have been listed separately. 6µg beta-carotene = 1µg retinol, which is called a "retinol equivalent."

The US National Cancer Institute has recommended a daily amount of 6,000µg beta-carotene, an amount that is not that difficult to obtain from five or more good portions of fruits and vegetables a day. The beta-carotene list here is not comprehensive; for more good sources, see the Food Charts at the end of the book. Beta-carotene is not thought to be toxic, although fairly high intakes of over 30 mg per day may make the skin orange-tinged, and high doses of beta-carotene supplements (not carotene-rich foods) may increase the risk of cancer in smokers.

■ Vitamin D
CHOLECALCIFEROL

USA RDI 10 µg **UK** RNI *no recommendation for non-pregnant adults under 65* **EC** RDA 5 µg
Vitamin D intake is important for the absorption of calcium and phosphorus in the body, helping to form bones and carry out other mineralization. One research trial has found that vitamin D can halt the progress of osteoarthritis.

Deficiency of vitamin D can lead to rickets in children and weakness and pain in adults. In excess, vitamin D can produce kidney damage by causing excess calcium to be deposited in the organs. Levels of 50 µg a day have been known to have this effect, so it is wise to regard the RDIs as a maximum as well as a minimum.

Sunlight and milk are the primary sources of vitamin D. Fifteen to thirty minutes' exposure to sunlight should provide adequate vitamin D synthesis, however this is not always possible (especially during the winter months in northern states and because we tend to spend our working days indoors). Thus, fortified milk represents the only significant and reliable source of vitamin D. It is important that the milk be fortified because there are few natural food sources of vitamin D. Other dietary sources are fortified margarines, dairy products, oily fish, and fortified breakfast cereals.

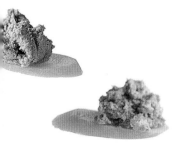

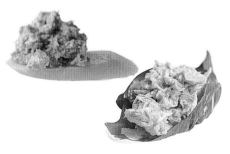

■ Vitamin E

TOCOPHEROLS

USA RDI 20 mg **UK** RNI 5 mg **EC** RDA 10 mg

The most active vitamin E compound is (d) alpha-tocopherol, which is though to be a powerful antioxidant, protecting the cell membranes from oxidation damage and helping to prevent the build-up of plaques in the arteries, as well as "thinning" the blood, thus helping to protect against heart disease and aging. In one large European study published in 1997, vitamin E from 268 mg up to 537 mg per day reduced the risk of non-fatal heart attacks by a massive 77%.

Vitamin E has also been shown to increase the body's immune response and therefore may protect against disease and cancer. A new study has shown that smokers who took vitamin E supplements were nearly one-third less likely to get prostate cancer. It can also help reduce the pain of osteoarthritis. Vitamin E is important for maintaining healthy skin and for helping the healing process of all damaged tissue, including skin wounds, and one trial found that 600 mg per day supplements significantly improved levels of sperm activity in males with low fertility.

SELECTED BEST SOURCES OF VITAMIN E (mg per 100 g)

Food	mg	Food	mg
Wheat germ oil	145	Soybean oil	16
Canola margarine	57	Peanut oil	15
Sunflower oil	44	Pine nuts	13.5
Sunflower seeds	38	Popcorn, plain	11
Safflower oil	32	Marzipan, homemade	11
Hazelnuts, shelled	25	Peanuts, plain	10
Sun-dried tomatoes	24	Brazil nuts, shelled	7
Almonds	24	Low-fat spread	6.3
Canola oil	22	Sweet potato, baked	6
Cod liver oil	20	Potato chips	5.8
Mayonnaise	19	Pistachios, dried	5.4
Corn oil	17	Tomato paste	5.4

It is very rare for adults to show clinical symptoms of vitamin E deficiency. Occasionally, malabsorption can occur, though, leading to deficiency. Optimum levels for the full antioxidant effect are, however, thought by some experts actually to be much greater than the RDIs and so it may be wise to increase your intake of vitamin E-rich foods to offer optimum protection. A supplement may be of benefit (see page 146). In trials, supplements from 70 mg up to 540 mg per day have been used. Vitamin E excess rarely causes any problems, although people on anti-coagulant drugs, such as Warfarin, should avoid very high intakes, as vitamin E also acts to thin the blood.

The higher the diet is in polyunsaturated fats (PUFAs), which are quite vulnerable to oxidation in the body, the more vitamin E the diet should contain. Luckily, foods that are rich in PUFAs also tend to be rich in vitamin E. For people consuming half their fat calories as PUFAs, 20 mg per day of vitamin E is easily achievable.

Best sources of vitamin E are vegetable oils, nuts, avocados and other vegetables, and cereals.

See the chart above and the Food Charts at the end of the book.

ANTIOXIDANTS

The vitamins C, E, and beta-carotene, along with the mineral selenium, and many of the phytochemicals discussed later, are antioxidants, which protect our bodies against the damaging effects of an excess of substances called "free radicals."

Everyone produces free radicals in the process of creating energy and this is quite normal. However, excess may be produced by various factors, such as stress, tobacco smoking, pollution, sunlight, radiation, illness, and so on. These surplus free radicals may cause cell damage and this may predispose to cancer and other illnesses, and is thought to be how the aging process takes place. Free radicals can also oxidize polyunsaturated fats in the body, which can cause further damage. The oxidation of LDL cholesterol may be a factor in the build-up of plaque in the arteries, a factor in CHD (coronary heart disease, see Heart Disease, page 118).

The antioxidants present in our diet help to neutralize the free radicals in our body and stop them producing their damaging effects. For example, vitamin E protects polyunsaturated fats from oxidation; vitamin C helps the body's natural defences against the free radicals and interacts with vitamin E. Much more research still needs to be done for us to understand exactly how antioxidants work and their full range of effects.

A diet high in fresh fruits, vegetables, and other plant foods will be naturally high in the antioxidant vitamins. Research to date seems to show that it is better to get your antioxidants as part of your natural diet rather than as supplements, particularly in the case of beta-carotene. The antioxidant minerals and phytochemicals are discussed in more detail in the pages ahead.

■ Vitamin K

The last of the fat-soluble vitamins, vitamin K is essential for the normal clotting of blood.

It is widespread in food in small quantities, but best sources are dark green leafy vegetables and the skins of fruit and vegetables.

It can also be synthesized in the intestines, so deficiency in adults is extremely rare and for this reason no RDIs or RNIs have been set. Infants are generally born with low levels so vitamin K is usually given at birth.

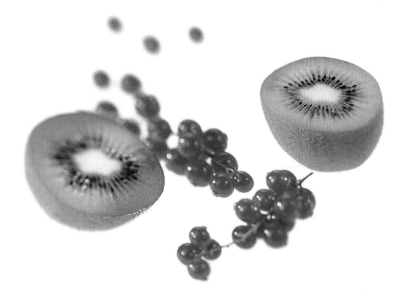

■ Vitamin C

ASCORBIC ACID

USA RDI 60 mg **UK** RNI 40 mg **EC** RDA 60 mg

Another important antioxidant vitamin, vitamin C has a protective role for the body, helping to maintain a healthy immune system. It is necessary for building healthy connective tissue, bones, and teeth, and helps the healing of wounds and fractures. It also helps in the absorption of iron. Extra vitamin C may be needed at certain times, for example when the body is under stress (e.g. illness, high workload) and for certain people (e.g. smokers, heavy drinkers, people working in heavily polluted atmospheres). Many experts believe that the RDIs and RNIs are too low for modern living, but that is a subject of considerable debate.

As an antioxidant (see the box opposite), vitamin C appears to help cut the risk of coronary heart disease. Low levels of vitamin C are associated both with high blood pressure and with increased risk of heart attack; however, one large study concluded that, once vitamin C intake is adequate, high-dose supplements will probably not be associated with lessened risk. Other trials have shown that vitamin C can dilate the arteries and help blood-flow in heart patients.

Vitamin C may also help to reduce

SELECTED BEST SOURCES OF VITAMIN C	(mg per 100 g)		
Rosehip syrup	295	Brussels sprouts, lightly boiled	60
Guava	230	Kiwi fruit	59
Chili peppers, red	225	Cabbage, red	55
Bell peppers, red	140	Snow peas	54
Black currants, stewed	130	Oranges	54
Bell peppers, yellow	130	Broccoli, lightly boiled	44
Bell peppers, green	120	Baby corn, lightly boiled	39
Chili peppers, green	120	Nectarines	37
Collard greens, lightly boiled	77	Mangoes	37
Strawberries	77	Grapefruit	36
Kale, lightly boiled	71	Green salad	36
Papaya	60		

the length and severity of colds if taken in doses up to 2,000 mg (2 g). New research indicates it may also reduce the risk of osteoarthritis.

A deficiency of vitamin C results in poor wound healing, bleeding gums, lowered resistance to infection, nosebleeds, and in the long term can result in scurvy, although this is rare.

An excess of the vitamin can give a laxative effect, including diarrhea and gastric upset. It has often been said that high intakes may also increase the

production of oxalic acid and, hence, kidney stones in susceptible individuals, but this has not been substantiated.

Vitamin C is found mainly in fruits and vegetables, and is easily lost in storage, processing, preparation, and cooking (see page 208). For example, fresh peas contain approximately 24 mg vitamin C per 100 g; canned garden peas only 1 mg.

The only plants that contain no vitamin C are unsprouted grains and dried legumes.

■ The B Vitamins

The B vitamins are a group of six water-soluble vitamins that work together in the body and are essential for growth and the proper development of a healthy nervous system; for body maintenance and food digestion and the metabolism. Each, however, has its own role to play.

As they can't be stored in the body, it is important that adequate amounts of the B vitamins are eaten on a regular basis. Certain people will need more of the B group than others—for example, smoking, alcohol, illness, and stress deplete the body's levels.

The vitamins in the B group, like vitamin C, are depleted through the storage, processing, preparation, and cooking of food (see pages 208–9 for notes on how best to retain the water-soluble vitamins in food).

In general, it isn't advisable to take high doses of just one of the B vitamins, unless with medical advice, as the group works synergistically together.

■ Vitamin B1

THIAMIN

USA RDI 1.5 mg **UK** RNI 0.8 mg (females), 1.0 mg (males) **EC** RDA 1.4 mg

Vitamin B1 is needed to release the energy from carbohydrate foods and helps to ensure that the brain and nerves have adequate glucose for their needs. A lack of B1 can lead to the deficiency disease beri beri. Heavy drinkers may be short of B1. An excess isn't harmful as it is excreted. B1 is found in a variety of foods, especially pork, bacon, and nuts.

■ Vitamin B2

RIBOFLAVIN

USA RDI 1.7 mg **UK** RNI 1.1 mg (females), 1.3 mg (males) **EC** RDA 1.6 mg

This B vitamin is involved in the release of energy, too, but more from fat and protein than carbohydrate. Adequate vitamin B2 is needed to maintain healthy skin and mucous membrane (e.g. inside

SELECTED BEST SOURCES OF B VITAMINS

Vitamin B1 (mg per 100 g)

Sunflower seeds	1.6	Bran flakes, Fruit 'n Fiber	1.0
Special K	1.3	Whole-wheat spaghetti, dry	1.0
Canadian bacon, broiled	1.2	Granda cereal	0.8
Peanuts, unsalted	1.1	Raisin bran	0.8
Pork, lean tenderloin	1.0		

Vitamin B2 (mg per 100 g)

Liver	4.6	Oatmeal	1.3
Total cereal	2.2	Liver pâté	1.2
Special K	1.8	Venison, roasted	0.7
Grapenuts	1.5	Goats'-milk cheese	0.6
Weetabix	1.5	Cheddar cheese	0.5
Nori seaweed, dried	1.3	Eggs	0.5
Bran flakes, oat bran flakes	1.3	Tomato sauce for pasta	0.5
Vegetable pâté	1.3		

Vitamin B3 (mg per 100 g)

Total cereal	24	Peanuts, plain	19
Special K	23	Pork tenderloin, lean	18
Chicken breast, no skin	22	Fruit 'n Fiber, Corn Flakes	17
Lambs' liver	21	Ovaltine powder	17
Tuna canned in oil, drained	21	Tuna, fresh	17
Branflakes	20	Shiitake mushrooms, dried	15
Grapenuts	20	Swordfish, broiled	14
Turkey, light meat, roasted	20	Mackerel, broiled	13

Vitamin B6 (mg per 100 g)

Wheat germ	3.3	Squid	0.7
Turbot, broiled	2.5	Walnuts, shelled	0.7
Fruit 'n Fiber	1.8	Beef steak, lean	0.7
All Bran	1.3	Chicken breast, no skin, broiled	0.6
Lentils, dry	0.9	Hazelnuts, shelled	0.6
Salmon, broiled	0.8	Swordfish, broiled	0.6
Turkey, light meat	0.8	Baked potato	0.5

Vitamin B12 (mg per 100g)

Liver	54	Scallops, steamed	9
Seaweed, nori, dried	27.5	Shrimp, cooked	8
Mussels, steamed, shelled weight	22	Skate, broiled	8
Oysters, shucked weight	17	Salmon, steamed	6
Sardines, canned in oil, drained	15	Tuna, canned in oil, drained	5
Herring, broiled	15	Eggs	2.5
Anchovies, canned, drained	11	Lean beef	2
Rabbit meat	10	Cheddar cheese	1.1

the mouth and nose) and if deficiency occurs symptoms may include a sore mouth. Excess B2 is excreted in the urine, so there is no safe upper limit recommended. B2 is found in many foods; particularly rich sources are variety meats, dairy products, and fortified breakfast cereals.

■ Vitamin B3
NIACIN

USA RDI 20 mg **UK** RNI 13mg (females), 17 mg (males) **EC** RDA 18 mg

Vitamin B3 is also involved in the release of energy from food and can be manufactured from the amino acid tryptophan within the body, but the FDA has still offered RDIs to ensure adequate niacin. A deficiency results in the disease pellagra, which initially affects the skin and can be very serious if left untreated. Excess B3 (over 3 g a day) can cause liver damage, dilation of the blood vessels, and kidney damage. Niacin is found in meat, fish, and fortified breakfast cereals, as well as a variety of other foods.

■ Vitamin B6
PYRIDOXINE

USA RDI 2 mg **UK** RNI 1.2 mg (females), 1.4 mg (males) **EC** RDA 2 mg

B6 is important for the metabolization of protein, is also involved in the production of B3 from tryptophan, and is necessary for healthy blood. In recent years vitamin B6 has been used by nutritionists to help ease PMS, often in conjunction with evening primrose oil, but, in 1997, the UK government banned over-the-counter sales of supplements containing more than 10 mg of B6 (levels up to 50 mg are allowed under medical supervision), as high levels can cause nerve damage.

Some European governments report that damage can occur at levels over 50 mg per day. Obvious symptoms of deficiency of B6 are rare, but the latest research into heart disease indicates that a deficiency of B6, along with deficiencies of folic acid and B12, may cause high levels of the amino acid homocysteine in the body, now believed to be an important cause of coronary heart disease. Richest sources of B6 are meats, fish, eggs, whole grains, fortified cereals, and some vegetables.

■ Vitamin B12

USA RDI 6 µg **UK** RNI 1.5 µg (male and female) **EC** RDA 1 µg

Vitamin B12 is necessary for the formation of blood cells and nerves, and a deficiency leads to the form of anemia called pernicious anemia and can also lead to nerve damage. It is now also known that low intake of B12, along with low intakes of B6 and folic acid, can lead to high levels of homocysteine, which is linked with coronary heart disease.

Vegans often take supplements of B12, as the vitamin is only found naturally in animal produce and seaweed. A little can be synthesized in the body by bacteria. High intakes appear to have no toxic effects. Excellent sources of B12 in the diet are variety meats and meat; dairy products also contains some.

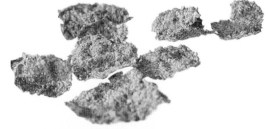

■ Folate
FOLIC ACID
USA RDI 400 µg **UK** RNI 200 µg (males and females) **EC** RDA 200 µg

Folic acid is necessary for the formation of blood cells and for proper development of infants. It is routinely given to pregnant women as a supplement, to help prevent birth defects such as spina bifida. Deficiency can lead to megaloblastic anemia and, along with deficiencies of B6 and B12, can cause high levels of homocysteine, which is linked to coronary heart disease (see Vitamin B6 on page 27). About 35% of the US is deficient in folate. Since January 1998 enriched bread, pasta, flour, cereal, crackers, and rice have been fortified with folate.

There are no known toxic effects of high levels, but they may hinder zinc absorption, and the FDA recommends no more than 1,000 µg per day. Folic acid is found in variety meats, leafy green vegetables, whole grains, nuts, legumes, and fortified breakfast cereals, among many types of foods.

SELECTED BEST SOURCES OF FOLATE (µg per 100 g)

Chicken livers	995
Black-eyed peas, dry weight	630
Soybeans, dry weight	370
Grapenuts	350
Soy flour	345
Wheat germ	331
Special K	330
Cornflakes (and most other commercial breakfast cereals)	250
Lambs' liver	205
Lentils, boiled	179
Chickpeas, boiled	172
Asparagus, lightly boiled	155
Baby corn, lightly boiled	152
Broccoli, lightly boiled	140
Swiss-style muesli	140
Red kidney beans, dry weight	130
Brussels sprouts, lightly boiled	110

Minerals

Minerals are inorganic substances, and various vital body processes—as well as normal development—are reliant on adequate intakes of them. Altogether 15 minerals have been classed as essential in the diet. The major minerals, needed in larger quantities, are calcium, magnesium, potassium, sodium, and phosphorus. Iron and zinc, although needed in milligrams rather than grams (1,000 mg = 1 gram) are also usually classed as major minerals. The "trace elements," needed in much smaller (but equally essential) quantities, are selenium, copper, fluoride, iodine, manganese, chromium, and cobalt.

In general, the three main functions of minerals are as constituents of bones and teeth (particularly calcium, magnesium, and phosphorus); as salts regulating body fluids (sodium, potassium, and chloride); and as components of enzymes and hormones, regulating or helping all the functions of the body, including the nervous system, blood supply, and energy release (most minerals).

A deficiency of certain minerals may result in all kinds of health problems, such as anemia (iron), osteoporosis (calcium), and weak immune system (zinc). Research over the last few years is also finding strong evidence that optimum intake of certain minerals can help to prevent heart disease—for example, calcium, magnesium, and the antioxidant mineral selenium.

Minerals are present in most foods and drinks, in varying quantities. A varied healthy diet, providing adequate calories, should ensure intake is at least the minimum recommended by the FDA, but this isn't always the case. One reason is that levels of minerals in even an apparently healthy diet may vary. For example, some minerals in both plants and animal produce are dependent upon the soil in which the plants are grown or on which the animals graze, and mineral content of soil varies in different parts of the country. Another reason is that minerals are not always easily absorbed by the body (calcium needs vitamin D, for example, and absorption of several minerals can be hindered by certain acids in other foods). A third reason is that some people may need more than the minimum recommended levels of minerals at certain times; for example, women with heavy periods may need extra iron, and so on. In the pages ahead we look at the main minerals that may be lacking in our diet.

For more information on minerals and the body's requirements throughout every stage of life, see Section Three. For notes on recommended daily amounts and the pitfalls of supplementation, see the introduction to Vitamins on page 22. The Food Charts at the back of the book list significant mineral content of about 400 foods.

■ Calcium
USA RDI 1,000 mg **UK** RNI 700 mg (males and females) **EC** RDA 800 mg

Calcium, as the major constituent of bone and tooth mineral, is the mineral needed in greatest quantities. The average human body contains about 1 kilo of calcium and around a gram a day is needed to maintain that level.

Adequate calcium intake is vital throughout life. In infants and through to adulthood, it is vital to ensure peak bone mass is reached. In women it is important to help prevent osteoporosis in later life. Calcium is also important for the smooth functioning of the muscles, including the heart, for blood clotting, for nerve function, and other activities. There is some evidence that low calcium levels may be linked with coronary heart disease, as hardness of tap water is related to lower incidence. Symptoms of deficiency include muscle cramps and disease caused by calcium (or calcium absorption) deficiency.

Only about 40% of the calcium that we eat is absorbed. Adequate vitamin D is needed for this process (see Vitamins, page 23) and absorption can also be affected by certain foods. Essential fatty acids may help absorption, and exercise helps maintain bone mass. Foods high in insoluble fiber, such as wheat bran and whole grains, can hinder absorption (if taken at the same time), due to the phytates they contain (although this effect may be temporary), and so can oxalates, found in spinach, rhubarb, chard, chocolate, and beets, and the tannin in tea and coffee. If you drink tea or coffee, leave a gap between your meal and your drink. A diet containing high levels of protein (120 g a day or more) may cause bone demineralization and calcium to be excreted in the urine.

For all these reasons, milk and milk products are included in the USDA's food pyramid guide to healthy eating. Calcium works closely in the body with magnesium, and a high calcium intake may require additional magnesium. Calcium needs of special groups of people (e.g. pregnant women, children, and the elderly) are discussed in Section Three. Calcium in a vegetarian diet is discussed on page 63.

Rich sources of calcium include cheese, yogurt and milk, dark green leafy vegetables, white bread and flour (fortified). Canned fish (such as sardines and salmon) can be a rich source, but only if the bones are eaten.

SELECTED BEST SOURCES OF CALCIUM (mg per 100 g)

Food	mg	Food	mg
Poppy seeds	1,580	Muesli	200
Parmesan cheese	1,200	Low-fat plain yogurt	190
Swiss cheese	975	Goats'-milk soft cheese	190
Gruyère cheese	950	Navy beans, dry weight	180
Kombu seaweed, dried	900	Spinach	170
Cheddar, low-fat	840	Brazil nuts, shelled	170
Edam	770	Chickpeas, dry weight	160
Cheddar, full-fat	740	Naan bread	160
Sesame seeds	670	Kale, lightly boiled	150
Sardines canned in brine, drained, including bones	540	Corn tortilla	130
Brie	540	Vanilla ice cream	130
Mozzarella	530	White bread, French	130
Tofu, steamed	510	Low-fat 2% milk	120
Danish blue	500	Skim or nonfat milk	120
Sardines, canned in oil, drained, including bones	500	Tilapia fish	120
		White bread	120
Nori seaweed, dried	430	Whole milk	115
Feta cheese	360	Shrimp, cooked and peeled	110
White chocolate	270	Collard greens, lightly boiled	75
Almonds, shelled	240	Cottage cheese, low-fat	75
Soybeans, dry weight	240	White cabbage	49
Figs, dried	230	Broccoli, lightly boiled	40
Milk chocolate	220		

SELECTED BEST SOURCES OF IRON (mg per 100 g)

Total cereal	60	Peaches, dried, no-soak	6.8
Curry powder	58.3	Navy beans, dry weight	6.7
Ground ginger	46.3	Most commercial cereals	6.7
Nori seaweed, dried	19.6	Red kidney beans, dry weight	6.4
Special K	16	Cashew nuts, plain	6.2
Rasin bran	16	Whole-grain barley, dry weight	6.0
All Bran	12.0	Couscous, dry weight	5.0
Lentils, green or brown, dry weight	11.1	Bulgur wheat, dry weight	4.9
Cocoa powder, unsweetened	10.5	Apricots, dried	3.4
Sesame seeds	10.4	Beef, lean	2.1
Pumpkin seeds	10.0	Kale, lightly boiled	2.0
Soybeans, dry weight	9.7	Eggs	1.9
Chicken liver	9.2	Lamb, lean	1.6
Textured soy protein or TVP	9.0	Canadian bacon, broiled	1.6
Lentils, red, dry weight	7.6	Brown rice, dry weight	1.4
Lambs' liver	7.5	Baked beans in tomato sauce	1.4
Liver pâté	7.4	Collard greens, lightly boiled	1.4
Weetabix	7.4	Broccoli, lightly boiled	1.0

◼ Iron

USA RDI 18 mg **UK** RNI 14.8 mg (females), 8.7 mg (males) **EC** RDA 14 mg

Iron's main function is to carry oxygen from the lungs to all the cells of the body. Half of the body's iron store is used to make hemoglobin, which acts as the carrier. Iron can also increase resistance to infection and help the healing process. Lack of adequate iron (or iron absorption) leads to anemia, with symptoms including tiredness, pallor, weakness, and lack of energy. Women, in particular, need to ensure their diet is high enough in iron as it is lost in the blood through menstruation. It is thought that many women are iron-deficient.

Iron is supplied in the diet by both animal foods and plants. Iron from meat sources is better absorbed than that from plant sources, but if body stores of iron are depleted, or when needs are great, then absorption from plants increases.

Absorption is affected by other factors, including intake of phytates, oxalates, and tannins (see Calcium, page 29), and also by calcium itself, which can bind with iron in plant sources, though it is thought that in these circumstances the body adapts to absorb extra as needed.

Vitamin C aids iron absorption—certain foods, such as dark leafy greens, contain both iron and vitamin C. Other iron-rich foods should be eaten if possible with foods rich in vitamin C (e.g. a glass of orange juice with lentil soup).

Excess iron can cause stomach upsets, constipation, and kidney damage. Good iron sources are variety and red meats, dark green vegetables, legumes and whole grains, nuts and seeds, and fortified cereals. Many dried herbs are excellent sources, but are not often used in sufficient quantity to make much contribution to the diet. Ground spices can do so, though—e.g. 1 teaspoon of ground ginger gives nearly 1 mg of iron, and curry powder slightly more.

◼ Zinc

USA RDI 15 mg **UK** RNI 7 mg (females), 9.5 mg (males) **EC** RDA 15 mg

Zinc is present throughout the body tissues and helps the activities of a wide variety of enzymes. It is essential for normal growth and development; for a healthy reproductive system and fertility; and for healthy fetal development. It helps to keep skin healthy, helps wound healing, regulates the sense of taste, and is important for immune system strength. It also helps destroy surplus free radicals in the body (see Antioxidants, page 24).

A deficiency of zinc during pregnancy and infancy can cause retarded growth and sexual development. A deficiency in adulthood can cause increased risk of infections, skin and hair problems, slow wound healing, impaired sense of taste and smell, low sperm count, night blindness, and other problems. There is also some evidence that low zinc coupled with high copper levels is linked to violent behavior.

Zinc levels may be affected by smoking and alcohol. It is found in greatest quantities in meat and dairy products. It is also found in good amounts in whole-grain cereals and

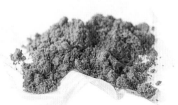

SELECTED BEST SOURCES OF ZINC (mg per 100 g)

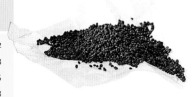

Calves' liver	14.2
Wheat germ	12.3
Poppy seeds	8.5
Oysters, raw, weight including shells	8.3
Cocoa powder, unsweetened	6.9
All Bran	6.7
Pumpkin seeds	6.6
Pine nuts	6.5
Seaweed, nori, dried	6.4
Beef steak	6.0
Cashew nuts, plain	5.9
Crab, canned in brine, drained	5.7
Corned beef, canned	5.5
Fresh crab, meat only	5.5
Sesame seeds	5.3
Parmesan cheese	5.3
Pecan nuts, shelled	5.3
Lamb leg, roasted, lean	5.2
Sunflower seeds	5.1

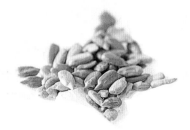

legumes, but—like calcium and iron—its absorption may be hindered by eating foods rich in phytates, oxalates, and tannins (see page 29). Both calcium and iron can also interfere with absorption, though it is thought that this is only of relevance at doses supplied in supplements.

People at risk from zinc deficiency may then be smokers and heavy drinkers, some vegetarians, people with long-term illness, and anyone who eats a poor or meager diet. Excess zinc (over 50 mg a day) can hinder copper absorption and possibly iron, too.

Selenium

USA RDI none UK RNI 60µg (females), 75µg (males) EC RDA none

Selenium is an important trace element—it is an antioxidant (see page 24) and, as such, helps to protect us from heart disease, some cancers, and premature aging. In one large recent American study, selenium supplementation at 200 µg per day was associated with a 50% drop in deaths from cancers of the lung, prostate, and colon. Deficiency may increase the risk of these diseases.

Working with vitamin E, it helps control the production of hormone-like substances called prostaglandins, and is important for normal growth, fertility, thyroid action, healthy skin and hair, and more. One study showed that women with low levels of selenium had increased risk of miscarriage; and other tests show that selenium levels are often low in people with rheumatoid arthritis and that selenium supplements may reduce pain and inflammation. Yet another recent study has linked low selenium in HIV sufferers with a twenty-fold increased risk of dying of HIV-related causes.

Because selenuim comes from plants or plant-eating animals, the amount in the food that we eat relates to the amount in the soil—the US dietary intake levels are high so at present there is no RDI. Unlike other minerals, the amounts in the food we eat can't be guaranteed (depending on where it comes from), but brazil nuts are a very rich source and fish, seeds, and variety meats should all be good sources. The levels listed here are, therefore, a guide only.

Selenium is, however, toxic in excess, producing nerve disorder and hair- and nail-loss. Up to 1,000 µg per day should be safe, however toxicity is most likely to be a consequence of occupational exposure. For notes on supplementation, see page 146.

SELECTED BEST SOURCES OF SELENIUM (µg per 100 g)

Brazil nuts, shelled	1,530	Wheat flour, whole-wheat	53
Mixed unsalted nuts and raisins	170	Sardines, canned in oil, drained	49
Lambs' kidneys	160	Sunflower seeds	49
Dried mushrooms	110	Swordfish	45
Lentils, green or brown, dry weight	105	Mussels, cooked	43
Tuna, canned in oil, drained	90	Lambs' liver	42
Wheat germ	79	Sardines, broiled	38
Tuna, canned in water, drained	78	Whole-wheat bread	35
Squid	66	Cod	33
Lemon sole	60	Salmon	31
Tuna, fresh	57	Cashew nuts, plain	29
		Shrimp, cooked	23
		Pork, lean, roast	21
		Walnuts, shelled	19

■ Magnesium

USA RDI 400 mg **UK** RNI 270 mg (women), 300 mg (men) **EC** RDA 300 mg

Magnesium is present throughout our bodies. It works with calcium to maintain healthy bones, it helps release energy and to absorb nutrients, as well as regulating temperature, nerves, and muscle function. Adequate levels are important to maintain a healthy heart, and lower levels of coronary heart disease have been noted in hard-water (calcium- and magnesium-rich) areas. There is evidence that magnesium can help relieve PMS and prevent osteoporosis.

If magnesium is deficient, symptoms include muscle weakness and abnormal heart rhythms, tiredness, appetite loss, fits, and cramps. Absorption can be hindered by heavy alcohol consumption.

Magnesium-rich foods include whole grains, nuts and seeds, and green vegetables. Tap water can also be a good source if you live in a hard-water area.

■ Potassium

USA RDI 3.5 g **UK** RNI 3.5 g (3,500 mg) (males and females) **EC** RDA none

Potassium works with sodium to regulate body fluids and is essential for correct functioning of the cells. It regulates nerves, heart-beat, and blood pressure. If the diet is high in sodium, more potassium will be needed to help prevent fluid retention. In trials, young men who had a low potassium intake (390 mg per day) were less able to excrete excess sodium—and their blood pressure was higher—than when they took the RDI. High blood pressure can be lowered by a diet low in sodium and high in potassium.

Potassium is found in a wide range of foods, and clinical deficiency is unusual, but diets low in fresh fruit and vegetables (good sources) and high in salty snack foods may create a potassium/sodium imbalance. Also, people who take diuretics or laxatives, or who are on some types of drug (e.g. steroids), may excrete too much potassium. Severe potassium deficiency can result in serious heart problems—even heart attack. Excess is unlikely in a normal diet, though very high levels of supplementation would be toxic. Low-sodium, potassium-rich foods include dried fruits, legumes, nuts, potatoes, bananas, garlic, onions, and many other fruits and vegetables.

■ Phosphorus

USA RDI 1 g **UK** RNI 550 mg (males and females) **EC** RDA 800 mg

About 1 kilo of body weight is phosphorus and most is in the skeleton. It is an essential part of all body cells, helping in the release of energy and regulating protein activity. As it is a major constituent of all plant and animal cells, and added to many commercial foods, deficiency in the diet is not likely and, on average, our diets are above the RDI.

High intakes of phosphorus without adequate calcium may upset the body's phosphorus/calcium balance and cause bone demineralization, and so may be a factor in osteoporosis. Luckily, many foods high in phosphorus are also high in calcium—milk and cheese are rich natural sources of both. Other foods high in phosphorus include meats, fish, and eggs. For women with risk factors for osteoporosis, it may be wise to keep a watch on phosphorus intake, but not by cutting back on a nutritious diet.

■ Sodium

USA Daily Recommended Value (DRV) less than 2,400 mg/day **UK** Lower RNI 575 mg (males and females) **UK** Upper RNI 1,600 mg/day (males and females)

Sodium is unlike all the other minerals necessary to humans in that it is the only one we have come to recognize as a particular taste in the diet (as part of salt, sodium chloride), adding it to foods in the home and buying large amounts of added-salt processed products. Sodium also occurs naturally—usually in much lower amounts—in foods, including meat, fish, vegetables, and even fruit.

Sodium, with potassium and chloride,

SELECTED BEST SOURCES OF MAGNESIUM (mg per 100 g)	
Cocoa powder, unsweetened	520
Brazil nuts, shelled	410
Sunflower seeds	390
Sesame seeds	370
Instant coffee (dry weight)	330
Pine nuts	270
Cashew nuts, plain	270
Textured soy protein	270
Soybeans, dry weight	250
Licorice	170
Hazelnuts and walnuts, shelled	160
Shredded Wheat	130

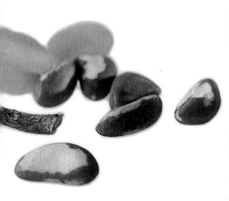

helps to regulate the body's fluid balance and is present in all body fluids, especially outside the cells, such as blood. Sodium is also necessary for nerve and muscle activity, but most of us eat far more than we need—in 1996, we averaged 3.5 g per day. As salt, or sodium chloride, is 40% sodium and 60% chloride, that represents over 9 g of salt a day. Since our bodies can function with a wide range of dietary sodium, the RDA developed by the National Academy of Science, estimates that levels as low as 1.1 g may be sufficient.

The problem with high intake of sodium is that it is linked with high blood pressure and heart disease. Not everyone is susceptible to raised blood pressure through high sodium intake, but it is estimated that 10–25% of the population are. One research has shown that reducing sodium intake from 3.9 g (9.75 g salt) a day to the recommended levels significantly reduces raised blood pressure.

Excess sodium in the diet is also linked with fluid retention (edema) and kidney stones, and a diet high in sodium and also low in potassium can exacerbate potential problems. A high-sodium diet increases the need for potassium.

Sodium deficiency in the US is not common, but may happen during heavy and/or prolonged exercise, due to loss in the sweat, and in high temperatures. Signs of sodium deficiency are cramps, weakness, fatigue, nausea, and thirst.

Main sources of sodium in the diet are salt used in cooking and at the table (approximately 20% of the sodium we eat), bouillon cubes, canned and packaged soups, bottled and canned sauces, cured and smoked foods, pickles, snacks such as potato chips, fast food, hard and processed cheeses, spreading fats, and breakfast cereals (which account for another 25% of daily salt eaten). Many other processed foods contain fairly high amounts of salt, though—baked beans, canned spaghetti, and cookies; even bread is higher in salt than you might realize, at 175 mg an average slice.

To reach your day's maximum DRV of 2,400 mg sodium or 6 g salt, you would need to eat no more than, say, one average portion of bacon, an average Cheddar cheese sandwich and a dab of pickle relish, plus a portion of Cornflakes. Or just half a bouillon cube and 2 tablespoons soy sauce in your stir-fry could take you to the limit. People wanting to cut down their salt intake should limit the amount of processed foods they eat, choosing reduced-salt versions if available. Less salt should be added at table and in cooking (salt substitutes are available).

■ Other minerals

A *fluoride* deficiency will encourage tooth decay, but these days deficiency symptoms are rare as most of our dietary fluoride comes from fluoridated tap water and toothpaste.

Iodine is required for the functioning of the thyroid gland and deficiency can cause goiter, but in the US average intakes are well above the RDI of 150 µg per day. Iodine is found most abundantly in milk and seafood.

Chromium is important for helping to control glucose levels in the blood, including insulin function, and may help to control blood cholesterol. The RDI for chromium is 120 µg per day. Meat and variety meats, eggs and seafood, cheese and whole grains are good sources.

Deficiencies of the trace elements *copper, sulfur,* and *manganese* are rare, although a diet very high in zinc may inhibit absorption of copper.

SELECTED FOODS AND THEIR SODIUM CONTENT (mg per 100 g)

Food	mg	Food	mg
Salt	39,300	French-style dressing	1,320
Chicken bouillon cubes	16,300	Processed cheese slices	1,320
Salted dried cod	7,530	Dill pickle	1,282
Soy sauce, light or dark	7,120	Danish blue cheese	1,260
Minestrone soup, dry pack	6,400	Smoked cod	1,200
Textured soy protein, dry	4,420	Cornflakes	1,100
Chili condiment, oily	4,050	Edam cheese	1,020
Anchovies (oily)	3,670	Canned cook-in sauce	940
Bacon slices, broiled	2,700	Tortilla chips	860
Black bean sauce	2,150	Potato chips	840
Prosciutto	2,000	Canned creamed tomato soup	830
Smoked salmon	1,880	Margarine, average	800
Salami	1,800	Butter, average	
Pretzels	1,720	(not low-salt)	750
Tomato ketchup	1,630		

Phytochemicals— the 21st-century food pharmacy

The food scientists are now discovering that, for your health's sake, it may be even more important to eat a diet rich in fruits, vegetables, and other plant foods than it is to cut down on the saturated fat, junk foods, or calories. Here we look at the whole new world of the phytochemicals and how they can protect your health.

Just as vitamins were discovered in the first half of the 20th century, scientists are now uncovering a wealth of new health-protecting compounds in plant foods. These compounds are not nutrients as such, but have been described as "biologically active non-nutrients." The scientists have called them phytochemicals (from "phyto" meaning plant).

There are literally thousands of different phytochemicals and they can be present in plants in quite high amounts—maybe several percent. They include the substances responsible for giving the plant its color, flavor, odor— its particular unique characteristics, you could say.

A lot of research has been done in the past few years to try to discover the health-giving properties of these compounds and it now seems that they have much to offer in the fight against many types of cancer, heart disease, and various health problems.

Many are antioxidants, while others help to block or suppress harmful cell reactions, for example. Many help the body in more than one way—and more is being discovered about the phytochemicals all the time. One thing is for certain—if you want to protect your health, you MUST eat up your fruits and vegetables, just like your mother always used to tell you to do.

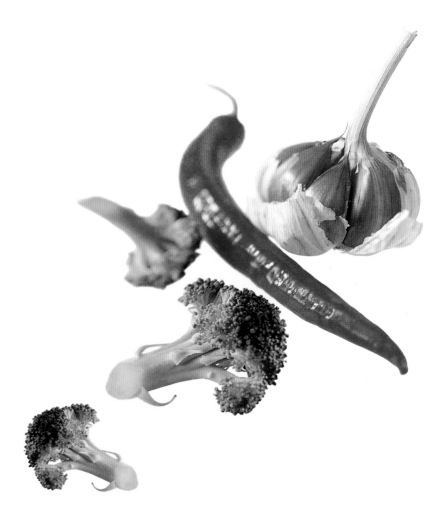

■ Carotenoids
Probably the first phytochemical to be linked with health was beta-carotene, the orange pigment in carrots, sweet potatoes, and other plants, which can convert to vitamin A and which was cited as one of the first antioxidants, along with vitamins C and E. In fact, the carotenoid group of compounds in foods numbers about 600, many of which are also potent antioxidants. Here are just some of them.

Lycopene is the red pigment found mainly in tomatoes, red grapefruit, and watermelon. Cooked tomatoes, including those in ketchup and bottled pasta sauces, are a particularly active source. It has been found that adequate intake of lycopene can reduce incidence of heart attacks by 50%, by antioxidant activity and possibly by lowering LDL blood cholesterol levels. It may also help prevent cervical, prostate, and several other types of cancers.

More carotenoids with promising anti-carcinogenic properties are lutein, found in dark green leafy vegetables, black currants and potatoes; beta-cryptoxanthin, found in mangoes; capsanthin, in red bell peppers; phytoene, in winter squash, and pumpkin; and canthaxanthin, in mushrooms.

■ Bioflavonoids
These are a group of no less than 6,000 (or so!) polyphenolic compounds, which many years ago were classed as "vitamin P"

and then more or less dismissed as of no significance. Now we know better.

The flavonoids usually appear to be most potent in fruits or in sweet vegetables, probably because the sugars help the flavonoids to be absorbed. Providing the orange and yellow colors in citrus fruits (for example), the flavonoids are antioxidants and also help the absorption of vitamin C. The main discovery to date is that they seem to help prevent cancers, but different flavonoids have different roles.

Taxifolin and rutin are two important flavonoids in citrus fruits, including oranges and grapefruits. Ellagic acid, found in greatest amounts in strawberries, blackberries, cherries, and grapes, blocks the action of cancer-inducing cells.

There is a sub-group of flavonoids called flavonols, of which one of the most researched, and probably the most abundant in foods, is quercetin—an antioxidant found in black tea and red wine as well as in onions, tomatoes, apples, potatoes, grapes, and fava beans. Studies have linked high quercetin intake with lower risk of heart disease. Quercetin may also help to prevent eye cataracts and hay fever as it has antihistamine properties.

Green tea (the unfermented form of black tea) contains catechins, the antioxidant effects of which may include the slowing down of the aging process as well as protecting the circulatory system from damage.

■ Glucosinolates
These phytochemicals, which were once thought to be toxic to humans and act as natural pesticides, are found mainly in cruciferous and green vegetables; among the best sources seem to be broccoli, Brussels sprouts, cabbage, kale, and cauliflower.

Broccoli is a particularly rich source of glucosinolates, which break down into a substance called sulforaphane that appears to have a strong anti-cancer effect by stimulating our natural defenses—so much so that food scientists are attempting genetically to inject it into other vegetables so that their benefit is spread wider.

Another glucosinolate is sinigrin, found in large quantities in sprouts, which has a different anti-cancer effect by suppressing the growth of pre-cancerous cells.

Watercress is rich in isothiocyanate, which can break down and render harmless one of the main cancer-causing agents in tobacco smoke.

■ Organosulfides
Garlic, onions, and the other members of the allium family—leeks and chives—are the main providers of these sulfides which seem to stimulate the immune system, are antioxidant, and appear to fight many cancers, particularly stomach cancer, ulcers, and heart disease.

Garlic is rich in allicin, which is antibiotic and antiviral. Its content of diallyl disulfide appears to shrink cancerous tumors, and other phytochemicals it contains may help prevent pre-cancerous cells from forming, as well as helping to lower LDL blood cholesterol, raise HDL blood cholesterol, and helping in the prevention of blood clots.

■ Phytoestrogens
These are a group of phytochemicals with a structure similar in effect to estrogen, the female hormone that protects against heart disease and osteoporosis. They also appear to be linked with a reduction in risk of the hormone-dependent cancers, such as cancer of the breast and womb.

There are two main types of phyto-estrogen, isoflavones and lignans. Isoflavones are found in legumes, particularly soybeans, and several trials have shown a link between low incidence of breast cancer development and high soy intake. The particular isoflavone equol appears to confer the most benefit.

Soy isoflavones also appear to reduce hot flashes and night sweats in menopausal women.

Lignans are found in various plant foods, especially flax seeds, whole grains, and berries. The lignan enterolactone in this case appears to be the most potent form in helping to prevent breast cancer. The phyto-estrogens may also be antioxidant.

Other phytochemicals that may help to fight hormone-related cancers are limonene, found in citrus oils, and certain members of the glucosinolate family (see above) found in sprouts, broccoli, etc. called indoles.

■ Other interesting phytochemicals
Bromelain, found in pineapples, aids digestion but may also clear blocked arteries and thin the blood. Similarly, papain, found in papaya, aids digestion, and is also a pain-reliever.

Capsaicin, found in chili peppers, is an antioxidant, pain reliever, and anti-inflammatory and can reduce LDL blood cholesterol.

Resveratrol, found in red wine and grape juice, appears to offer protection against coronary heart disease. Coumarins, found in various fruits and vegetables, as well as in licorice, help thin the blood and thus may help in the prevention of stroke and heart disease.

See also: Supplements, Heart Disease, Cancer, and Antioxidants.

Alcohol

Approximately 67% of Americans over the age of 21 claim to have drunk alcohol in the past year. In Europe the average is higher at about 80%. Recent news stories report that drinking alcoholic beverages has health benefits. Other stories say abuse of alcohol is related to many of the major causes of death in the US.

Of course, some people drink rarely, or only occasionally, and others drink much more—approximately one-tenth of men and one-sixteenth of women probably drink over safe limits.

So what is alcohol? It is a drug and an intoxicant with the power to kill—three-quarters of a bottle of scotch whisky (16 drinks or 24 units of alcohol) drunk rapidly would produce coma and death in many people. It is also a source of energy, containing 7 calories a gram, which is more than protein or carbohydrate but less than fat.

Some alcoholic drinks do contain a few nutrients (beer contains some B vitamins, red wine contains some iron, but spirits are totally nutrient-free); unlike fats, proteins, and carbohydrates, however, alcohol is not an essential part of our diet.

At high levels of intake it has many drawbacks, both major and minor, including the short-term effects of intoxication, risk of accident, increased risk of some cancers, liver damage, weight gain and/or nutritional deficiencies, heart damage, and so on (see Alcohol Abuse, page 86).

At low levels of intake, however, alcohol does appear to pose no health problems and there is increasing evidence that there are identifiable health benefits from recommended levels of alcohol consumption (see right) in regard to stroke, heart disease, and gallstones. The consensus of opinion is that moderate drinkers appear to live longer and have less incidence of heart disease than people who don't drink at all.

The link between lower risk of heart disease and alcohol intake has been found in several studies. These benefits appear to be linked with polyphenolic compounds found in alcohol (see page 35)—flavonoids such as quercetin and resveratrol in red wine, for example.

In fact, most experts agree that red wine is probably the "healthiest" alcoholic drink to take (more potent than others because of the concentration and type of polyphenols in the grape skins), but that all alcohol in moderation incurs protective effects against coronary heart disease, by reducing the levels of "bad" blood cholesterol LDL and increasing the "good" kind, HDL.

However, what do you do if you don't WANT to drink? Well, it is likely that red grape juice would probably have a similar effect to red wine ...

What are safe limits?

In the US the USDA's "Dietary Guidelines for Americans" recommends that *only* those who consume alcohol do so in moderation. By moderation they mean no more than one drink a day for women and no more than two a day for men. These are general guidelines and exclude the following: children and adolescents; women who are trying to conceive or are pregnant; individuals who cannot restrict their alcohol intake; individuals who plan to drive or that take part in activities that require skill or attention; individuals using prescriptions and over-the-counter medications.

In the UK units calculate accepted safe alcohol intake. The guidelines for safe drinking levels are 21 units a week for women and 28 units for men. The UK's Department of Health published an interdepartmental government report called "The Sensible Drinking Message," which is summarized below.

WHAT IS IN A "DRINK"? WHAT IS IN A UNIT?

USA

1 drink
* 12 fl oz (360 ml) standard beer
* 1.5 fl oz (45 ml) spirits
* 5 fl oz (150 ml) 12% wine
* 3 fl oz (90 ml) 20% wine

UK

1 unit
* 4 fl oz (125 ml) low-alcohol wine
* 10 fl oz (300 ml) standard beer
* 8 fl oz (25 ml) spirits, port or sherry

1½ units
* 4 fl oz (125 ml) 12% wine or champagne

2 units
* 10 fl oz (300 ml) strong beer

---

* 1–2 units of alcohol a day gives a significant health benefit in reducing heart disease for men over 40 and for post-menopausal women.
* It is better to drink the units regularly rather than save them up and binge.
* Men who drink 3–4 units a day and women who drink 2–3 units a day do not face significant health risks. Women's lower recommendation is because they generally have a smaller liver (which processes the alcohol and turns it into energy) and so they metabolize alcohol less well than men.
* Consistently drinking four or more units a day for men or three or more for women is not advisable, due to increasing health risks associated with higher levels of alcohol intake. Individual reactions to alcohol vary, so this can only be a benchmark.
* Pregnant women should not drink more than one or two units once or twice a week, and should avoid getting drunk.

So whether you measure your alcohol intake in drinks or units, the key to drinking for health seems to be "little and often." One large 1997 Australian survey found that there was a "major coronary event" risk reduction in men who regularly drank 1–4 units on five or six days a week, but they only drank their maximum units over one or two days a week.

Apart from your sex, other factors can affect how well or badly you tolerate alcohol. Short people and overweight people tolerate it less well. Alcohol on an "empty stomach" will make you drunk faster as it is absorbed into the bloodstream more quickly. Long term, it may also cause stomach upsets such as gastritis or ulcers. Alcohol with "fizz" also goes into the bloodstream quicker, whether it is champagne or a gin and tonic. If you are run-down, weak, ill, tired, or stressed, your alcohol tolerance may also be significantly affected.

Alcohol units—a guide

An "average drink" as defined by the USDA guidelines contains approximately 12 g of pure alcohol and a unit of alcohol contains 8 g. Thus, one drink in the US would be almost equal to 1½ units in the UK. A drink or a unit of alcohol is based on standard measures used in the individual countries, such as a glass of wine or a serving of beer. However with wine, and to a lesser extent with beer, there can be problems in working out exactly how much alcohol you are drinking.

Many people think they are drinking one "drink" or one unit when they have a "glass of wine," or reckon that half a bottle is two "drinks" or three units, but sadly this is not often the case—a glass of wine can easily be 2 "drinks", and half a bottle of wine can be more than 3 "drinks" or 5 units.

Why? Well, what is a "glass" of wine? A standard glass is 150 ml in the US and 125 ml in the UK. It is quite small, and you get five to six glasses to the 750 ml bottle of wine. Restaurants and private homes do usually use much bigger glasses, so a glass then might quite easily be two "drinks" or more than two units.

A bigger problem, though, is that a standard glass of wine can have different levels of alcohol. Average alcohol by volume is nearer 11–12%, the exception being some light Hock-style wines, which can be as low as 8–9%, and low-alcohol wines, which are usually 3–5%. Some wines can go as high as 14–18% alcohol by volume.

If you're drinking wine out of a bigger glass than standard, and having high-strength wine, you can see how easy it would be actually to be drinking more than you think you are.

Beers also vary tremendously in alcohol by volume, a "drink" or a unit of beer is based on alcohol by volume of 3–4%. Some strong beers go up to 10%! 12 oz of such a strong beer would not be one "drink" or one unit, but can be more than two. Mixed drinks can also be misleading. A martini, Manhattan, or a Black Russian can be more than two "drinks" or three units!

So when you're trying to keep drinking to safe limits, check the labels—and stick to small glasses for wine.

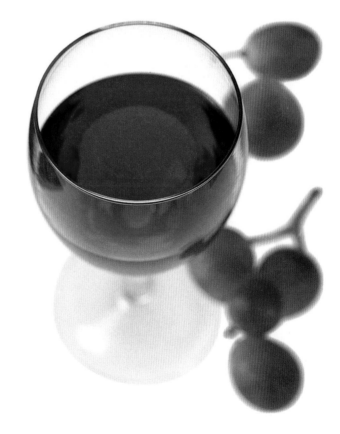

PUTTING IT ALL TOGETHER

Surprising though it may seem, putting together all the theoretical information into a practical eating plan for yourself isn't difficult. In the next few pages we look at different meals, your preferences, and how they can fit into a healthy lifestyle. There is no real need to worry about the exact nutritional content of every morsel of food you eat— trying to count grams of fat or the protein or carbohydrate in every meal, for example, would not only be time-consuming but almost impossible. The fact is that almost any kind of meal can be adapted to form part of a healthy diet if you follow a few easy guidelines.

Use your eyes! Studying the photograph opposite, you can see the proportions of the different types of food that will ensure your healthy meals.

■ Carbohydrates

To get the recommended sixty percent or so of carbohydrates, you need to ensure that at every meal you have a good-sized portion of (preferably unrefined) starchy carbohydrate food such as rice, pasta, potatoes, or bread—the bottom layer of the illustration opposite.

At most meals you also need about two portions of fruit and/or vegetables in good-sized portions (next layer up).

■ Proteins

Most meals should include a low- or moderate-fat protein (the third layer of the illustration opposite). That means choosing fish, game, poultry, legumes, extra-lean meats, milk, or low-fat cheeses. Portions of these can be quite small.

Remember, if you choose legumes they also have an excellent starch content and will count toward your carbohydrate intake. High-fat proteins, such as hard cheese, high-fat dairy products, and fatty meats, should be eaten in even smaller portions and less frequently.

■ Fats

As you've seen, fat is present in a great many foods, and as all fat is a calorie-dense food, it is easy to eat too much without realizing. Choosing plenty of complex carbohydrate, vegetables, and fruit and adding low-fat protein to this will ensure that you keep the fat content of your meal low. That means you can add small quantities of the fats YOU choose—ideally, healthy plant oils most of the time, such as olive or corn oil, perhaps some vegetable fat spread, and a little butter now and then when it helps the taste of the dish. Don't forget that some carbohydrates, such as certain breads, contain more fat than you think.

A FEW USEFUL TIPS

* Some types of meals lend themselves particularly well to the high-carb, medium-protein, lower-fat balancing act. You will find it easy with Italian pasta meals, and with eastern Mediterranean meals based on bulgur, other grains, and legumes. Indian and Asian meals using rice and noodles are ideal, too.
* When planning meals and snacks, keep thinking "carbohydrate foods" first. Then consider what protein foods you need to add. The traditional way of planning meals in the affluent West has been to think "protein" first and then add carbohydrates and vegetables as an afterthought. The other way around will ensure a much better balance.
* Split your meals up fairly evenly throughout the day in terms of both calorie content and times at which you eat them. This ensures more even blood sugar levels, avoidance of hunger, and a happier digestive system.
* If you feel hungry, eat. But eat a good-quality food, not a high-fat, high-sugar snack.
* Remember that calorie needs vary from person to person, and depend on many factors (see Section Four, Food for Weight Control), so use the meal portion sizes and nutrient guidelines here as just that—guidelines.

■ Drinks and snacks

Use what you drink as another chance to get nutrients—vitamin C from juices, calcium from low-fat milk or fortified soy milk, even phytochemicals from tea—but don't forget that one of the best drinks of all is water, tap or bottled. Look on snacks as a good excuse for obtaining some extra nutrients, rather than feeling guilty.

■ Sugars and alcohol

As by far the largest part of your daily calorie needs have now been taken up, you will only have a little room left for the sugars and for alcohol... add these to your diet in moderation, if at all. As a general guideline, an occasional drink or dessert can be added to your diet; however, they add little in the way of important nutrients to your diet.

■ The importance of variety

Balancing most of your meals this way forms the basis of a healthy diet for life. There is, however, one other very important tip, which will also ensure that most people will get adequate amounts of all the necessary vitamins, minerals, and phytochemicals. The message is "variety." Eat as wide a variety of foods as you can—different sources of carbohydrate, varying types of protein, and lots of different vegetables, salads, and fruits. Not only does this prevent boredom, it also ensures that you get all the micronutrients you need.

This is because even foods of the same group are not all good sources of the same things. For example, protein-rich cod is a good source of some B vitamins and selenium, but contains little calcium; while low-fat cheese is a good calcium source—and so on.

The last guideline of good nutrition is this: Don't believe that by cutting out things from your diet, you are necessarily doing your body a favor. Variety and balance are the most important elements, and within this framework there can be room for all kinds of food. Restriction isn't always a good thing. Good nutrition isn't just about cutting down items perceived to be "bad." Don't cut nutritious foods from your diet or restrict yourself unnecessarily unless you have a particular health complaint that needs such a restricted diet (see Section Two).

"Five a day" — interpreting the fruit and vegetable guidelines

Departments of health throughout the Western world are advising us to eat at least five portions of fruits and vegetables a day for good health. Based on all the research to date, that is sensible advice no one should ignore. In fact, we should aim for "five" as a minimum.

However, many people are confused as to what exactly the five portions means. For example, does it include potatoes? How big is a portion? Do the five portions all have to be different? And does everything have to be fresh? Here are the answers.

1 Total weight of all five portions should be at least 14 oz (400 g) of edible fruit or vegetable.

2 Vary your choices as much as possible. Different fruits and vegetables have differing nutritional qualities—e.g. avocados are high in fat and vitamin E, while carrots are high in beta-carotene and low in fat. So try to eat five different fruits and vegetables each day.

3 Items can be cooked, but it is best to cook them without too much added fat or sugar (though vegetables cooked with a little oil are fine). Try to eat one raw salad a day.

4 Potatoes, sweet potatoes, and yams are excluded as they are starchy carbohydrates and should be counted toward the day's complex carbohydrate intake. However, other root vegetables such as rutabaga, turnip, parsnip, and carrot can be included in the five a day.

5 Legumes like kidney beans, lentils, and soybeans can be included (and that includes baked beans), but as they also count as a protein source and contain good amounts of starchy carbohydrate, it is best to try to get the "five a day" from other sources and think of legumes as low-fat protein and starch. Unlike most other vegetables, legumes also contain no vitamin C unless sprouted.

6 Fruit and vegetable juice can be included, but is best counted toward only one portion a day as the fiber from the fruit is lost and the fruit sugars in juice are more likely to produce tooth decay if high quantities of juice are taken. Fruit juice is best freshly squeezed rather than bought. Fruit drinks are excluded.

7 Dried fruit can be counted, but the rest of the day's five should come from other fruits and vegetables as, although dried fruit is usually high in fiber and can contain useful minerals and vitamins, it contains no vitamin C, and is energy-dense and high in sugar.

8 Frozen and canned fruits and vegetables are included. Frozen items have a similar nutritional profile to their fresh counterparts—and sometimes can actually contain more vitamin C if picked and frozen immediately (see Food from Farm to Table, page 80). Canned produce is usually not as useful as fresh, and produce chosen should be canned without sugar or salt and preferably thought of as an occasional replacement for fresh or frozen items.

9 Nuts and seeds are excluded.

10 Composite (recipe) foods can be included as long as they include enough fruit or vegetables to constitute a portion (see the box below). A homemade apple pie will probably count, as will the vegetables in a casserole or pie. (Mixed fruits or vegetables reaching the required weight for one portion will count as one portion.) Many processed foods are unlikely to meet the portion size requirement. Items such as packaged pasta sauces and soups should not count. Commercially made salads, such as coleslaw, will count if portion size is met, but you need to be aware that their fat content may be high.

11 All other fruits and vegetables not mentioned above will count (as long as portion size guidelines opposite are followed).

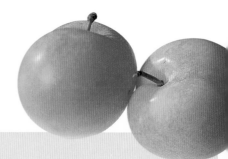

EASY WAYS TO GET YOUR "FIVE A DAY"

Here are some examples of how easy it is to incorporate "five a day" into your menus:

Example 1:
* Portion of fruit juice at breakfast time
* Handful of dried fruits mid-morning
* Bowlful of salad with bread and cheese at lunchtime
* Portion of root vegetables and portion of green vegetables with roasted chicken in the evening

Example 2:
* Portion of berry fruits with breakfast yogurt
* Glass of fruit juice with baked beans on toast at lunchtime
* Double serving of mixed stir-fried Mediterranean vegetables in evening with baked fish

Example 3:
* Glass of fruit juice on waking
* 1 apple and 1 banana chopped into breakfast cereal
* Homemade carrot soup for lunch
* Large bowlful of salad with venison steak for evening meal

■ Portion sizes

Portion size of your "five a day" is important. A couple of lettuce leaves or the two or three slices of tomato in a sandwich won't be enough to count—most salad items weigh very little and you need a really good bowlful of them. All the portion sizes are minimums—larger portions may be preferable, depending on your size, age, appetite, and own needs. The table below gives portion-size guidelines (which do not necessarily match the FDA guidelines) per person, and throughout this book, unless otherwise stated, a "portion" is as listed here.

Food	Portion size	Example
✱ Very large fruits	¹⁄₂ cup (one 100 g slice)	Melon
✱ Large fruits	One fruit, edible part at least ¹⁄₂ cup (100 g)	Peeled orange, cored apple, peeled banana
✱ Medium fruit	Two fruits, total edible parts approx. 1 cup (100 g)	Two kiwis or two plums
✱ Fresh berries or cherries	Approx. 1 cup (100 g)	1 cup raspberries or small fruits
✱ Cooked fruits	Approx. 1 cup (90 g)	Stewed apples, plums
✱ Dried fruits	Handful—approx. 40 g	Apricots, peaches
(dry ready to eat weight—stewed dried fruits count as cooked fruits for weight)		
✱ Fruit or vegetable juice	¹⁄₂ cup (100 ml)	Orange, tomato
✱ Green vegetables	Minimum 1 cup (90 g) cooked weight	Cabbage, broccoli
✱ Root vegetables	Minimum ³⁄₄ cup (80 g) cooked weight	Carrot, rutabaga
✱ Small vegetables	Minimum ²⁄₃ cup (70 g) cooked weight	Peas, corn, mixed frozen vegetables
✱ Other vegetables	¹⁄₂ cup (100 g) raw weight or ³⁄₄ cup (80 g) cooked	Onions, bell peppers, zucchini, eggplant, tomato
✱ Vegetable compotes	Minimum ³⁄₄ cup (80 g) cooked weight	Ratatouille, vegetable stir-fry
✱ Legumes	Minimum ³⁄₄ cup (80 g) cooked weight	Baked beans, kidney beans
✱ Salad	Large bowlful	Lettuce, tomato, cucumber

Power breakfasts

Some reports say that up to a quarter of us don't eat breakfast at all—yet it is a very important meal. Here's how to get it right.

Breakfast... it says what it is. A meal that breaks the fast your body has endured, probably for at least 12 hours, since your evening meal on the previous day. Looked at that way, it is surprising that so many of us don't bother with breakfast at all, but prefer to cram all our food intake into a few short hours every day, from lunch until a big burst in the evening.

■ Why do I need breakfast?

There are at least three good reasons why having a healthy and balanced breakfast is important for you and your well-being.

One: After a long period without eating your blood sugar levels will be dangerously low. As you attempt to go through the morning without eating you may suffer various symptoms such as headache, shakiness, weakness, lack of concentration, and even reduced brain power, research suggests. Performance of any kind of strenuous physical activity could also be quite significantly impaired in these circumstances.

QUICK BREAKFAST

A typical quick breakfast, but not ideal

1 cup (30 g) cornflakes, ½ cup (125 ml) low-fat 2% milk, 1 oz (30 g) slice of white toast with 1 teaspoon (5 g) soft margarine and 2 teaspoons marmalade.
299 calories, 6.8 g total fat, 2.7 g saturated fat, 9 g protein, 53.75 g carbohydrate.

This breakfast of cereal and toast is the kind that millions of people eat every day and one which most people would consider healthy. Yes, it is low in fat and saturated fat and contains just about the right amount of protein, a good amount of calcium (and other vitamins and minerals, because cornflakes are fortified), and plenty of carbohydrate. Yet it has several drawbacks.

It is very short on complex carbohydrate and fiber, containing only 0.75 g in the whole breakfast, which is just 4% of a day's average adequate intake, and would have you feeling hungry again much sooner than the healthy breakfasts. There is no fresh fruit or juice or vitamin C, and the amount of energy it provides would be quite low for most people.

Even quicker, and a better bet for most ★ ★ ★ ★

1 cup (75 g) no-added-sugar-or-salt muesli, ½ cup (125 ml) skim or nonfat milk, ¾ cup (110 g) fresh raspberries, ½ cup (125 ml) orange juice.
388 calories, 6.2 g total fat, 1.4 g saturated fat, 14.25 g protein, 73.25 g carbohydrate.

This breakfast is better than the first one on several counts. It, too, is low in total fat and even lower in saturated fat, but contains more essential fatty acids in the muesli. It is very high in carbohydrate (at 71% of the meal), most of which is complex carbohydrate, and high in fiber at 6.5 g (nearly a third of average daily needs), which means that it will keep hunger at bay well into the morning and help regulate blood sugar. Protein content is higher than the breakfast on the left, at nearly 15% of the meal—an ideal amount for early in the day. The breakfast gives two portions of fruit toward the day's five portions of fruit and vegetables, and contains more than the recommended daily needs of vitamin C (at 84 mg) as well as providing calcium, iron, and vitamin E. It provides more energy, which is good. Males, teenagers, and active people could add bread or serve extra muesli.

Two: Breakfast is an ideal opportunity to get certain nutrients into your diet that you may not find space for later in the day—fresh or dried fruits and fruit juice, for example, can help you attain the "five a day" and boost your vitamin C levels.

Yogurt or milk can provide important calcium, especially for women—many people only take these foods at breakfast, and things like oatmeal and cereals can be a good opportunity to eat fiber and oats, which can help lower LDL blood cholesterol.

Breakfast also provides calories, of course—important for children and teens, active adults, and anyone who has a problem maintaining body fat (thin people). Even for overweight people trying to lose fat, breakfast is still vital—see the next point and Section Four.
Three: If you miss breakfast you will probably suddenly feel very hungry around mid- to late-morning and crave something sweet, such as a doughnut. This, in effect, is your body telling you, you didn't give it breakfast and it needs glucose—fast! Highly refined sweet food will provide that within minutes, so you eat the sugary snack—which also often happens to contain a lot of fat and few nutrients. In other words, you are swapping a balanced nutritious meal for a less balanced, less nutritious snack.

COOKED BREAKFAST

A typical cooked breakfast

2 large eggs fried in 2 teaspoons oil, 2 slices of Canadian bacon, lightly broiled, ½ cup hash browns made with 4–6 oz (115–150 g) potato and 4 teaspoons vegetable oil, 1 cup (200 ml) orange drink.
808 calories, 64.4 g total fat, 16.5 g saturated fat, 17.9 g protein, 39 g carbohydrate.

72% of the calories in this breakfast come from fat and 18% from saturated fat—that's about twice the recommended level for both. Both figures could have been even higher if it were commercial bacon and fried in lard, not broiled. However, this is still far too high for a normal meal. Although the protein content isn't too bad and there is plenty of iron and B vitamins here, basically the balance of the meal is all wrong. Carbohydrate represents only 19% of the calories in the meal, when we should be aiming for an average of 55–60%. There is less than a gram of fiber here—only about 3% of a day's requirement. The meal is high in salt. The high fat content is reflected in the fairly high calorie content, as fat is twice as calorific as either carbohydrate or protein.

The healthier version ★★★★

1 large poached egg, fried in 1 teaspoon oil, 2 slices of Canadian bacon, broiled to crisp, 1 whole-wheat English muffin (1¾ oz/52 g), 2 slices (1¾ oz/50 g) wheat bread with 2 teaspoons of low-fat margarine (60%), and 1 teaspoon marmalade, 1 cup (200 ml) fresh orange juice.
675 calories, 22.5 g total fat, 6.1 g saturated fat, 40 g protein, 78 g carbohydrate (without optional orange juice).

Fat content is reduced considerably, mainly by using leaner bacon and cooking it to a crisp. You actually have more food on your plate by weight because fat has been replaced by high-carbohydrate foods, such as bread. The plate's fiber content is about 7 g, and only just over 3% as fat (under 10% saturated)—a much better balance. Vitamin C is close to the RDIs for the day and the dish is also high in protein and a variety of vitamins and minerals. However, salt content is still high (because of the processed foods, such as bacon) and the rest of the day should reflect a lower salt content. Many people opt to include milk at breakfast, since there is little calcium here, make sure other meals have higher sources of calcium.

■ What is a healthy breakfast?

A good breakfast should contribute to your day's diet enough calories, some protein, a reasonable amount of complex carbohydrate, a little fat, and a variety of vitamins and minerals. Within that broad outline there is plenty of scope, as the ten healthy breakfasts on the right show.

Most people don't allow enough calories for their breakfast. A quarter of your day's calorie intake—that would be around 500 for women and 650 for men—would be a good amount to aim for most days. Exactly what proportion of carbohydrate, protein, and fat those calories should consist of is a matter of debate among researchers. Some have shown that a high-carbohydrate, low-fat breakfast makes you more alert and assertive and that a high-fat meal slows down the brain; others that it is a high-protein breakfast that helps brain power and that too much carbohydrate slows you down.

The key seems to be a sensible balance of all three main nutrients. A breakfast including at least one-third of your day's protein needs is certainly a good idea; whether or not protein helps you power through your morning's work, it certainly helps to stave off hunger pangs, because it takes longer to be digested than carbohydrate. And, of course, if you get little protein at breakfast-time you will need to make up that shortfall later in the day. Try to pick at least one calcium-rich protein food, such as milk or yogurt, on most days.

The breakfast should also include a small amount of fat which, like protein, helps to keep hunger at bay and regulate blood sugar levels. This is a good opportunity to give your essential fatty acid intake a boost, perhaps with nuts and seeds added to a cereal. A pure vegetable oil spread on any bread would add a little more fat. By using skim milk and low-fat yogurts, saturated fat intake can be kept to a minimum.

Breakfast should provide a good mix of both starch and sugars. Sugar is best provided in the form of fruit or fruit juice, which will soon (within 20 minutes or so) break down into glucose and raise the blood sugar levels, as well as providing your first vitamin C of the day. Starch is ideally provided in bread and/or cereals, and for morning-long sustenance at least some of this should be as unrefined as possible, for example, whole-grain cereals and whole-grain breads. There is nothing wrong with a slice of white bread spread with some jam, but on its own it will quickly have you hungry again, as the refined flour and sugary jam are quickly digested. Moreover, a breakfast high in refined carbohydrate won't boost your fiber.

A balanced breakfast will provide a good range of vitamins and minerals and make an important contribution to your day's intake.

■ So is it good-bye to the Sunday brunch?

Lovers of bacon and eggs may by now be feeling slightly depressed, but there is no need. Although the traditional cooked breakfast is extremely high in fat (see previous page), there is no need to give it up completely. A cooked breakfast can fit quite easily into your diet once a week or so. Even "reworked," such a breakfast is still not perfect—containing a bit too little carbohydrate and too much protein—but it is very easy to balance that out during the rest of the day by having a lowish-protein lunch and a very-high-carbohydrate evening meal, for example.

A cooked breakfast, higher in calories than you may normally eat, is actually a very good idea if you have an active physical day ahead—say a long brisk Sunday walk. Such a breakfast a few hours before a traditional Sunday lunch, however, would not be a good idea. Remember—good nutrition is mainly about common sense and balance.

■ Top ten quick and healthy breakfasts

1 ⅔ cup (150 g) low-fat yogurt with 1 small banana chopped in, ½ grapefruit or glass of grapefruit juice, large slice of whole-wheat bread with a little olive oil margarine and honey.
2 ⅔ cup (150 g) low-fat yogurt topped with 2 oz (50 g) no-added-sugar luxury muesli and a portion of strawberries, small slice of bread with olive oil margarine.
3 Multigrain cereal with 2 teaspoons of chopped walnuts and skim milk to cover, handful of dried ready-to-eat apricots, 1 slice of bread, olive oil margarine and honey, glass of orange juice.
4 Two Shredded Wheat with 2 teaspoons sunflower or pumpkin seeds and skim milk to cover, 1 pear, small slice of whole-wheat bread with olive oil margarine and marmalade.
5 A cup of plain low-fat cottage cheese with 1 teaspoon of brown sugar and a slice of cantaloupe melon, chopped, plus 2 teaspoons of chopped toasted almonds, 1 slice of bread, olive oil margarine or peanut butter.
6 A large bowl of oatmeal made with half low-fat 2% milk and half water, 2 teaspoons honey, 2 teaspoons golden raisins, 1 glass of orange juice.
7 6 oz (175 g) low-sugar, low-salt baked beans on 1 large slice whole-wheat toast with a little olive oil margarine, 1 orange or glass of orange juice, second slice of bread with spread and marmalade.
8 All Bran with 1 chopped apple and skim milk, ½ grapefruit ,1 slice of bread with olive oil margarine and honey.
9 1 large banana mashed with 1 kiwi fruit and 1 teaspoon of lemon juice on 1 large slice of whole-wheat bread with olive oil margarine, glass of low-fat 2% milk.
10 Milkshake: blend 1 cup (200 ml) low-fat 2% milk with 1 small banana, 3 tablespoons of orange juice, 2 teaspoons of honey and 1 teaspoon of wheat germ, drink chilled; 1 large slice of whole-wheat bread with peanut butter.

Desserts

Desserts can be a good opportunity to get vitamin C and/or calcium and/or fiber into your diet.

■ For vitamin C
* Fresh fruit, especially strawberries, kiwi, citrus, mango
* Fruit salad
* Low-calorie jello with fruit bits
* Fresh fruit compote, especially black currants, berries
* Any of the desserts in this book

■ For calcium
(but remember ice cream can be high in fat)
* Yogurt
* Ice cream
* Low-fat frozen yogurt
* Low-fat rice pudding

■ For fiber
* Any of the fresh fruit desserts mentioned above
* Dried fruits
* Dried fruit compote
* Fruit crisp with oat, nut, and whole-wheat flour topping
* Baked apple with chopped nuts

Many people save truly indulgent desserts for when they go out or entertain (see Eating Out section, page 64). Layer cakes, tarts, and pies, as well as most rich chocolate desserts, are all heavy on calories and fat. Here, though, are some ideas for more indulgent and quick desserts that won't do too much damage to the overall balance of your diet:
* Small portions of jello
* Fruit desserts topped with aerosol cream
* Angel food cake
* Individual fruit trifle or mousse
* Fresh fruit salad and low-fat yogurt

Drinks

We should drink about 9 cups (2.25 liters) of liquid a day. If you increase your fiber intake you should also increase the amount you drink, as you should if you are physically active or eat high-salt foods.

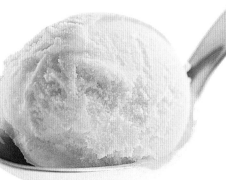

The optimum drink for most of us would be plain water, but most of us tend to drink sodas and caffeinated beverages. Below we look at the advantages and drawbacks of the most popular drinks. For more detailed information on particular drinks see the Food Charts on pages 260–317.

■ Milk
This is one of our main sources of calcium, as well as providing protein. Whole milk is high in saturated fat; low-fat 2% and skim or nonfat are better alternatives for most people. Milk taken as a late-night hot drink can help sleep (see Insomnia, page 123). For people with a lactose intolerance or vegans, calcium-fortified soy milk is a good alternative.

■ Fruit juice
These are usually good sources of vitamin C, but they can contribute to tooth decay. They are higher in calories than most people realize, at around 80 calories for a 7 fl oz/200 ml glassful. It is best to dilute them with some water.

■ Tea and coffee
In moderate amounts, these are both good antioxidants, as well as being stimulating. In excess, they may no longer act as stimulants and can cause tiredness. They are virtually calorie-free provided cream and sugar is limited, but don't take either with a meal as they can hinder absorption of some nutrients. They can also act as diuretics, particularly coffee. Herb teas are a good alternative (see page 255).

■ Fruit and carbonated drinks
These are usually sources of many additives and are often very sweet. They contain few nutrients unless they are added by the manufacturer. Low-calorie versions are similar, but with artificial sweetener. Sparkling mineral water with a dash of fruit juice would be preferable—and nicer?

■ Alcoholic drinks
Don't use these as thirst quenchers, and don't drink alcohol during the day. If you have any, have a little for your evening meal, when it can aid digestion and is less quickly absorbed into the bloodstream.

See also: Constipation, Hangover, Weight Control, Alcohol Abuse, Alcohol, Food Charts.

A new look at lunch

For most of us, lunch needs to be something quick and easy—even when we're not working, there's usually little time to spare. But it doesn't HAVE to be a cheese sandwich every day.

Even if you've had a good breakfast, you shouldn't skip lunch. If you do, you'll probably find that around 4–5pm you are so hungry you'll eat a candy bar or something similarly high in fat and sugar.

Hunger isn't the only consideration, though. Lunch is an ideal time to pack in some powerful nutrients to help you to health... to get your quota of fish or legumes; to eat plenty of salad and fruit; to get ahead on your vegetable intake with big bowls of soup.

Like breakfast, your lunch should be a sensible balance of carbohydrates and proteins, plus a little fat. Because your evening meal is going to be higher in carbohydrate and lower in protein (see overleaf), your lunch can contain a large proportion of your day's protein intake while being slightly lower in carbohydrate. Research shows that a high-carbohydrate lunch can result in sluggish performance in the afternoon.

Before deciding what you will have for your lunch, it's a good idea to plan out also what your evening meal will be, so that you don't "double up" on certain things and miss out on others. For example, if you are going to have meat as part of your evening meal, avoid having meat at lunch and choose a vegetable protein instead, such as legumes, or have fish. If you're having pasta in the evening, don't also have pasta salad at lunch, and so on.

When choosing a lunch for speed, beware of the possible nutritional pitfalls.

SOME SUGGESTIONS FOR HEALTHY QUICK LUNCHES

* Double portion of Canellini Bean and Basil Spread (page 213); 3½ oz (100 g) Italian bread; large salad of mixed leaves; 1 orange.
* 3½ oz (100 g) rollmop herring; portion of new potatoes; mixed salad with vinaigrette dressing; Apple and Apricot Shake (page 254).
* Portion of Tuna, Avocado, and Tomato Salad (page 223) with added cooked whole-wheat pasta; 1 apple.
* 1 portion of Hummus (page 212) with 1 whole-wheat pita bread; 1 banana; Water-melon Refresher (page 253).
* 1 portion of Lentil and Cilantro Soup (page 218); rye bread; 1 orange.
* 1 portion of Counry Pea Soup (page 219); whole-wheat bread; dried figs, 1 banana.
* 1 warmed chapati; 1 portion Feta and Pepper Spread (page 212); selection of crudités; 1 apple; handful of dried apricots.

PACK A PUNCH

Before

Baloney and cheese sandwich (3¼ oz/90 g sliced bologna meat, 1¾ oz/50 g cheese, 1¾ oz/50 g white bread with 2 tsp mayonnaise, lettuce, mustard), one (1½ oz/45 g) chocolate bar, 1 oz (30 g) light potato chips, 1 apple, ¾ cup (200 ml) diet cola. *980 calories, 52 g total fat, 22.5 g saturated fat, 30 g protein, 98 g carbohydrate, 4.8 g fiber:*

This typical lunchbox—despite the "diet" cola, "light" chips and apple is not all that well balanced. It is high in saturates and salt, and low in complex carbs and fiber, while not being a particularly good source of vitamins. The cheese is a good source of calcium, but a lower-fat hard cheese would also supply this.

After ★★★★★

1¾ oz (50 g) lean cooked chicken (no skin) in 7 oz (200 g) French bread with 2 tsp Tofu Mayonnaise (page 246); 1 cup (140 g) mixed salad (tomato, cucumber, bell pepper, red onion, corn, celery); 1 apple; ¼ cup (30 g) ready-to-eat dried apricots; 1 Oat-Apricot Bar (page 251); ¾ cup (200 ml) orange juice. *963 calories; 18 g total fat, 3.5 g saturated fat, 42 g protein, 158 g carbohydrate, 8.5 g fiber.*

Just as appetizing and even more to eat, this lunch offers roughly the same calories, but is lower in saturated fat and artificial additives, and high in vitamin C, iron, fiber, EFAs, and a good range of other vitamins and minerals.

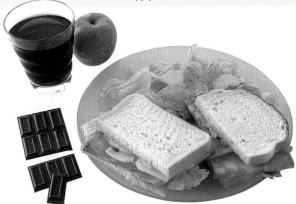

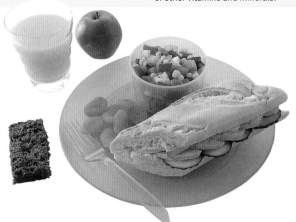

Many ready-made soups are high in salt and can be low on "real" ingredients'—if you're going to choose ready-made, choose chilled rather than canned or packaged soups. In fact, almost anything that needs reconstituting or comes out of a can should be limited to an occasional stand-by. However, there is nothing wrong with baked beans on toast—a high-fiber, low-fat, and filling meal—but choose the low-salt, low-sugar kind.

Anything in pastry is probably very high in fat, saturated fat, and calories, so limit items like pies and sausage rolls to very occasional use.

Many sandwiches are high in fat, but calorie-counted ones containing plenty of fresh salad can be fine, though this wouldn't be enough for an average person's lunch. When making your own sandwiches, garnish with lots of salad, go easy on the spread, and, if choosing high-fat Cheddar cheese, grate it to go further.

Vary the types of bread you use, too—there is nothing wrong with decent white bread sometimes, although wholewheat will boost your day's fiber intake. With some fillings you will need no butter or other spread on your bread, but if you do, go for an unsaturated spread containing no or few hydrogenated (trans) fats.

Deli counter salads and pre-packed supermarket ones are often very high in fat—slaws, potato, pasta, and rice salads are the worst culprits. The other problem with a "salad" lunch is that often the true fresh salad part of the meal is nothing more than a couple of lettuce leaves, a few thin slices of tomato, and a sprig of parsley. This weighs next to nothing and will contain virtually no nutrients. To be a real working part of your healthy meal, salad has to come BIG.

Think "lots of things" when you think about salad. Add some nuts, seeds, cold cooked vegetable items like beans, chunky bits of carrot or bell pepper, dried or fresh fruits.

Pub and bar lunches are often high-fat affairs—quiche and salad or Brie and French bread are typical saturated-fat-laden fare. For tips on eating out at lunchtime, see page 64.

Home-packed lunches can be a healthy alternative to a lunchtime cafeteria meal or take-out, but even so it is all too easy to put together a packed meal that's very high in salt, fat, and sugar, and low in fiber and vitamins. They can also get boring, so if you eat—or could eat—a packed lunch regularly, invest in suitable plastic containers and vacuum flasks for salads, desserts, and soups. Dressings and utensils can usually be kept at work.

LUNCH AT HOME

Before

10 oz (295 g) can of low-cal veggie soup; 1½ oz (45 g) white roll spread with 1 tsp margarine; 1¾ oz (50 g) lean ham; ¾ oz (25 g) mortadella; 2 tbsp coleslaw; small green salad (lettuce, some garden cress, cucumber); 2 tsp light mayonnaise. *483 calories, 25.8 g total fat, 6.6 g saturated fat, 19.8 g protein, 38.4 g carbohydrate, 2.7 g fiber.*

A typical quick lunch for the calorie-conscious, with lean ham and light mayo. Yet, it has over a day's salt, at nearly 6 g (soup is particularly high), nearly half calories are from fat at 48% (mortadella and coleslaw the main culprits), and carb are too low at under 30%. There is little complex carbs and fiber is only 15% of a recommended day's intake.

After ★★★★★

1 whole-wheat pita, with 1¾ oz (50 g) lean ham, ¼ cup (50 g) canned chickpeas, 1 tomato, 1¾ oz (50 g) lettuce, 1 oz (25 g) watercress and 1 tbsp vinaigrette dressing (made with olive oil); 1 low-calorie fruit yogurt, 1 kiwi fruit. *462 calories, 13 g total fat, 1.7 g saturated fat, 27.5 g protein, 60 g carbohydrate, 9.6 g fiber.*

Similar with about the same calories, but only 26% from fat, now fatty mortadella and coleslaw are replaced by chickpeas and more fresh salad and fruit. Only 3.3% saturates, plus useful amount of essential fatty acids from olive oil dressing and chickpeas. 50% carbs, with protein at 24%. Salt is much lower at 3 g; chickpeas and pita have added fiber to give 53% of day's needs.

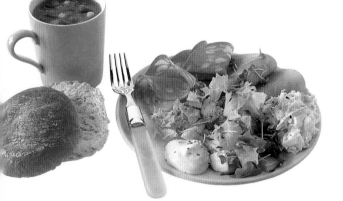

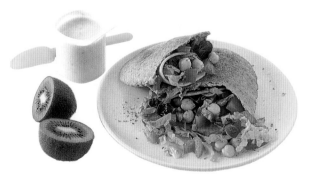

Evening meals

Though there may be a fragment of truth in the saying that we should breakfast like kings and dine like paupers, most of us look forward to our evening meal and treat it as the main food event of the day.

Although many people do, it's wise not to blow all your day's calories in the evening. The digestive system usually responds best to a "little and often" approach—three similarly sized meals and two small snacks are ideal. However, most of us prefer our largest meal in the evening when there is time to relax. Certainly, there is no harm in allotting around 35–40% of your calories to the evening. However, do try to eat such a meal no later than two hours before bed.

Like breakfast and lunch, dinner should provide a mix of nutrients. However, this is the best time of the day really to go to town with your carbohydrates. These have a calming effect and may help your brain to "slow down," to relax and get a good night's sleep.

A meal rich in complex carbohydrates, such as whole grains, pasta, potatoes, or legumes, will also sustain you through the night. And yet, so often, we prepare a supper based mainly on a high-protein food. Most of us still don't say "let's have rice tonight," we say "let's have a steak," and only as an afterthought do we consider accompaniments.

For healthy eating in the evening, the single most important rule you should bear in mind is to think of the protein element of your meal—especially animal or dairy protein—as a SMALL PART of the meal, the "accompaniment", and think of starches and vegetables as the LARGE

MEAL MAKEOVER

Before

7 oz (200 g) roasted chicken, including crispy skin, 3 roast potatoes (5¼ oz/ 150 g); ⅓ cup (70 g) peas and carrots; 4 tbsp unskimmed gravy; ⅓ cup (50 g) ready-made parsley stuffing. *798 calories, 41.5 g total fat, 11.2 g saturated fat, 53.6 g protein, 55.5 g carbohydrate.*

This plateful contains just about the right proportion of a day's calories for a main meal at 41% (women), 31% (men), but contains 41.5 g of fat, which is 47% of the meal and 64% of the recommended daily max intake for females and nearly 50% for a man. Saturated fat and protein content are very high, too, compared with the meal's low carb content, which provides just 26% of the calories. Also low in vegetables and has only 5 g of fiber. If a woman ate this meal plus the cereal "before" breakfast on page 42 and the salad "before" lunch on page 47, and nothing else, she would be 14% over the max recommended day's fat intake at a total of 74 g, while her carb intake would have given only 57% of her needs and her fiber intake would be merely 8.5 g, or less than half a day's adequate intake.

After ★★★★★

4½ oz (125 g) lean roasted chicken (no skin); 8 oz (225 g) new potatoes in skins and ½ cup (100 g) butternut squash, brushed with 2 tsp olive oil and baked; ⅓ cup (70 g) peas; ¾ cup (100 g) dark leafy greens; ½ cup (50 g) homemade rice, apricot, and nut stuffing; 5 tsp pan juices made into sauce with a little wine and cornstarch. *631.5 calories, 21 g total fat, 4 g saturated fat, 45.7 g protein, 68.5 g carbohydrate.*

Removing skin from chicken, brushing veggies with oil, and using skimmed pan juices for gravy reduces fat easily, although essential fatty acid (EFA) content is higher. Less chicken is compensated for by more vegetables, providing carbs, vitamin C, beta-carotene, and iron. By eating this, plus "after" breakfast and lunch, a woman would have consumed 1,480 calories or 64% of day's energy needs; used up only 68% of her day's recommended max fat intake and only 33% of her max saturates intake. She would have attained 78% of her min carb needs and a total fiber intake of 28 g and would have eaten 7 portions of fruit and veggies. EFA and micronutrient requirements will have all been supplied.

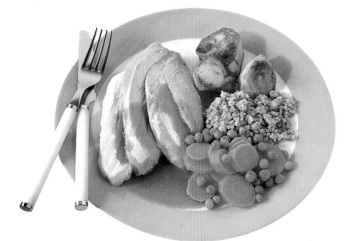

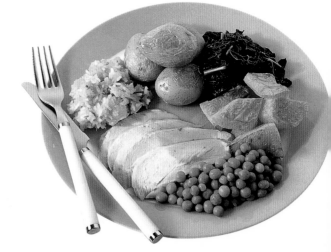

TIPS FOR HEALTHY EVENING EATING

✱ Limit meat to once or twice a week maximum.

✱ Have fish at least twice a week.

✱ Have a vegetarian or vegan night at least twice a week, not relying heavily on cheese.

✱ Have poultry or game once or twice a week.

✱ Remember that full-fat hard, blue, and creamy cheeses are high in saturated fat and calories, and best used sparingly.

✱ Remember pastry is very high in fat, saturated fat, and calories—keep for occasional use.
Phyllo is better than other pastries, as you add your own fat, so can use less, and can use olive oil.

✱ Only use as much fat when cooking as absolutely necessary.
If following a recipe, you can reduce the fat used in many of them without detriment.

✱ Check out how many portions of fruit and vegetables you've had in the day and use your evening meal to make up the total to at least five portions.

✱ Add a glass or two of wine some evenings if you like.

✱ If your main meal is large, instead of having a dessert, have a snack during the day instead or a late-night milk drink, so that you don't have too many calories all at one time.

treat (overleaf). Her protein needs have already been well met and she needs no more fat as the fat intakes are maximums not minimums.

NOTE: A man would need to increase portion sizes by about a third on all the "made-over" meals to get enough calories and nutrients.

■ *Swap this* ... 6 oz (175 g) lamb steak, new potatoes, small salad
For this ... Large portion of whole-wheat noodles stir-fried with 3¼ oz (90 g) sliced lamb, 1½ cups (200 g) mixed vegetables, oriental sesame oil, and light soy sauce.

■ *Swap this* ... Deep-fried fish and chips
For this ... Large portion of brown rice with salmon and red bell pepper brochettes and tomato sauce.

■ *Swap this* ... Cottage pie and peas
For this ... Large baked potato with small portion of chile con carne, large salad.

■ *Swap this* ... three-egg cheese omelet
For this ... rice kedgeree with smoked haddock and one hard-boiled egg, peas.

PART of the meal, the "stars." By cutting back on animal protein, you not only allow more room for the healthy carbs and vegetables, but you also naturally cut back on fat and saturated fat.

You can fit even traditional meals, such as roasts—if not exactly, then at least partially—into this ideal simply by altering the balance on your plate—less meat or poultry, more vegetables. (See the example on the left.)

To reinforce the message that you don't need to worry about getting enough protein in your evening meal this way, let's look back at the breakfasts and lunches we've analyzed in the previous pages. In the "after" muesli and salad lunch there was 41.75 g of protein altogether. An average woman has a minimum daily need of about 50 g protein and a maximum daily need of about 73 g, so she will need only between 8 and 31 g more protein after that breakfast and that lunch to fall within a suitable intake range. An

average man's needs are about 64–95 g a day, so he will need only another 22–53 g.

As a mere 3½ oz (100 g) small portion of lean meat contains 1¼ oz (35 g) of pure protein, and as protein is present in many of the other foods on your plate, you can see that perhaps that half-pound steak (1½ oz/50 g pure protein) isn't such a good idea after all. Even after tweaking the roast meal opposite to a better balance, it still contains 45.7 g protein—bringing the day's intake to more than enough for a woman and enough for a man.

The meal now provides under 30% of its calories as fat and the carbohydrate content has gone up to over 40%. This last figure is still low, as we're aiming for 50% as a minimum—but by choosing the right dessert and other daily snacks we can boost the day's carbohydrate intake even further.

A woman could make up her day's calorie intake with a carbohydrate-rich dessert (see page 45) and a snack or

DAY'S TALLY SO FAR

Before Cereal and toast breakfast, cold cuts lunch, first roasted chicken dinner.
1,580 calories, 74 g total fat, 20.5 g saturated fat, 82.5 g protein, 148 g carbohydrate, 8.5 g fiber.

After Muesli breakfast, pita and yogurt lunch, second roasted chicken dinner.
1,480 calories, 40.25 g total fat, 7.1 g saturated fat, 87.5 g protein, 201.5 g carbohydrate, 28 g fiber.

Snacks and treats

If your regular meals are nutritionally well balanced, as we've seen in the last few pages, it is actually quite easy to make room for a daily dessert or extra snack without pushing your fat, calorie, or sugar levels too high.

Here we look at ways to fit your favorites into your daily diet and offer suggestions for healthier alternatives to high-fat, high-sugar treats.

Most of us consume a fair proportion of our daily calories in the form of snacks, desserts, drinks, and "extras." So, even if your actual "meals" are fairly well balanced, it is easy to put your total diet out of balance with a poor choice in these extras. Too many high-calorie high-fat snacks can contribute toward weight gain, as well as being likely to increase your intake of saturated fats and trans fats, and possibly sugar. Over-indulgence in such snacks can also fill you up and reduce your motivation to eat fresh and nutritious foods.

On the other hand, a carefully chosen day's eating will give you room to indulge in one or two favorite treats, such as a slice of cake, some cookies, a candy bar, or an alcoholic drink.

It is wise to allow no more than 10% of your total day's calorie intake for such items—that would be about 200 calories for women and 250 for men. Alternatively, if the day's eating hasn't been ideal, one or two well-chosen healthy snacks can actually help to improve the day's total nutritional profile. Let us look at some examples of both sensible and not-so-sensible choices of these little "extras."

The boxes opposite give the calorie and fat content of some typical "indulgence" foods, so you can fit them into your overall diet now and then if you like.

For comparison, there follow some suggestions for healthier snack alternatives.

EXAMPLE 1

This is a woman who has eaten the "before" breakfast, lunch, and evening meal on the past few pages, and has notched up 1,580 calories, leaving her 420 to "play with" (because of low activity her needs are about 2,000 calories a day). However, she has already eaten 14% OVER her day's fat allowance at 74 g and is nearly at her saturated fat limit—and she's still low on carbohydrate (particularly complex) and fiber. She decides to opt for these extras:

¾ cup (200 ml) skim milk for her tea and coffee—66 calories, virtually no fat.

One ½ cup (100 g) portion of vanilla icecream bar—250 calories, 12 g fat, 8 g saturated fat.

1 plain scone—174 calories, 7 g fat, 2.4 g saturated fat.

1 double Scotch whisky—96 calories, fat-free.

Not exactly an excessive list, but one that finishes her day's eating profile like this:

2,166 calories—which is 9% more than she needs, so she may slowly gain weight on such a diet.

93 g of total fat—which is 43% too much.

31 g saturated fat—which is 43% too much.

222 g of carbohydrate—which is 30% too little and is also far too low in complex carbs.

10.5 g fiber—which is less than half average needs.

One snack of fresh fruit and one of dried fruit would have been a better bet than the icecream and scone, while keeping the milk (for calcium) and the whisky, bringing the day's calorie and fat total to reasonable levels, increasing complex carbs and fiber, and raising her tally of fruits and veggies for the day to four—still low, but better than the two she managed with her main meals.

EXAMPLE 2 ★★★★★

This woman eats the "after" breakfast, lunch, and main meal and has so far eaten: 1,480 calories, 40.25 g total fat, 7.1 g saturated fat, 201.5 g carbohydrate, and 28 g fiber.

She has 460 calories left to use up, has plenty of room for maneuver on her fat intake, is already well on the way to getting her day's carbohydrate intake, and has eaten lots of fiber, plus seven portions of fruits and vegetables. She opts to add:

¾ cup (200 ml) skim milk—66 calories, virtually fat-free.

1 Oat-Apricot Bar (page 251)—189 calories, 8.7 g fat, 1.8 g saturated fat.

1 portion of Citrus Granita (page 249)—142 calories, virtually fat-free.

5 fl oz (150 ml) Bloody Mary—116 calories, fat-free.

Her final profile for the day then is:

1,993 calories—almost exactly spot-on for average weight maintenance.

49 g total fat—only three-quarters of what she could have eaten according to health guidelines, representing 22% of her total day's calorie intake, but still plenty to give her all her essential fatty acids.

9 g saturated fat—less than half what she could have eaten according to health guidelines, representing 4.1% of her total day's calorie intake.

If this second woman had wanted to indulge in a candy bar or similar rather than the seemingly healthier citrus granita, she could have done so and still been within her day's allowance for fat and only marginally over her day's calorie target.

SNACK COMPARISONS

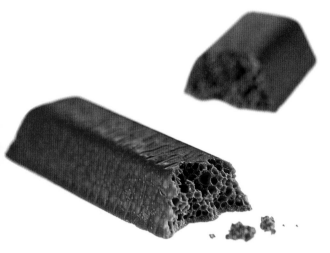

the usual indulgences	Calories	Fat (g)
Standard bar of milk chocolate	255	14.8
Kit-Kat	244	13.2
Sundae	320	9.9
Hot dog	214	14
Cream donut	180	11.5
Chocolate eclair	260	18.0
Average 3½ oz (100 g) slice of chocolate fudge cake	400	20.0
Salted peanuts, 1½ oz (50 g) pack	295	24.0

better ...	Calories	Fat (g)
1 muffin, lightly spread with low-fat spread and 1 teaspoon low-sugar jam	110	2.5
½ cup (100 ml) vanilla ice milk	92	2.8
1 low-calorie instant hot chocolate drink, plus 1 small chocolate chip cookie	98	3.6
1 light individual chocolate pudding and 1 small banana	160	3.5

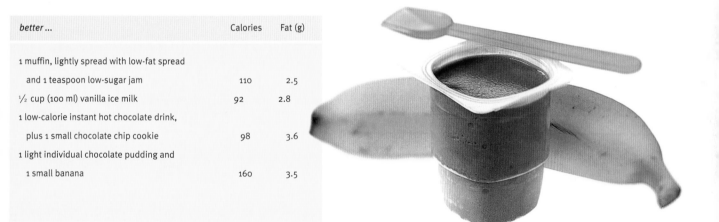

best ... ★★★★★	Calories	Fat (g)
One 4 fl oz (125 ml) tub of low-fat yogurt and 1 medium piece of fresh fruit	140	2.0
1 whole-wheat English muffin with a little spread and honey	180	4.0
1½ oz (50 g) ready-to-eat dried apricots, 1 banana	190	0.6
2 dark rye crispbreads spread with ¾ oz (25 g) homemade guacamole (spiced mashed avocado)	82	3.6
One 1 oz (30 g) slice of dark rye bread, spread with 1 portion Canellini Bean and Basil Spread (page 213)	152	3.5

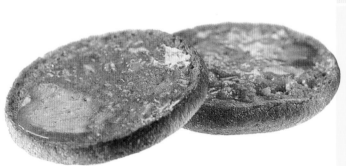

Ensuring a basic healthy diet

The seven-day diet plan opposite shows how a healthy adult could put together all the preceding information into a delicious healthy everyday diet. Recipes picked out with capitals appear in Section Five.

With the help of the recipe section later in the book plus the healthy eating tips you've learned in this section it won't be difficult to eat well indefinitely. Let's summarize those guidelines as follows:

1 Eat more complex carbohydrates—bread, potatoes, pasta, cereals, grains, legumes.

2 Eat at least five portions of fruit and vegetables a day. Include plenty of leafy greens, and red and orange fruits and vegetables. Eat them raw, or cooked lightly, and don't smother them in too much butter or commercial dressings.

3 Eat less fat, especially saturated and trans fats. Cook with less fat and go easy on bought foods high in fat, such as pastries, cakes, pies, cream and full-fat cheese, and fatty cuts of meat.

4 Eat natural oily fats such as those found in pure vegetable, seed, and grain oils, nuts, grains and seeds. These provide essential fatty acids. Use oils on salad and in cooking.

5 Eat less sugary and salty foods. For sweetness go for naturally sweet items like fresh and dried fruits. Use herbs, spices, and so on for taste and use less salt in your cooking and at the table.

6 Eat more plant- and fish-based meals and less meat.

7 Get as wide a variety of foods as possible into your diet.

8 Eat the best quality foods that you can—fresh, wholesome, unadulterated food is best for your body.

9 Eat regularly throughout the day, having a breakfast, lunch, main meal, and snacks.

10 Drink plenty of fluids and don't forget that water is one of the best drinks of all.

Most importantly—relax and enjoy your food. Make some time to plan your mealtimes ahead and enjoy the pleasures of cooking.

The next section of the book contains special guidelines for diets to suit different lifestyles.

■ The basic healthy diet

This diet is a guideline only, to help you plan your own eating. No precise portion sizes are given because this isn't a weight-loss diet—it is a healthy eating diet. If "medium" portions are eaten, plus the milk and "extras" allowance detailed below, you will be getting approximately the right amount for a maintenance diet.

Eat to suit your sex, size, activity levels, and appetite. As a guide, if you are female, sedentary, and/or small you will eat smaller portions. If you are male, tall and/or active you will need to eat more. Try to get in touch with your appetite and be sensible about portion sizes. Eating more than you need will result in weight gain, even if your diet is healthy.

Unlimiteds

Unlimited are water, any leafy green vegetables and salad items, herbs and spices, herb and "no added sugar" fruit teas, lemon juice. Tea and instant or filtered coffee can be taken in reasonable amounts (using milk from the allowance below, if you wish). Fizzy calorie-free drinks should be limited to occasional use.

Milk

In addition to any milk mentioned in the plan opposite, you should have about 1 cup (200 ml) skim milk or calcium-enriched soy milk every day. If you don't want this, have a 4 fl oz (125 ml) plain low-fat yogurt instead.

Extras

Allow yourself, in addition, 200 calories or so a day for a little indulgence. This could be a little alcohol or something chocolatey. It could even be something like extra bread, or potato, or a milk drink at bedtime. It is up to you.

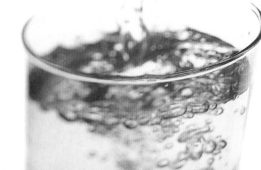

THE BASIC HEALTHY DIET

DAY ONE
Breakfast
2 Shredded Wheat with skim milk, sprinkled
with chopped nuts and sesame seeds
1 slice of whole-wheat bread with
sunflower spread and honey
glass of orange juice , 1 apple
Lunch
Spiced Lentil and Mixed Green Vegetable
Salad
7 oz (200 g), cooked weight, couscous
1 satsuma
Evening
Pasta with Milanese Sauce
large bowlful of mixed salad leaves with a
little olive oil and lemon dressing
portion of thick strained yogurt with
honey
Snack
1 Oat-Apricot bar

DAY TWO
Breakfast
Mango and Peach Booster
multigrain roll with sunflower spread and
low-sugar marmalade
handful of ready-to-eat dried apricots
Lunch
Anchoïade as a dip
whole-wheat pita crudités
Tomato and Bean Salsa
portion of vanilla ice cream
Evening
Spanish-Style Baked Trout
green beans, French bread, 1 banana
Snack
handful of dried fruit and nuts

DAY THREE
Breakfast
portion no-added-sugar muesli
skim milk, 1 orange
slice of whole-wheat bread with sunflower
spread and honey
Lunch
Squash, Potato, and Butter Bean Soup
large bread roll, 1 banana
thick strained yogurt
Evening
Spiced Chicken and Greens
portion of brown rice
Stir-Fried Fruit Salad
Snack
1 Oat-Apricot Bar

DAY FOUR
Breakfast
low-fat plain yogurt
portion of blackberries
whole-wheat English muffin with
sunflower spread and honey, peach juice
Lunch
large hunk of French or Italian country bread
with Feta and Pepper Spread
bowlful of mixed salad, red grapes
Evening
Winter Squash with Lentils and Ginger
portion of potato mashed with a little olive oil
portion of kale and portion of green beans
fresh figs
Snack
cottage cheese with honey

DAY FIVE
Breakfast
Boiled egg
large slice of whole-wheat bread with
sunflower spread, 1 satsuma
Apple and Apricot Shake
Lunch
Panzanella Salad, 1 banana
portion of low-fat yogurt
Evening
Turkish Lamb Stew
large portion of bulgur wheat, broccoli
Mango Phyllo Tart
Snack
mixed dried fruit and nuts

DAY SIX
Breakfast
1 whole-wheat English muffin with sunflower
spread and low-sugar marmalade
thick strained yogurt with chopped apple
and pistachio nuts
Lunch
Carrot and Orange Soup
Canellini Bean and Basil Spread
French baguette, 2 tomatoes
Evening
Pasta with Olives and Sardines
large mixed salad
Snack
ready-to-eat dried apricots and prunes

DAY SEVEN
Breakfast
Banana and Strawberry Smoothie
large slice of whole-wheat bread with
sunflower spread and honey
Lunch
Thai Salmon Salad, kiwi fruit
Evening
Chickpea and Vegetable Crumble
baked potato, collard greens
Snack
1 Oat-Apricot Bar

CHOOSING A DIET TO SUIT YOUR LIFESTYLE

So we've seen what the ideal diet is like—but how can you translate that into the way YOU live? In the next few pages we look at how healthy eating can fit into any lifestyle, from those of students on a budget to busy family cooks, to executive dining.

Fast food for busy people

When your life is so busy that you can hardly find time to sleep, it is often "proper" eating that suffers. Food is grabbed on the run, chocolate bars are a principal source of "instant energy" and main meals always come carton-shaped. Here we look at what can be done to get your eating back into balance.

If you're busy, the chances are that you are busy earning money! If so, it is worth paying a small premium for time-saving food ideas from the supermarket.

For example: ready-peeled and -chopped vegetables; ready-prepared fruits, such as pineapple and oranges; ready-made chilled stocks, soups, and sauces, and so on. All these can help you to eat healthily for only a little extra cost.

Much time can be saved if you freeze meals, sauces, soups, etc., that you have made yourself in batches on one of those rare less-busy days—it really is almost as quick to cook double or treble quantities.

If even the quickest and easiest cooking is out of the question most of the time, that doesn't matter. The trick is to swap fast fatty or low-nutrient food for fast healthy, high-nutrient food. Luckily, many foods you can eat with virtually no preparation are widely available. Fruits, salads, yogurts, cottage cheese, cheeses, milks, juices, bread, cereals—make these a sizeable part of your diet and who needs the take-out—a plate of whole-wheat bread, goat's cheese, and tomatoes is a fast food feast!

■ A head start in the morning

Breakfast is the meal most often missed by busy people; and yet, as we saw on page 42, breakfast is very important. A good breakfast can help your energy, your concentration, your memory, and your alertness. So, for anyone pushed for time with a demanding lifestyle and decisions to be made all day, breakfast makes sense. It doesn't, though, necessarily have to be

FAST AND HEALTHY BREAKFASTS

* Muesli with milk, and berry fruits
* Bread with spread, milk, and nectarine or peach
* Bio yogurt, shelled nuts, orange juice, and banana
* Oat-Apricot Bar (see page 251), orange juice, and banana

cooked, or large, or time-consuming. You simply need a fix of carbohydrate and protein, with a little fat and a good range of vitamins and minerals.

Try one or more of these strategies:

* Get ahead. Get your breakfast organized the night before. Put out cereals in their dish and cover them; pour out your juice into a glass and put it in the refrigerator. Thaw a frozen bread roll. Do whatever you can so that in the morning rush you can still have some food.
* Pick a portable breakfast. Choose something you can eat on the way to work or as soon as you get there. Something based on bread or a pot of yogurt and a banana is better than eating nothing. If you take a packed lunch to work, pack extra and eat earlier in the day.
* Choose a shake. There are several shakes based on milk or yogurt in the recipe section. Any one will provide a quick breakfast, which you can make up the night before.

■ Time limits for lunch

The obvious answer for busy people is to persuade someone else to make you a healthy packed lunch—failing that, make it yourself. It will still save time on going to the deli or sandwich shop in between meetings, or whatever. The bonus of a packed lunch is that you know what is in it, you know when it was prepared, and you can tweak it to suit your own needs. You can also eat it at a desk, although it is best not to try to eat while working as that is a sure way to digestive problems.

You need to take a short relaxing break in which to enjoy your lunch, even if it is only 15 minutes.

■ Here is the blueprint for the contents of a healthy packed meal:

* Something high in complex carbohydrate. This can be bread for sandwiches, which is by far the quickest option. Cold cooked rice, bulgur, couscous, or pasta are alternatives, which may be quick if you have some leftovers from, say, the previous evening's meal. Cooked new potatoes on their own make a tasty treat.
* Something with low- or moderate-fat protein. Fill bread, baguette, or pita with low-fat cheese or ham, vegetable pâté, or tuna, or add to the rice, etc., for a salad.
* Add a dressing, if you like—keep a jar of ready-made vinaigrette handy. A little homemade mayonnaise also acts as a good spread, instead of butter.
* Add fresh vegetables. If you haven't time to chop, add items to your lunchbox whole—tomatoes, scallions, peeled carrots. In cold weather, try a vacuum flask of vegetable soup.
* Choice of shelled nuts, fruit, dried fruit.
* A pot of yogurt or cottage cheese. This will be enough for many people, but men or very active people can also add:
* Graham crackers, bagel, muffin, or other semi-sweet bakery item.

■ If a packed lunch is impossible, here

are some guidelines for other options:
Sandwich shop or deli: Order along the guidelines above. Pitfalls: lots of sandwich fillings are heavy on mayonnaise or vinaigrette-type dressings. Go for dressings made with olive oil and, at least some days, ask for fillings and salad without dressing.
Fast-food outlet: Most burger bars can supply at least one or two items lower in fat—perhaps a fish or chicken patty on a whole-wheat bun. Many fast-food bars provide little or nothing in the way of salads, vegetables, or fruits, so pack your own fruit in your pocket.

■ Working from home

Many more people nowadays use the home as their workplace and find fitting in a healthy lunch just as much of a problem.

In summer, think "everything basic," such as the breads, cheeses, yogurts, fruits, tomatoes, and so on, outlined above. In winter, think a bowl of soup, a hunk of bread, and a piece of fruit. However busy you are, it is vital to stop for a break and something sustaining to eat. You will work better afterward if you do.

■ Fast tracks to an evening meal

Don't always rely on a take-out or pizza delivery for your evening meal! The main secret to having yourself a delicious and healthy meal ready to eat within half an hour or so of coming home—and with not a great deal of effort on your part— is to have a well-stocked pantry. If you're busy, stocking it up is best planned as a once-a-month exercise, which will save you time in the long run.

Items you must have include:

* Dried pastas of various shapes and at least some whole-wheat versions.
* Instant whole-wheat noodles.
* Couscous and instant rice.
* Brown and green lentils.
* Ready-to-eat dried fruits, shelled nuts, and seeds.
* Cans of fish, such as tuna, salmon, and sardines.
* Jars of black olives, pimientos, artichoke hearts (all canned in water if possible or, if using those canned in oil, well drained).
* Cans of beans, such as mixed beans, chickpeas, red kidney beans, canellini beans, and pinto beans. Even baked beans in tomato sauce are fine.
* Lots of tomatoey-things, such as jars of purée, tubes of tomato paste, packs of sun-dried tomatoes, tubs of sun-dried tomato paste, and cans of crushed and whole tomatoes.

QUICK DO-IT-YOURSELF SOUP

This soup will almost make itself while you do something else, and it can be varied according to what you have in the pantry.

To make 4 servings, take 3 cups (750 ml) ready-made vegetable or chicken stock. Take a package of ready-prepared and chopped supermarket vegetables, e.g. carrot, onion, parsnip (even leftovers from your own refrigerator), about 1 lb (450 g) in all, and add them to the stock in a pan with a 1 lb (400 g) can of crushed tomatoes. Simmer for 30 minutes. Drain a can of mixed beans and tip them in. Heat through. If you have time, purée half the soup in a blender and return to the pan. If not, it doesn't matter. Stir in 1 tablespoon ready-made pesto and add sea salt and pepper to taste before serving. Leftover potatoes are also very nice in this soup.

* Packages of dried Italian and Chinese mushrooms.
* Herbs and spices, and a few bottles of seasonings and sauces, such as light soy sauce, Worcestershire sauce, chili sauce, plum sauce, oyster sauce, and so on. These can be high in salt, but are used in small quantities.
* Low-sodium vegetable bouillon cubes, which are useful as standbys when you haven't got any fresh stock.

If your freezer contains a selection of the following, then you have the basis of a very healthy quick evening meal most nights of the week, especially if you have a microwave oven for quick thawing:
* Frozen vegetables, a good selection, including peas, broccoli, corn.
* Ready-made tomato sauce.
* Ready-diced, -sliced or -ground chicken, turkey, or lamb.
* Pizza bases.
* Ready-grated low-fat mozzarella cheese and some home-grated Parmesan.

In the refrigerator, the following will keep for weeks rather than days and will be welcome additions to your diet:
* Fresh chili peppers, ginger, and garlic. Keep in the salad crisper.
* Yogurt, cottage cheese, eggs, cheeses.

Tomatoes, bell peppers, and Napa cabbage will all keep well in the refrigerator for a week or more, as will fresh carrots, zucchini, and white cabbage. So will oranges, satsumas,

kiwis, and other fruits, depending on the condition they are in when you buy them. If you add these to your basic quick meals you will also be getting more vitamin C.

A large bag of potatoes will last a long time in cool dark conditions, so if you have a microwave you can add baked potatoes to your list of quickie dishes.

From all of this you can make dozens of different dishes. Here are just a few ideas (you will also find plenty of quick recipes in the recipe section on pages 207–255):
* Pasta with tomato sauce, with added black olives, and Parmesan.
* Pasta with a sauce made from cottage cheese, re-hydrated Italian dried mushrooms, and grated mozzarella cheese.
* Pasta with (frozen or jar) pesto.
* Noodles with a stir-fry of diced chicken, frozen stir-fried vegetables, ginger, garlic, and soy sauce.
* Pizza topped with tomato sauce, grated cheese, sliced olives, and re-hydrated dried mushrooms.
* Rice or baked potato served with quick chili, made from tomato sauce mixed with canned beans, fresh chopped chili peppers (lean ground meat can be added if desired).
* Couscous reconstituted and topped with a jar of drained pimientos in oil, heated with drained canned chickpeas in 1 tablespoon of the pimiento oil.

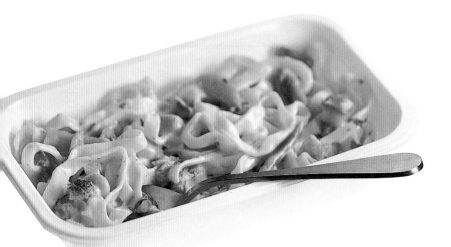

COTTAGE PIE: LOW IN FIBER
AND VEGGIES, AND QUITE HIGH IN FAT—
TRY TO ADD SOME HIGH-FIBER VEGETABLES SUCH
AS CABBAGE, WHICH WILL ALSO ADD VITAMIN C.

PASTA PRIMAVERA: HIGHER IN FIBER, CARBOHYDRATE, AND
VEGETABLES, AND LOWER IN FAT. A MIXED SIDE SALAD MAKES THE
DISH EVEN HEALTHIER.

CONVENIENCE MEALS

Many people rely on ready-cooked, chilled, or frozen convenience meals for their dinner—anything from a chicken curry to a Chinese meal for one or a roast dinner. But are they any good for you?

Of course, the answer is that they vary tremendously in nutritional content. For an average person (not trying to lose weight) many are too low in calories to satisfy the appetite. The main problem, however, is that many of them don't contain a reasonable balance of carbohydrate to protein and fat, although some manufacturers are making an effort in this respect.

If you need to rely on such meals more than occasionally, look for:
* The label. It should tell you how much fat the meal contains, and what proportion is saturated.

As a guide, under 10 g fat in the whole meal is low, 10–20 g is medium, and over 20 g is quite high. More than 25 g for women or 30 g for men per portion is probably too much, though this obviously depends on what else is eaten during the day. Look also for words on the package like "healthy eating" or "low in fat," which will be another guide, though not infallible.
* Vegetables included in the meal.
* A good carbohydrate content (if appropriate), such as rice, pasta, or noodles. (If you buy a meal that is just, say, meat or chicken in sauce, then you need to add some carbohydrate, even if it is just bread, and some fresh fruit or vegetables, (just a couple of tomatoes will do). If you choose wisely, you can fit prepared meals into your diet—but try to fill the freezer with homemade soup and casseroles, so that you don't have to rely on them too often.

Take-outs

Billions of US dollars are spent every year on just three kinds of take-out meals—burgers, pizzas, and fried chicken. This is equivalent to every single person in the country eating one of these types of take-out at least once a week. Add to that total the number of other kinds of take-out—Chinese food, for example, and you begin to see that the nutritional quality of the take-out foods is a matter of importance.

It is not possible to make many generalizations about take-out food as there are so many varieties, but one major European survey found that up to 60% of the total calories in take-out meals comes from fat, with three-quarters of meals analyzed over the recommended fat limits. Saturated fat is also likely to be high, and over half are high in salt. Considering that many take-out meals are high in calories, many also fall significantly short on a wide variety of nutrients, especially fiber, vitamin C, B group, and E.

Here we look in more detail at some of the most popular types of take-out meal, examine their nutritional content, and make some suggestions for the most balanced options to be found in each kind.

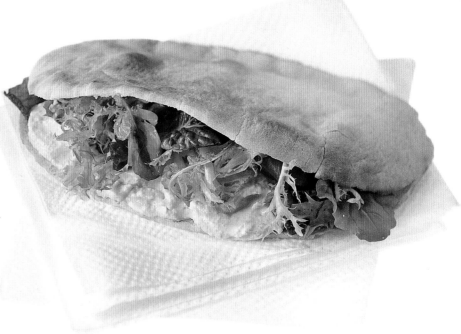

Burger in a bun with fries Hamburgers in a bun tend to be high in total fats, saturates, and calories, and are low in fiber, vitamin C, and some other vitamins, but are good sources of protein, iron, calcium, and zinc. A medium portion of French fries is also high in fat, with a little fiber and vitamin C. The complete meal will also contain, on average, almost a whole day's recommended salt intake.

A typical quarter-pounder burger in a bun with medium fries would give you around 800 calories and 50 g of total fat, of which approximately 25 g will be saturated, depending upon the fat used.

Adding cheese to the burger increases the calorie, salt, and fat content. Other types of burgers available at fast-food chains, such as chicken, fish, and vegetable burgers, are as high—or nearly as high—in fat as hamburgers. If you add a milkshake and a portion of apple pie to your meal, the fat content could reach a total of nearly 75 g—over the whole day's maximum intake.

Wisest choices at a burger take-out are plain small burgers in a bun (about 250 calories, 10 g fat), with orange juice, side salad and light vinaigrette, or a low calorie dressing. A beanburger, if available, is a reasonable choice.

Pizza Pizzas can be a reasonably good bet for healthy eating, depending on which you choose and size of portion. An average whole take-out pizza can be over 1,000 calories and would thus be hard to fit into a weight-loss diet, but would be fine for an average hungry man. Most pizzas are quite high in salt, especially deep pan pizza.

WATCH TAKE-OUTS IF ...

* You are vegetarian. Many seemingly vegetarian take-outs contain animal fat (e.g. French fries fried in lard).
* You suffer from allergic reactions. Some take-outs contain, for example, dyes (pilau rice, perhaps fish batter, even fries), flavor enhancers such as monosodium glutamate (Chinese meals), and soy products (batters, burgers) and other additives.
* You should be following a low-fat diet.
* You are trying to lose weight. Only a few take-outs are suitable for a diet if eaten regularly.
* You rely on them more than occasionally. A diet high in all but the most carefully chosen of take-outs is likely to be high in calories and fat and low in fiber, fresh fruits and vegetables, and certain vitamins, such as C and E. Some fresh fruit or salad added to any take-out will increase its nutritional profile.

FOOD FOR A BALANCED DIET

Pizzas contain plenty of carbohydrate in the base, the cheese provides protein, and both provide calcium. The tomato sauce is a good source of carotenoids, including lycopene. An average single-portion of cheese pizza will contain around 750 calories and 20–25 g fat. Any pizza with a generous portion of vegetables on top—bell peppers, for example—is a good bet, as are seafood pizzas. One of these pizzas, plus a side salad without added fat, would provide a reasonably balanced meal.

Fish and chips If you can find a fish-and-chip shop that serves generous portions of white fish encased in a light homemade batter fried in fresh vegetable oil to order, along with fries made out of good-quality potatoes and fried, again, to order—then a fish-and-chip meal can be quite nutritious, if high in calories and fat (though not saturated fat). The meal contains protein, carbohydrate, fiber, and a good range of vitamins and minerals, including some vitamin C in the fries. You could make it better balanced by adding a salad.

Sadly, however, much take-out fish and chips isn't carefully made. The fish and/or fries will often be twice fried, increasing fat and decreasing vitamin C. The proportion of fish to batter may be low, again increasing fat content. The fat used to fry may be lard, high in saturates, or it may be vegetable oil that has oxidized through over-use to a trans fat.

An average portion of fish and chips weighing 1 lb (450 g) may contain around 1,000 calories and 50 g fat.

Chinese Many of the choices on the Chinese take-out menu are high in fat, calories, and salt. Some of the higher-fat dishes include sweet-and-sour pork in batter, duck dishes, and special fried rice. Dishes lower in fat and calories may include stir-fried vegetable dishes (with or without shrimp or chicken), chop suey,

beef or chicken with green bell peppers, shrimp in a chili sauce, and barbecued spare ribs, plain boiled rice, and noodles.

For a balanced meal go for plainly cooked rice or noodles with a vegetable dish containing some lower-fat protein, such as shrimp, chicken, or tofu.
■ Some average values per portion:
Beef chow mein: 600 calories, 25 g fat
Chicken chop suey: 500 calories, 15 g fat
Spare ribs in sauce: 800 calories, 50 g fat
King prawns in ginger and chili sauce: 250 calories, 10 g fat
Large spring roll: 450 calories, 25 g fat

Indian/Thai There are still many take-out "curry" shops that will sell you a dish literally covered in oil. All the meat, onions, other vegetables, and spices have been fried in oil, which later rises to the surface. Some "curry houses" are trying to use less oil in their cooking; if you can find one that does and/or skims off fat, some curries can be quite good nutritional value. Balti curries may be lower in fat because of the method of cooking; they are also a good source of iron.

Curries based on vegetables and legumes are a good choice as they are high in fiber—for the regular take-out eater, this can be important as most take-outs are not. Shrimp or chicken curries (chicken off the bone and without skin) can also be good—but with chicken, choose a tandoori (dry) curry or one with a stock-and-tomato-based sauce rather than the high-fat "tikka masala" or any curry with coconut cream. Meat curries tend to be high in fat, as do many of the "snack type" Indian take-out foods, such as bhajis and samosas. Naan bread is high in fat and calories—a better bet is chapati, which is cooked without fat.

Pilau rice is fried and contains about a third more calories than plain. A good side dish is a lentil dhal, providing fiber, protein, and iron—in fact an ideal Indian take-out would be dhal with plain rice or

chapati and a small vegetable curry.
■ Some average values per portion:
Tandoori chicken: 350 calories, 15 g fat
Chicken tikka masala: 700 calories, 30 g fat
Vegetable curry: 400 calories, 20 g fat
Chapati: 150 calories, 1 g fat
Naan: 300 calories, 16 g fat
Lentil dhal: 200 calories, 8 g fat

Baked potato A take-out baked potato is high in fiber and carbohydrate and low in fat, with moderate calories. Lower-fat toppings are tuna in low-fat dressing, cottage cheese, baked beans, chile beans or cottage cheese with chives. All contain protein, helping to a better balance. An average 9 oz (250 g) baked potato with a high-fat topping has about 350 calories; with a lower-fat topping, about 250 calories. A salad balances the meal.

Gyros A gyro made from lean lamb and stuffed into pita bread, with a generous portion of salad, can be a fairly well-balanced meal, containing carbs, protein, and fat in reasonable proportions, as well as iron, fiber, calcium, and other vitamins and minerals. However, it may be high in salt and, if the lamb is fatty and a high-fat dressing is added, fat content may increase to 40 g or more.

For those wishing to avoid meat, a pita stuffed with salad and hummus is a good idea—the hummus contains a lot of fat, but mostly unsaturated, and the chickpeas are nutritious.

Fried chicken This is usually breaded (with fatty skin on) and then deep-fried, turning a low-fat source of protein into high-fat. An average small piece (90 g with bone) contains around 200–250 calories and about 10–15 g fat.

Side dishes may include coleslaw, high in fat, around 11 g, and in calories, with 120 per small portion, or baked or barbecued beans, which are a better bet, around 100 calories and only 1–2 g fat per portion, plus plenty of fiber and iron.

CHOOSING A DIET TO SUIT YOUR LIFESTYLE *59*

Vegetarian eating

A vegetarian diet is typically thought of as very healthy—and, certainly, that can be true. However, if you—or any of your family—are thinking of becoming a vegetarian, it is important to understand the possible pitfalls, as well as to enjoy the nutritional benefits that giving up meat may bring.

Only about 1% of the US population are full-time vegetarians. However, there is an increasing number of people who have reduced their meat intake and are seeking vegetarian options. Statistically, if you choose to go vegetarian—eating no meat, poultry, fish, or flesh of any kind—you are choosing an option that should boost your chances of living a long and healthy life.

Large research studies conducted over the past decade agree that, compared to non-vegetarians, vegetarians have up to 30% less heart disease, up to 40% less cancer, 20% less premature mortality, less obesity, lower blood pressure, and less occurrence of several other disorders.

However, statistics are not always as straightforward as they may seem—these results may also reflect the fact that most vegetarians have other lifestyle factors that may influence their health. For example, many are non-smokers and the level of alcoholism among them is low.

Vegetarians may generally be more health-conscious—for example, taking more exercise.

The health-giving properties of a typical vegetarian diet may also not simply be due to it containing no flesh. The benefits may be, for example, from eating more plant foods, such as fresh fruits and vegetables, grains and legumes, thus bringing the diet more in line with the healthy blueprint outlined in the previous pages of this section—more carbohydrate, more fiber, more vitamin C, more phytochemicals. Vegetarians, on average, have a lower body weight than non-vegetarians, and lower calorie intake has also been linked with longer lifespan. The vegetarian diet will also probably be higher in unsaturated fats (though this isn't always the case) and higher in essential fatty acids than that of a meat eater.

Indeed, other statistics back up the theory that it isn't just giving up meat that procures the health benefits for the vegetarian. For example, health benefits similar to the vegetarian diet have been found in non-vegetarians who tend to eat high amounts of fruit and vegetables and little dairy products.

The population of the Greek island of Crete in the Mediterranean has extremely low rates of heart disease, cancer, obesity, and early death, while eating meat in moderation and above average amounts of fish.

That is significant because there are certainly many vegetarians who, despite getting no saturated fat from meat, will be getting just as much saturated fat as meat eaters by replacing meat protein with an increased intake of dairy-based protein foods, such as cheese, milk, and eggs. There are also unknown numbers of vegetarians who eat little fresh fruit and vegetables and exist on a vegetarian version of a junk-food diet. Teenage vegetarians seem particularly prone to eating an unbalanced and/or unvaried diet (see the Teenage Section, page 166).

The moral here appears to be that a healthy diet—whether vegetarian or non-vegetarian—is one high in natural plant foods (fresh fruits and vegetables, grains, nuts, seeds, legumes), low-fat and non-animal fat sources of protein, and natural oils. If a vegetarian diet fits in with this blueprint then it will be healthy. The things to watch out for when starting a vegetarian diet are:

* Don't just give up meat without replacing it with other sources of the important nutrients it contains, particularly protein, selenium, iron, and B vitamins.

* Don't just use dairy products as a meat replacement—if you do, you are likely to be eating too much saturated fat. However, low-fat dairy products, such as skim milk and

VEGETARIAN SOURCES OF:

Iron: curry powder, cast-iron cooking utensils, ground ginger, seaweed, fortified breakfast cereals, lentils, unsweetened cocoa powder, sesame seeds, pumpkin seeds, soybeans, textured soy protein, dried peaches, navy beans, red kidney beans, cashew nuts, whole-grain barley, couscous, bulgur wheat, dried apricots, dark green leafy vegetables, eggs, brown rice, baked beans in tomato sauce, broccoli.
Selenium: Brazil nuts, lentils, sunflower seeds, whole-wheat bread, cashew nuts, walnuts.
Calcium: poppy seeds, Parmesan cheese, cottage cheese, Cheddar cheese, Edam, sesame seeds, mozzarella, Brie, tofu, Danish blue cheese, feta cheese, white chocolate, almonds, soybeans, figs, milk chocolate, yogurt, navy beans, spinach, brazil nuts, chickpeas, kale, white bread, milk, shrimp, broccoli, collard greens, white cabbage.

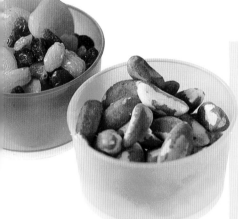

THE VEGETARIAN PANTRY

Here is a list of items you will find invaluable in your store if catering for a vegetarian or converting to vegetarianism yourself. Remember even pantry items deteriorate with time, so don't buy large packages for one person, as they may not be eaten soon enough. When buying for the pantry, as much as when buying fresh foods, buy the best quality you can.

* Dried legumes of several kinds, including various lentils and an assortment of differently colored and textured beans, plus chickpeas.
* Canned beans, chickpeas, and lentils as above; especially good if you are busy. Chickpeas are an ideal standby for a quick snack—puréed with olive oil and garlic, they make a quick and tasty hummus.
* Grains that don't take long to prepare, such as instant rice, couscous, bulgur.
* Other grains, such as barley and millet, which are useful for casseroles—or you can buy packages of mixed grains.
* Selection of pastas and noodles, at least some whole-wheat, and some instant polenta.
* Rolled oats and muesli.

* Flours of various kinds, such as buckwheat and whole-wheat (useful for crêpes, which can be made and frozen).
* Dried fruits, including peaches, apricots, prunes, figs, dates, raisins.
* Cans of tomatoes and other vegetables that are good in cans, such as pimientos and artichoke hearts.
* Cans of ready-made hummus, pasta and pizza sauces.
* Dried spices and herbs, chili sauce, soy sauce, black bean sauce.
* Jars or tubes of tomato paste, tomato purée, black and green pitted olives, olive pâté (tapenade), pesto.
* Vegetarian bouillon cubes and Worcestershire sauce.
* A good selection of oils and vinegars.
* Honey and good-quality unrefined sugar.

low-fat plain yogurt, are good—providing calcium as well as protein. Eggs are a good source of iron and vitamins, and also provide protein. Their saturated fat and cholesterol content mean that they shouldn't be relied on too heavily, especially for anyone who has been asked by their physician to follow a low-cholesterol, low-fat diet.

* Do eat plenty of plant sources of protein, such as legumes of all kinds and soy-based products, such as tofu, and, if you like it, textured soy protein. Nuts and seeds are also good sources of protein. However, they are high in oils and should not be eaten in excess.
* Do take care to eat plenty of vegetarian sources of iron, selenium, and calcium (see box opposite). Red meat is rich in easily-absorbed iron (heme iron); the iron from plant sources (non-heme iron) is less well absorbed, but with care a vegetarian diet can provide enough. In a recent survey, selenium levels have been found to be low in vegetarians and vegans, but this varies from area to area. Vegetarians cutting down on dairy products may have a problem, therefore, maintaining calcium intake and should eat lots of seeds, tofu, legumes, nuts, and leafy vegetables.
* Do be wary of eating too many sweet foods, such as pastries, cookies, cakes, and chocolate. These are all often high in fat, trans fats, and calories, and eating

too many of them will almost certainly mean you are less likely to be filling up on more nutritious foods.
* Do get plenty of the foods rich in essential fatty acids, such as nuts, seeds, and plant oils. If you don't eat fish you will be missing out on the omega-3 fatty acids EPA and DHA, but these can be converted in the body from alpha-linolenic acid, and linseeds (flaxseeds) and linseed oil are a particularly rich source of this. The healthiest vegetarian diets are those that:
* Follow the general principles for healthy eating as outlined in this section.
* Contain a wide variety of fresh, natural, and whole foods.

* Do not contain too much high-fat dairy products to replace meat poultry and fish.
* Do not rely on too many sweet low-nutrient foods.

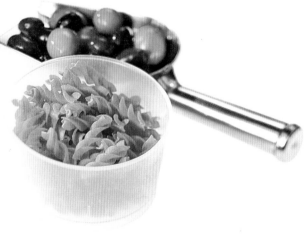

Plant protein versus animal protein

Until recently it was thought that, because most plant proteins (excluding soybeans) were "incomplete" (i.e., not containing all eight of the essential amino acids), vegetarians should combine different protein sources at each meal to obtain all eight amino acids to provide "complete" protein. The latest advice, though, says that a varied diet on a daily basis, containing a wide range of

DIFFERENT TYPES OF "VEGETARIAN"

Semi-vegetarian: Will (usually) eat everything except red meat. Sometimes poultry is also excluded, but fish is included, though may be eaten only infrequently.
Lacto-ovo-vegetarian: Will eat all dairy products and eggs, but no flesh of any kind.
Lacto-vegetarian: Will eat all dairy products, but no eggs, or flesh of any kind.
Vegan: Eats only plant foods—no dairy products, eggs, or flesh. (See The Vegan Diet opposite.)
Fruitarian: Eats only fruits (at least 75% of diet), uncooked vegetables (mostly leafy vegetables), raw nuts, seeds, and beansprouts.
Sproutarian: Eats mostly sprouted seeds, grains, legumes, and rice.
Macrobiotic: Excludes all meat, poultry, dairy products and eggs, but at initial levels may eat fish. Diet may progressively become more and more restricted, with the final level being a diet of brown rice only.

NOTE: These last three are not diets recommended by qualified nutritionists, as they will fall short of a variety of nutrients. The more restricted any diet is, the more chance that your full nutrient quota will not be met.

vegetarian protein foods, is sufficient, without worrying too much about providing "complete" protein at every meal.

However, some vegetarian groups make an exception for pre-school children, whose parents are advised to use the combining method at every meal, to ensure adequate protein intake. This method means mixing legumes with grains (e.g., beans on toast, pita and hummus, rice and bean salad), grains with a dairy product (e.g. cheese on toast, cereal and milk), or legumes plus starch (e.g., potato and lentil casserole).

Studies of adult vegetarians show that they tend to consume lower levels of protein than non-vegetarians. However, as we have seen earlier in Section One, many of us tend to eat more (sometimes much more) protein than we need.

For more on protein see page 20. For more on children and teenagers and a vegetarian diet, see page 168.

The lone vegetarian in the family

Catering for a sole vegetarian may seem daunting, and can create extra work. Here are some ideas to make catering easier:
* Gradually introduce more non-meat meals into the whole family's menus—many of the recipes at the back of the book could possibly inspire you. Meat lovers will appreciate the robust flavors and textures of brown or green lentils and several of the legumes, especially Egyptian brown beans, borlotti or pinto beans, and black beans.
* Make full use of pasta—you can cook pasta with a vegetarian sauce based on tomatoes or pesto, for example, freezing the surplus sauce in batches, and serve a sauce with added meat for the rest of the family. Again, vegetarian pasta dishes make an excellent dish for meat eaters anyway.
* Some vegetarian dishes are easy to cook ahead and freeze. Things like bean casseroles, curries based on potatoes,

eggplant, squash (freeze undercooked), nut and bean burgers and loaves all freeze successfully.
* Make main-course salads for the whole family and substitute non-vegetarian items for the lone veggie, e.g. salade Niçoise for the family, but use silken tofu instead of tuna for the vegetarian.
* For lunches or suppers, make chunky soups that are basically vegetarian and committed meat eaters can add chunks of chicken, ham, shrimp, etc.
* Pizzas please everyone—and, again, you can add small amounts of shellfish or meat topping as required.
* Legumes are an important nutritional source for vegetarians—canned, pre-cooked beans are fine, and widely available, but if you do soak and boil your own legumes you can freeze leftovers in individual bags for another occasion.
* The occasional convenience vegetarian meal is acceptable, particularly when served with fresh vegetables, but try not to rely on them too much.

It is important to find out just what a vegetarian will and will not eat before cooking anything for him or her.

See the box on the left for different types of vegetarian. See the second box on the right for a list of items which may also be on the "banned" list if the vegetarian is strict.

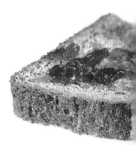

SAMPLE DIET

DAY ONE
Breakfast
muesli with skim milk
whole-wheat bread with olive oil margarine
and marmalade
1 orange
Lunch
Chunky Vegetable and Lentil Soup
pita bread
slice of vegetarian cake
banana and yogurt
Evening
Pasta with Basil and Ricotta
large mixed salad
Raspberry Gratin

DAY TWO
Breakfast
oatmeal with skim milk
whole-wheat bread with peanut butter
fruit juice
Lunch
Chickpea Salad with Bell Peppers
and Tomatoes
pita bread
Evening
Winter Squash with Lentils and Ginger
kale
1 orange

ALSO WATCH OUT FOR ...

Rennet: This enzyme from the stomach of animals is used in the production of many hard cheeses (as a curdling agent) and, therefore, these cheeses are unsuitable for most vegetarians. If a hard cheese isn't labeled "vegetarian," it probably does contain rennet. Many hard cheeses are now being produced without rennet, using plant curdling agents, and these are widely available.

Gelatin: Derived from the bones of animals (often cows) and therefore obviously unacceptable to most vegetarians. Can be present in any commercial dessert or product requiring a setting agent—e.g., mousses, fruit-flavored gelatins, even fruit yogurts. The vegetarian alternative is agar-agar, derived from seaweed and fairly easy to obtain.

Worcestershire sauce: Usually contains anchovies, but some brands don't, so read the label.

Bouillon cubes: Vegetable bouillon cubes are usually free of animal products, but it is worth reading the label.

Margarine: May contain fish oils. Read the label.

Honey: Some vegetarians and most vegans won't eat honey; best to check.

When catering for any type of vegetarian it is best to talk to them to discover just exactly how strict they are. Some vegetarians also require the use of organic produce and/or whole foods.

The vegan diet

Vegans eat no dairy products of any kind, or eggs, or anything from an animal, including honey. Those following a vegan diet are increasing in number and a high proportion of people who have been vegetarian for some time do eventually turn vegan. Vegans also often wear nothing made from leather or wool, and many also prefer organic products and whole foods.

Nutritionally, a vegan diet is quite restricted, but research shows that only a few nutrients (for adults—see Section Three for children) may find themselves short on a varied vegan diet, although calorie consumption is consistently lower in vegans than in non-vegetarians and in vegetarians, because the diet contains more high-bulk/low-calorie foods like fruits and vegetables, and protein intake is about 75% of average (but still within acceptable limits). The nutrients that may be in shortfall are calcium, selenium, iodine, vitamin B12, and vitamin D, plus possibly riboflavin, though, surprisingly, iron intake is not lower than the average.

However, the average vegan diet provides MORE than the national average of vitamin C, magnesium, copper, folate, beta-carotene, and essential fatty acids. Total fat intake is about 25% lower than average and saturate intake is 50% lower than average, while average carbohydrate intake is nearly 55%—an optimum level, and fiber intake is also higher than the national average and higher, indeed, than in ordinary vegetarian diets.

✱ Vegan sources of:
Calcium: Fortified soy milk, white bread, baked beans, dried figs, leafy green vegetables, tofu, nuts, muesli, legumes.
Selenium: Brazil nuts, lentils, sunflower seeds, whole-wheat bread, cashew nuts.
Iodine: Seaweed, kelp supplements.
Vitamin B12: fortified breakfast cereals, fortified soy milk, fortified bread.
Vitamin D: Fortified vegetarian margarines, fortified breakfast cereals, fortified soy milk, sunlight.
Riboflavin: fortified breakfast cereal, soy milk, fortified soy milk, and tomato sauce.

Eating out and entertaining

As eating out and having friends over to dinner are such enjoyable things to do, it is a shame that special-occasion meals so often seem to incur guilt and result in several pounds of weight-gain. Here's how to pick the wisest choices from the menu or the cook book—and still have fun.

The degree to which eating out or entertaining affect your nutritional status—and your size—is dependent upon two factors. First, how often you do it. If your eating out is restricted to a few times a year, then it really doesn't matter a great deal what you choose or how much you eat (with the proviso that, if you suddenly indulge in an over-rich large meal after a lengthy period of eating more healthily, your digestive system may well complain, see Heartburn and Indigestion, page 117).

However, many people find that if they add up business lunches and dinners, private invitations, and restaurant meals, they are eating out almost as often as they eat at home. In such a case, it is very important to pick and choose from what is on offer to please your health as well as your taste buds. This is the second factor—making sensible choices.

For those who experience "special occasion" eating all too frequently, the next few pages of this section really are required reading.

■ Lunching

Eating out at lunch is much more likely to be a "duty" lunch these days than a long, lingering pleasure lunch. If the latter, read the notes about restaurant meals below.

The average business lunch, luckily for our waistlines, no longer needs to be an overindulgent, overlong affair. For most occasions, it is perfectly acceptable to restrict the meal to one—or, possibly, two—light course(s), usually avoiding a dessert. Alcohol figures less and less at lunch; if you are doing the entertaining, always offer alcohol but don't feel obliged to indulge too—ice water is fine.

If you are choosing the lunch venue and are lucky enough to have a wide choice nearby, suitably light menus can be found at fish restaurants, Japanese restaurants, modern American or French restaurants. Most top chefs, whose ideas are often multinational, are very aware of the demand for light and healthy meals.

When picking from any lunch menu, try to remember the guidelines for healthy eating at lunch (see page 46), remembering that a starchy high-carbohydrate meal, such as a large pasta dish, may leave you less than alert all afternoon. A salad or light fish dish would be ideal, with a fruit first course and some good bread.

Consider also what you will be eating later in the day, if you know, and choose a lunch to balance that out.

For further guidelines on specific healthy and less healthy choices, read the tips below.

■ Evening eating

It has been estimated that the average person who goes to a restaurant or to someone else's house for an evening meal, will eat in that one meal at least a whole day's normal calorie intake and probably more. Statistics also show that food eaten outside the home contains, on average, more fat and saturated fat than that eaten inside the home—an average of 50% of the calories in "outside" food comes from fat. So anyone who eats out regularly will almost certainly be putting on weight and eating a diet unhealthily high in fat and saturated fat.

The two major considerations, then, may be to restrict the calories in your restaurant meals and to cut the fat. Protein needs are normally more than adequately met by the average restaurant meal, but, as with take-outs, some thought may be needed to pick a meal that contains adequate fiber and fresh fruit and/or vegetables.

Here are some general tips that will help you to achieve this:

✳ Take some plain bread from the bread basket, but avoid the butter.

✳ Vow to pick only one rich course at any meal; make the others light.

✳ Unless unavoidable, have only two courses.

✳ Try to pick at least one course based on fruit and/or salad—e.g., a salad first course, a fruit dessert.

✳ Choose plenty of vegetables with your main course. Avoid restaurants where vegetable portions are minuscule.

✳ Watch out for added butter, fats, cream, and cheese in each course. Anything fried, sautéed, or sauced may be very high in fat.

✳ If enjoying a private informal occasion, many calories and much fat can be saved without lessening enjoyment if you share a dish. For example, there are six of you at a restaurant meal. None of you are hungry after your main course, but you want to taste dessert. You choose just two or three different desserts and hand them around. Most restaurants accept this solution with good grace.

✳ If the meal is the kind where you serve yourself, serve small portions of the high-fat items.

■ Now we look at some popular types of restaurant and pick out the best choices for health, and the less good.

French Traditional French cuisine has always been very heavy in calories and fat: everything cooked in butter, and cream and buttery sauces. More modern French chefs are moving away from this and producing lighter, healthier versions

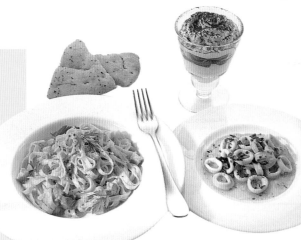

TYPICAL ITALIAN RESTAURANT MEAL

2,050 calories; 100 g fat (approx.).
Choose this meal—45% of which is fat—and you will be eating most of a day's calories (for women) and more than a day's fat allowance for women OR men all at once. The meal is also low on fresh fruits and vegetables and fiber.
Italian garlic flat bread, 75 g (approx. 350 calories, 12 g fat).
First course: Portion of fried squid (approx. 300 calories, 15 g fat).
Main course: Portion of Pasta Carbonara (approx. 900 calories, 45 g fat). This dish of pasta with a sauce made from eggs, cream, and bacon is very high in fat and saturates.
Dessert: Portion of tiramisu (approx. 500 calories, 30 g fat). Made from eggs and mascarpone cheese, this trifle is a typically rich Italian dessert.

HEALTHIER ITALIAN MEAL ★★★★★

1,150 calories, 41 g fat, (approx.).
Almost half the calories and less than half the fat and plenty of fresh fruit/salad.
Plain bread, 75 g (approx. 240 calories, 5 g fat).
First course: Melon and prosciutto (approx 150 calories, 5 g fat). Melon provides vitamin C and fiber, and an average portion prosciutto weighs only 50 g or so, so fat content is relatively low.
Main course: Spaghetti Napoletana (approx. 450 calories, 10 g fat). Large mixed side salad with olive oil dressing (120 calories, 10 g fat). Sauces based on tomato are ideal Italian food—seafood or a little grated cheese can be added for protein. The salad provides vitamin C, and fiber. The dressing provides healthy olive oil.
Dessert: Portion zabaglione (200 calories, 11 g fat). A fairly low-calorie treat.

of old favorites. In general, however, many French restaurants still seem reluctant to give decent amounts of vegetables and rely too heavily on the "protein first, forget the carbohydrates" approach. The further south the influence, the healthier a French meal may be, becoming more Mediterranean in outlook.

* Go for: "Provençal" cooking, e.g. dishes rich in tomatoes, bell peppers, or onions, for example. These may be high in olive oil and therefore calories, though, so choose a very light first course or dessert to balance the calories. Broiled fish and mussels marinière are also good choices.

* Think twice: anything "meunière"; in a rich butter sauce; cream sauces, creamy mousses; hearty French casseroles made with lardons of bacon or pork; cream puffs, rich cakes.

Italian Northern Italian food can also be high in fat and calories—it is the southern Italian food that is healthier, although high in calorie-rich olive oil. Many of the Italian restaurants found in the US mix the cuisine of both northern and southern Italy, but the good news is that in almost all Italian cafés there will be a good choice of healthy alternatives.

* Go for: vegetable and fruit first courses, such as grilled vegetables or artichoke salad, figs and prosciutto or a healthy bean soup; pasta dishes without a creamy sauce, e.g., tomato-based sauces, seafood sauces, pesto; chicken cacciatore, tuna and white bean salad; grilled calves' liver and broccoli, squid (casseroled not deep-fried).

* Think twice: pasta dishes laden with cream and cheese, such as Alfredo or carbonara; pasta dishes with meat, such as Bolognese; deep-fried calamari; antipasto platters heavy with fatty deli meats. Most risottos in restaurants are very high in butter and/or oil and perhaps cheese, too.

Pizzas are extremely variable—meat and cheese toppings are high in fat and calories, but tomato and seafood and vegetable toppings are better. Many Italian desserts are extremely high in calories and fat, so stick with Italian ices, fresh fruit, or baked peaches most of the time.

Asian Chinese, Thai, and most Asian cooking will be able to provide you with a reasonable amount of healthy choices, but you need to be careful. You may find portion sizes quite large and fat content may be high, especially in Thai cooking, which uses a lot of coconut milk. However, many dishes are rich in vegetables, fiber, and vitamin C, although many Asian dishes are high in salt.

✳ Go for: chicken and corn or hot-and-sour soup; stir-fries of vegetables and shrimp, pork, tofu, or chicken, rice or noodles; casseroles of chicken, tofu, or shrimp and vegetables; spare ribs (dry), plain cooked rice, chili shrimp or crab; sushi; lychees.

✳ Think twice: spring or egg rolls, deep-fried dumplings, deep-fried pork (etc.) in batter; special fried rice, spare ribs in wet sauce; coconut curries; caramel bananas.

Indian Much traditional Indian cuisine is well balanced nutritionally, with plenty of complex carbohydrate and vegetables and much protein coming from plant sources. However, many Westernized Indian restaurants cater to the Western taste and offer more dishes rich in animal proteins, fat, and cream. Try to find Indian restaurants that base their cooking on traditional lines. Even so, if you are watching your weight, be aware that many Indian dishes may be very high in oil. Spices can be good for the digestion, stimulating and metabolism-boosting.

✳ Go for: vegetable-based curries, lentil dhal, rice, flat breads including chapati; tandooris, fresh fruit salads, mangoes.

✳ Think twice: masalas and korma curries containing cream; coconut curries; deep-fried samosas, bhajis.

Family-style restaurants If you often eat at hotel dining rooms and other traditional restaurants you will, unless you are very careful, be getting an unbalanced diet, high in protein, high in fat, low in carbohydrate, fruits, and

---

MENU IDEAS FOR ENTERTAINING:

Marinated herbed shiitake mushrooms
Seared tuna with lemon grass
Blackberry Ice

Baked baby tomatoes and basil
Turkish Lamb Stew
Stir-Fried Fruit Salad

Cucumber and Mint Soup
Parcels of Tilapia, Tomatoes, and Olives
Mango Phyllo Tarts

Mushroom and Red Pepper Skewers
Thai Guinea Fowl with Cashews and
    Pineapple
Citrus Granita

---

vegetables. A meal of shrimp cocktail, steak and French fries, and chocolate cake will probably contain at least a day's recommended maximum fat, saturated fat, and protein intake.

✳ Go for: melon; grilled/roast chicken, turkey, salmon, trout; baked potatoes; large salad bowl; sorbet; strawberries, ice cream.

✳ Think twice: pâté, shrimp cocktail; large steaks, French fries; apple pie, ice cream, and chocolate cake.

■ **Healthy eating at home**

If you like to entertain, you have total control over what you serve and so choosing a healthy but delicious menu shouldn't be a problem. People no longer feel cheated if they aren't served a meal rich with butter, cream, and thick sauces at every course. Tastes, colors, and presentation are important, and a well-planned ethnic-style meal will always be appreciated.

Many of the recipes in this book are ideal for entertaining and some suggested three-course menus appear in the panel above. Here are some more simple tips to help you plan a special, but

---

well balanced and nutritious meal.

✳ For pre-dinner nibbles, vegetable sticks, and perhaps Italian sesame breadsticks, with one of the dips that appear in the recipe section—such as anchoïade, skordalia, rouille, or baba ganoush. These are much less salty than most potato chips and salted nuts.

✳ Decide on your main course first and then plan a first course and dessert to balance it. For instance, a meat main course would require a vegetarian or light fish or shellfish appetizer. Whereas, if you are serving a high-carbohydrate main course, such as pasta, your first course could be a small portion of a high-protein food, such as crab or shrimp. Try to include salad/vegetables or fruit with every course—e.g. a crab salad appetizer, a roast vegetable and grain main course, and a fruit dessert.

✳ Quick, healthy and easy appetizers are grilled peppers in a vinaigrette on herb salad; asparagus spears with balsamic vinegar; artichoke hearts bottled in oil, drained and served with quail eggs.

✳ If you are short of time, don't bother to make a dessert—a selection of fresh fruits with goat's cheese and oat crackers is ideal. Quick hardly-any-cooking desserts are fresh fruit compotes (e.g. lightly cooked summer fruits simmered in wine) or flambéed pineapples and bananas.

■ **Before you think of drinking and driving**

If you eat out in the evening, it is easy to notch up several alcoholic drinks. If you have to drive, however, be wary of how much you drink, however sober you may feel. As we saw on page 36, a unit of alcohol contains 8 g of pure alcohol and safe limits for health are one drink a day for women and two for men. To most people, though, this means little in terms of how much they can drink before their blood alcohol concentration rises to a level that means it is unwise to drive.

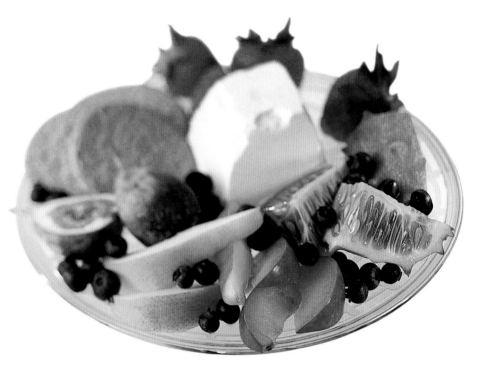

In the US, you are "over the limit" if your blood alcohol concentration is more than 80 mg alcohol per 100 ml blood (though "Healthy People 2000" proposes all states to lower it to 40 mg). As a guide, a man can have about three to four drinks in an evening (four hours) with food, and a woman two, before going over the limit. However, not everyone will have the same blood alcohol concentration after drinking the same amount. Generally, taller, heavier people can drink more than shorter, lighter people before reaching 80 mg/100 ml. Also, young people and people not used to drink will probably be more easily affected by the alcohol, and women are more quickly affected than men because they have a higher percentage of body fat and lower percentage of body fluid (for dilution of the alcohol) than men.

Moreover, if you drink quickly, your blood alcohol concentration will also go up more quickly. If a man takes three drinks, or a woman two drinks, in just one hour instead of in a whole evening, he or she will almost certainly be over the legal driving limit. It will then take a wait of 1 to 3 hours to get the levels below 80 mg/100 ml again.

The chart below gives a guide to what constitutes being "at the limit"—but remember, it is only a guide, and different people may reach their limit on less alcohol. Even after just one or two

drinks, judgment is impaired and, even though you may be below the legal limit for driving, it is safest not to drive after drinking any alcohol at all. The following tips may help you reduce your alcohol intake—and/or blood alcohol concentration—when eating socially:

✱ Remember that food slows down the absorption of alcohol. Try not to drink anything alcoholic before you start to eat; on an empty stomach it will rapidly cause a rise in your blood alcohol levels.

✱ Don't start the evening by quenching thirst with alcohol—quench it with

water. You will find that you drink much more slowly then.

✱ Drink slowly. Alternate alcohol with water as much as possible.

✱ For your own guests, make sure there are plenty of low-alcohol or alcohol-free drink alternatives available—in winter, a low-alcohol punch, in summer a low-alcohol sangria (see page 254), plus juices, mineral water, and alcohol-free beers and wine.

✱ Don't think that strong coffee will "sober you up" or lower blood alcohol levels. Neither will running around the block or drinking water or vitamin C. Once the alcohol is in your body, nothing can do this except time. A healthy liver "neutralizes" the alcohol at the rate of approximately one drink per hour (though this varies with individuals).

Alarmingly, this could mean that, if you have had a very heavy evening's drinking—say, two large gins, a bottle of 12% alcohol by volume wine and a large brandy (10 drinks altogether)—you would still be over the legal driving limit the following morning.

THAT'S THE LIMIT

You will probably reach your blood alcohol concentration limit if you drink:

Men			
140 lb	1.5 drinks in 1 hour	3.5 drinks in 3 hours	4 drinks in 4 hours
168 lb	2 drinks in 1 hour	4 drinks in 3 hours	4.5 drinks in 4 hours
Women			
112 lb	1 drink in 1 hour	1.5 drinks in 3 hours	2 drinks in 4 hours
140 lb	1 drink in 1 hour	2 drinks in 3 hours	2.5 drinks in 4 hours

FOOD FROM FARM TO TABLE

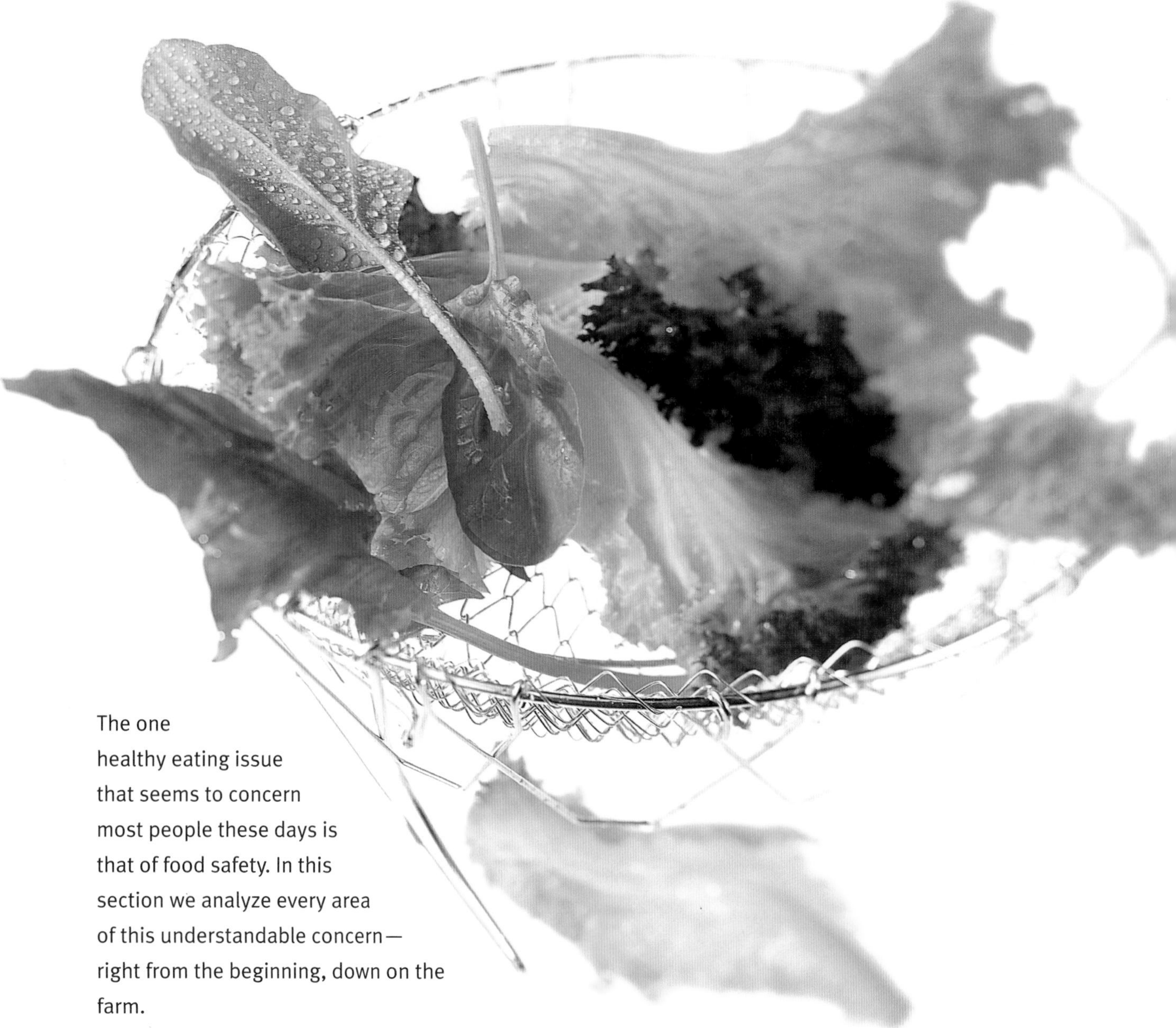

The one
healthy eating issue
that seems to concern
most people these days is
that of food safety. In this
section we analyze every area
of this understandable concern—
right from the beginning, down on the
farm.

Modern "factory farming" is the result of our international quest for cheap and plentiful foods, in the face of a growing population. However, such intensive farming has brought all kinds of problems and these do need to be faced.

We look at crop farming and the methods employed by the arable farmers in order to maximize their yields. Chemical farming is of increasing concern to many of us—so the facts and the alternatives are discussed. Similarly, especially since the BSE ("mad cow disease") crisis in Europe, people are worried about intensive animal farming, so we look at just how good or bad factory-farmed produce IS for your health, and offer alternatives where possible and if necessary.

Food preservation is another area of possible concern. We are all so keen on being able to buy a wide variety of produce out of season, all year round, that we may not always realize just how some foods look so fresh ...

And the ones that DON'T look fresh inside those packages and cans, shrink-wraps and jars—are they OK, or should we give them a miss? Are our governments protecting us enough from harmful additives.

The issue of food poisoning is discussed in detail and we look at ways to avoid the risks, again from farm to table. We also look at all the other food safety issues that each of us can help to prevent by buying, storing, preparing, and cooking our food properly. From the shop to YOUR table—food safety really is in your hands.

In fact, in a way all food safety is in our hands. The choices we make about the things that we buy, where we buy them, and how much we are prepared to pay, are what will make the difference to the quality and the safety of the food that we eat in the long term.

When it comes to food, the choice IS yours. Let it be the right one.

Food production

The way in which we grow our crops, raise cattle, and even fish the seas has changed dramatically in the last generation.

Crops

With mass production, the use of chemicals in the production of our food crops—everything from grains to vegetables, fruits, and salads, from field to orchard to greenhouse—quickly became standard procedure. It seemed nothing but a good idea to use pesticides to kill insects and other creatures that were damaging crops, herbicides to kill weeds that were choking them, and fungicides to cure diseases, as well as applying artificial fertilizers to help maintain the fertility of the new-style large-scale farms where, with the help of modern mechanization, food production could be vastly increased by growing just one type of crop on the same land, year after year.

In a very short time we had—almost miraculously—food that was plentiful, cheap, and widely available. Most crops were also better to look at and more regular in shape, and, as they appeared clean, they no longer needed scrubbing before use... "advantages" that most people now take for granted.

As the agri-industry took off, farms became vast and specialized; hedges, woods, ponds, and wildlife disappeared and, by the '60s, hundreds of different chemicals were being used to bring us our food as a matter of course, chemicals that often lingered on in the food that we ate but which were declared safe.

Nowadays, after being harvested many crops are still sprayed with preservatives and inhibitors to prolong their life for transportation, storage (sometimes for months), and shelf-life. Such sprays are even more likely to linger as residues on the food that we eat.

TIPS ON MINIMIZING RESIDUES

* Wash all fruits and vegetables thoroughly before eating
* Peel vegetables and fruits where appropriate
* Discard outer leaves of lettuce, cabbage, etc.
* Never eat the green end of a carrot—remove at least 1 inch of the carrot below the stalk and peel a thick layer off carrots before use; residues of toxic organophosphates have, in past years, been found to be over safe limits.

Only in the past few decades did the drawbacks of intensive farming become apparent. Many people did not enjoy the idea of eating foods that might well be contaminated with chemical residues. They also began to worry about the effect of the agricultural industry on the environment, as it became clear that it has destroyed much of our wildlife by killing off the insects at the lower end of the food chain, by denuding the countryside and destroying natural habitats, and by polluting rivers. It has also interfered with traditional natural processes, such as pollination, because pesticides can't tell the difference between "pests" and "good" insects such as bees. It has also helped to deplete the ozone layer.

Ironically, as the time progressed, it also became apparent that many common pesticides no longer actually worked—the pests and diseases were becoming resistant to the chemicals the industry used. Nowadays it can take only as little as two years for a pest to develop complete resistance to a new chemical. Fertilizers, too, often need to be used in larger and larger quantities to achieve the required results, and artificially fertilized soils may well be quite deficient in vital nutrients such as selenium.

What controls are there for our food safety?

In 1906 the Pure Foods Act began the modern era of consumer protection in the US. The Food, Drug, and Cosmetic Act, which is constantly being amended for increased food safety, followed this. In the US the Enviromental Protection Agency (EPA) is in charge of regulating the use and distribution of pesticides. Before any pesticide is approved, the EPA can require more than 100 tests to determine its safety. The EPA is also in charge of setting a tolerance level (the maximum residue level legally permitted in our food). On the other hand, the FDA and the USDA are the agencies who monitor the food supply. The tolerance levels set by the EPA are the guidelines used by the FDA's monitoring programs that ensure we all receive a safe food supply. The FDA enforces these tolerance levels for all foods—including imported foods—except for poultry, meat, and some egg products (enforced by the USDA). Every year the FDA spends more than $20 million on monitoring pesticide residues in our foods.

One way they monitor our food supply is through the Total Diet Study. This ongoing study is conducted by collecting and processing (i.e., cooking) commonly consumed foods throughout the US. The foods are then analyzed for about 200 pesticide residues. Any food found to contain residues above the EPA's tolerance levels cannot be sold in the US. The most recent study showed that about 98% of sampled foods did not exceed the tolerance levels. However, one problem with this system is that by the time offenders are found the crops have already been sold and eaten.

Another problem may be that, even if maximum levels are not being exceeded in isolation, if we take official advice and "eat more fruit and vegetables" and more plant foods to prevent diseases such as cancer and coronary heart disease (CHD), we will inevitably be consuming more and more of these toxic chemicals. The cumulative effect of a range of killer chemicals eaten over a lifetime, in doses individually declared officially safe, is yet to be assessed. Perhaps we should also remember that, from time to time, chemicals previously thought safe are withdrawn from use. So, what are the alternatives?

Integrated pest management (IPM)

This is a kind of "halfway house" between modern agrochemical and organic farming. Although the idea of IPM developed in the 1950s, only recently has it captured the US interest. In fact, in 1993 the Clinton Administration set a national goal of having 75% of all US farms using IPM techniques by the year 2000. IPM "borrows" organic and traditional ideas, such as crop rotation and using natural predators to control pests. It also uses innovations (with the help of gene technology, see opposite), such as disease- and pest-resistant varieties of crops, but doesn't ban the use of chemicals in certain circumstances (e.g., pesticides are still permitted on potatoes), simply trying to ensure "broad-spectrum" chemicals are avoided where possible and preventative mass crop spraying is discouraged.

The supermarkets say that IPM is no more expensive than chemical farming, therefore doesn't increase costs, but rewards in terms of the environment and pesticide levels in food are great.

Organic farming

Organic farming has always been around, but only due to increased interest on health and the environment have we turned to organic food as a safe alternative. From a small market it has grown to a $4 billion industry. A recent national poll showed 54% of American consumers stated their preferences were for organic production and over 5% of all new foods and drinks introduced in 1996 were made with organic ingredients.

ARE THERE DRAWBACKS TO ORGANIC PRODUCE?

Basically, the extra money it costs to buy. This is due to various reasons, including the more labor-intensive and less land-intensive style of farming. The more that people show that they want organic food, the more farms will convert to organic methods, and the more the cost will come down.

Other than price, organic produce appears to have no disadvantages. It often tastes better than mass-market produce, and tests have shown that it often contains higher amounts of nutrients. It may, of course, have a shorter shelf-life. However, because turnover is much more rapid than it was a decade ago, stale, shriveled organic fruit and veggies are rarely seen... these days, it even looks fairly uniform too.

No chemicals at all are allowed in organic farming and methods used are based on the traditional ones of keeping crops healthy with good soil, rotation and natural fertilizers, and choosing suitable crops for the local environment. Pests and weeds are controlled by means of natural predators and methods.

Genetic engineering

Huge multinationals have spent several years developing bio-technological ways to improve plants, so the need for chemicals will be minimized they say.

For example, crops can be genetically altered to become resistant to a particular disease or insect, or to store better without damage. However, the whole subject of genetic modification is causing much debate—its ethics, its safety, and so on. We look at the subject in detail later.

Animal and dairy production

As with crops, intensive farming of meat and other animal and dairy products has brought us relatively inexpensive and plentiful food. The idea of "factory farming," with animals kept in conditions far removed from nature, is now taken for granted by most of us. Even food sources once considered "wild," such as salmon, trout, and novel meats like ostrich and crocodile, are being farmed intensively all over the world. But is all this intensive meat, fish, and dairy production all right for our health?

■ Meat

How cheap meat is produced

Low-cost meat, in general, means animals that grow quickly and take up as little space, food and labor as possible in so doing. In order for this to happen, intensive farming may take on board several practices with which many people find they are becoming disenchanted.

* *Keeping feeding costs low*: To put animals out to graze on foods that are natural to them, such as grass, is highly space-consuming, and is not a fast way of adding weight. Therefore it is expensive. A much cheaper method is to keep them indoors and feed them on manufactured foods, such as pellets made from the ground-up remains of other animals. It is thought that such an unnatural diet may be one of the causes of BSE—popularly known as mad cow disease—in cattle.

* *Restricting space*: By feeding animals on man-made produce they no longer need to roam fields. They can be kept in small spaces, such as barns and pens, which obviously means much less land is needed. Unfortunately, the animals don't get enough exercise, so they become less healthy with weak muscles. They also become more prone to infections, which can quickly spread through a farm.

This means that antibiotics need to be used in blanket form, with sometimes alarming frequency. Antibiotic residues can last through the food chain until our meat and dairy food is on the plate.

Animals that do graze on "natural" pasture may be eating food that has been sprayed with chemical weed-killers and fertilizers, which may show up later in the meat and milk (see below).

Industry, too, may increase toxic residues, for instance the highly poisonous chemical dioxin, which is a by-product of several industrial processes or waste clearance. Radiation discharges from nuclear sites around the country also show up in all of our food, albeit in levels which the government has decreed as safe.

* *Speeding growth*: Intensively reared animals are often "force-fed" on a diet unnaturally high in calories, with added nutrients, given automatically and regularly so that weight is gained uniformly and quickly. Today this is often not seen as good enough, and hormones which speed growth-rate, such as clenbuterol, are often used by cattle men.

Legal drugs, such as antibiotic growth-promoters, are widely used in certain areas of meat farming. Waste products from intensive farming are also increasingly polluting our rivers.

All this means that it is impossible to prevent traces of toxic chemicals and drugs from arriving in the food chain, at least in some foods, some of the time. Residue levels are officially monitored, but there is concern, for example, that because we may unwittingly ingest antibiotics in our food, we too will become resistant to them.

For example, in 1997 it was reported that, in humans, over 80% of infections with a salmonella bug were resistant to a wide range of common antibiotics; a result, a leading European public health doctor was reported as saying, of farming practices rather than overuse in hospitals.

A variety of new, hormone-related illnesses and problems are being noted in humans, too, and these may be related to the food chain.

Food poisoning with bugs such as E. coli is another increasing problem—meat is frequently the culprit, sometimes because of unhygienic handling or storage anywhere from slaughterhouse to table. Much stricter rules are being enforced by governments to help beat this problem, but it will take some time. This subject is dealt with in detail on page 81.

Making the meat you eat safer

✻ Organic meat will be guaranteed free from residues of artificial chemicals, antibiotics and hormones. Production is increasing and, although it is 30% more expensive than mass-produced meat, a little tends to go a long way—an idea that helps us eat a better-balanced diet anyway. Organic meat is produced using natural traditional rearing and living methods.

Many supermarkets now stock organic meat or, at least, offer meat pro-duced using less intensive methods. Their customer desk should be able to give further information. Many farm shops sell organic produce and many organic pro-ducers will deliver to you by mail order.

✻ If you can't buy organic, eat lean meat. Toxins tend to accumulate in fatty tissue.

✻ If you like beef, and are afraid of BSE (mad cow disease), simple guidelines can help you to be fairly sure (though no one can guarantee 100% safety) it is BSE-free:

Buy organic beef—organic herds have very little incidence of BSE and only when cattle have been brought in from non-organic herds.

Buy only steaks and joints; avoid cheaper products, like steak pies and beef sausages.

■ Fish and seafood

Nothing could be more healthy than a portion of fish, could it? We are all being encouraged to eat more fish. It would be

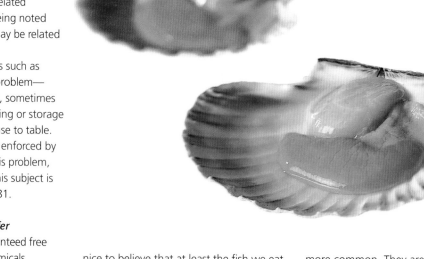

nice to believe that at least the fish we eat is clean, with no residues of poisons, antibiotics, hormone-disturbing chemicals, and so forth.

Sadly, this is no longer the case. The ocean and river outlets are increasingly polluted by industrial waste. For instance, high concentrations of cadmium have been found in the livers of fish in the North Sea in Britain. Investigators have found that one-third of plaice had skin complaints, which were probably pollution-related. Human waste in sewage can also cause some shellfish to harbor high levels of bacteria.

River fish are not faring any better. Very recent research has found that industrial estrogen-mimicking chemicals released into some of our river waters are causing up to 60% of male river fish to change sex!

Yet the alternative source of much of the fish that we eat—fish farming—also has its problems. For example, farmed salmon, now so cheap and plentiful, is raised in huge cages in lakes or coastal sea. These fish are often hosts to parasites, called sea lice, which are killed by means of antibiotics. The farmed salmon also live in conditions not dissimilar to intensively reared land animals, such as chickens, meaning that diseases and other pests are becoming

more common. They are also fed special dyes to make them look pinker. The main dye used, canthaxanthin, is toxic and, in 1990, the Food Advisory Committee of the UK recommended that it should no longer be used in animal feed; but, as the European Community had already issued approval, that advice has been withdrawn.

MAKING THE FISH YOU EAT SAFER

✻ White fish from the deeper waters, such as cod and haddock, is less likely to be affected by pollution than the fish that lives nearer the coasts.

✻ Crabs, lobsters, and the shrimp family are less likely to be affected by pollution or bacteria than the shellfish that live on the shoreline, such as mussels and oysters. These latter shellfish are cleaned before being sold, or cultured, in which case they should be sold as such and will be pollution-free naturally.

✻ Scallops are usually pollution- and disease-free.

✻ Sadly, oily fish and the livers of other fish are more likely to be affected because toxins such as cadmium and dioxins are stored in body fat and liver.

■ Dairy products and eggs

Largely because of increased concern by animal rights advocates there are various egg types found in the Western world. Nutritionally speaking, battery-raised eggs are not greatly different from free-range or organically-produced eggs. However, salmonella in eggs is still a big problem with intensively reared hens—according to the US Center of Disease Control about 40,000 cases of infection are reported yearly. Advice is still for the elderly, pregnant, and ill not to eat raw eggs. More on how to avoid food poisoning appears on page 81.

Egg types and what they mean

* *Battery eggs:* These won't be labeled as such on the package but most of eggs sold in the US are still from hens living in battery cages. These are the cheapest eggs to buy, and the hens are fed on a manufactured mixed diet that may include animal carcass by-products and medicines to keep diseases at bay.
* *Barn eggs:* These eggs come from hens live that live in barns and are free to move about, but may be overcrowded and their diet similar to the diet of caged hens.
* *Free-range eggs:* The conditions in which free-range hens are kept differ tremendously. Kept at the minimum standard required they may still only have cramped living conditions, with access to an outdoor area, but not necessarily to natural food. Their beaks may be clipped so they can't forage anyway. Perches and litter may or may not be provided; it isn't law. It is hard to tell from egg boxes just how free-range the hens who laid the eggs were.

Kept at a standard above the basics, free-range hens may lead a much more natural life, only going indoors at night and fed on fairly natural foodstuffs. The producers of this standard of egg will probably explain all this on the label as the eggs will be more expensive again.

MAKING DAIRY PRODUCTS SAFER

* Low-fat milk will contain fewer residues than full-fat milk because fat tends to store toxins. The same applies to other low-fat dairy products.
* Very fresh eggs, from whatever source, will contain fewer bacteria than older eggs, so try to find a source of eggs where the laying date can be established. Organic eggs and best-quality free-range eggs are also less likely to be contaminated, and some eggs are sold with a "salmonella-free" guarantee.
* Eggs shouldn't be eaten raw.

* *Four-grain eggs:* The hens who lay these eggs have been fed only on foods natural to hens, and not on animal protein. There is no medicine included in their food. They are still, however, likely to be barn hens rather than free-range.
* *Organic eggs:* These are hard to find for most of us, but will be from hens whose beaks aren't clipped and who live in a flock of less than 500. They lead natural lives, ranging over organic pasture, and all their other food is natural.

For more information on choosing healthy eggs, see page 77.

Milk and milk contaminants

Milk from any animal—and products such as cheese and yogurt—is similar to its meat in that any pollutants that the animal has eaten or been given or picked up elsewhere will show there, even if in minute amounts. Cows that graze on sprayed fields and who eat pelleted food containing contaminants will yield milk containing these items. One recent European survey showed a high percentage of milk containing the toxic pesticide lindane. Like other foods, milk is regularly monitored and declared safe by the US Government. However, many people are turning to milk from organic herds.

Pasteurization destroys harmful bacteria and virtually all milk on sale now is pasteurized. Raw (unpasteurized) milk, which can still be found in Europe, is about to be banned for sale, due to high levels of contamination with feces and other contaminants.

There has recently been much debate across the world about the use of BST, a man-made hormone which increases milk yield in cows. It is already in use in the US but is banned for use elsewhere until at least 2000.

Food processing and preserving

■ Fresh food—but is it?

Once food is harvested or slaughtered, much of it is sold unprocessed via the stores. When you go to buy it, however, all is not necessarily as it seems. How fresh is "fresh," for instance, and does it matter to your health? There are various ways the food industry can keep things looking fresh for weeks or even months.

✳ *Post-harvest spraying*: Many fruits, including apples, pears, and grapes, and some vegetables, including potatoes, may be treated with preservative sprays to prolong their life. There is no way of telling which have been sprayed, but as these chemical sprays are toxic—indeed, one has been banned in the US—a person eating a healthy diet rich in fruits and vegetables may be getting quite a dose of them.

✳ *Controlled-atmosphere storage and packaging:* The two biggest-selling fruits in the Western worlds, apples and bananas, are routinely harvested and then kept in a controlled atmosphere with the oxygen levels reduced and nitrogen and carbon dioxide levels increased. This prevents ripening and aging. When the fruits are needed they are artificially ripened with ethylene gas.

Many foods are also packed in a similar atmosphere for the shelf—e.g. prepared salads, fish, and meat. It extends shelf-life by up to five times and seems to be harmless.

✳ *Waxing*: Citrus fruits, apples, and various other fruits and vegetables are often wax-coated. This keeps natural moisture in, gives a shiny appearance, and extends shelf-life. Vegans will not be pleased to hear that a substance often used in waxing, shellac, is derived from insects. Various other waxes can be used and there is no obligatory labeling. However, "unwaxed" fruits are usually labeled as such.

✳ *Genetic engineering*: For more on this see page 82, but basically food scientists can now inject "long-life" genes into various foods, such as tomatoes, pineapples, and bananas. These raw foods first appeared on our table in the early 1990s.

✳ *Irradiation*: Food irradiation dates back to the early part of this century. Today it is used in about 40 countries and is said to kill more than 99% of food-borne bacteria. There is large public resistance against irradiated food, however the process (hitting fresh food with ionizing radiation to kill microorganisms that make food age and rot) is legal in the US and for more than five years certain foods—pork, poultry, white potatoes, fresh fruit, and spices—are being treated to extend shelf-life and decrease the risk of food-borne bacteria.

The main drawbacks of irradiated food, apart from "factor X" (unknown long-term effect of a diet high in irradiated products), are that they deplete vitamins in food by up to 90%, and destroy "good" bacteria along with the bad.

FOOD PRESERVATION METHODS COMPARED

Canned: can be stored up to several years.
pros: convenient, low cost, can be stored at room temperature.
cons: brine-canned foods high in salt; syrup-canned foods high in sugar. Vitamins B and C depleted. Coated cans may leach chemicals into foods.
Bottled: can be stored up to several years.
cons: vitamin depletion.
UHT: can be stored up to 6 months.
cons: vitamin depletion and taste change.
Ambient: (processed food stored at room temperature, such as jams) can be stored up to 3 months.
cons: generally high in chemical preservatives.
Chilled: can be stored up to a week
pros: fresh.
cons: cost, need to keep cool.
Frozen: can be stored from one month up to one year.
pros: similar nutritionally and in appearance to fresh.
cons: not suitable for all food; energy-costly.
Vacuum-wrapped: can be stored up to one month.
pros: convenient.
cons: may have preservatives added.
Dried: can be stored up to a year.
pros: convenience.
cons: destroys vitamin C and B, taste loss, texture change.

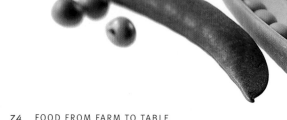

Processing

A large percentage of our basic food isn't sold "as is," though, but taken to food factories and processed into all the myriad different foods that are on the supermarket shelves—the cans and packages of soups, the bottled relishes and sauces, the packages of dessert and cake mixes; the convenience meals, the spreads for bread—and so on, and so on.

In general, the more a food is processed, the more it is likely to lose in terms of its natural nutrients, and the less "natural" it will be. As a very simple example, strawberries are high in vitamin C and fiber, but add them to sugar and make "economy" strawberry jam in a factory and you lose almost all of those two nutrients. Highly processed food, again in general, tends to lose its vitamins and fiber most frequently.

Where some things are taken away, however, others are added. Processed food is notoriously rich in high-calorie ingredients such as sugar, saturated fat, and trans fats. Cream is skimmed off milk (we are now drinking more skim milk than ever before, for our health's sake) and put into our bodies via processed food. We replace sugar in our coffee and sodas with artificial sweetener—only to eat even more of it in processed desserts, cakes, and cookies. And so on!

Processed food often contains fortifying ingredients to replace lost vitamins and minerals (as in many breakfast cereals, flours, crackers, breads, pasta, rice and grains), perhaps adding fiber and other "healthy" things (see

more about this in Functional Foods on page 83). Less welcome than these additions, though, are the ones that are put in the processing pot for other reasons.

Food additives
Processed food labels may contain a long list of additives and items that you will not recognize or consider necessary. Yet it is estimated that each of us eats about 5 pounds (2.25 kg) of additives a year.
* *Colors:* Used to make perhaps less-than-attractive foods look better or to restore a "natural" color to items where color has been lost in processing.
* *Preservatives:* Used to prolong product life and prevent bacteria build-up. Even "healthy" foods, such as dried apricots, will probably contain preservative (in the case of dried fruit, usually sulfur dioxide, a known allergen).
* *Antioxidants:* Used to stop the product going rancid.
* *Emulsifiers, stabilizers, thickeners:* Used in products such as fat-reduced desserts, soups, and sauces to enhance texture and stop separation.
* *Processing aids:* Used for a variety of reasons.

* *Flavor-enhancers:* Used to improve flavor in processed foods.
* *Glazing agents:* Used to add glaze and shine, and attractive appearance to foods.
* *Flour-improvers and bleaches:* Used in baked goods and breads to improve texture, cooking quality, and whiteness.
* *Sweeteners:* To add sweetness in place of sugars.
* *Miscellaneous*
In addition to the above, your product may also contain added nutrients, flavorings, natural drug-like chemicals like caffeine, and a number of less commonly used additives.

For people without known reactions, the additives are deemed safe (at normal levels of intake) by the FDA. However, nobody really knows what long-term effects there might be on say, a person who eats a diet high in additives (a typical "junk food diet") from early life on, and research indicates that some additives can cause cancer in animals.

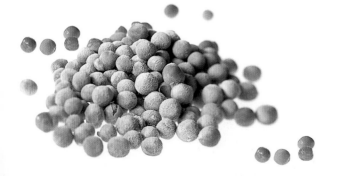

In Your Hands

Food and health from the store to the table

Healthy eating is not just about knowing your nutrients. The health issues of concern from shop to table are that the food we buy is the best quality we can find and/or afford; that it contains its full quota of nutrients and is safe to eat.

For instance, there is a world of difference in the nutritional content of a just-picked organically grown red pepper, displayed in cool conditions, taken home in a cool bag, stored and prepared correctly before being lightly cooked, and a red pepper of dubious origins which has been displayed too long on a sunlit counter, taken home in an overheated shopping bag and kept around on the vegetable rack for a week before being chopped too early and eaten too late. The first may contain its full quota of vitamin C (around 100 mg) while the latter will probably have none at all.

Also, cent for cent, there is much more vitamin C content in a top-of-the-range 100%-fruit long-life juice than there is in a lower-cost "juice drink," which—on reading the small print—contains only about 10% juice and a lot of sugar and additives.

Finally, there is a far greater chance of contracting food poisoning from a piece of chicken purchased just on its sell-by date, bought at the start of a day's shopping, and left in a warm kitchen before cooking in an old microwave than there is from a long sell-by date piece which is only out of cool conditions for minutes and is cooked thoroughly.

This section is all about being a sensible food shopper and handler.

■ Where to buy food

Corner store? Specialty store? Supermarket? Healthfood store or farmers' market? Where you buy your food is quite important. Here are a few checkpoints to help you decide:

* Pick stores with a high turnover of goods—the food will then be fresher.

* When it comes to fresh foods, avoid stores that keep their food on the road-side, in hot, light conditions (e.g., a display window for fruit and vegetables). Vitamin C and B content will be considerably diminished.

* With much food, you tend to get what you pay for, so consider how much you can pay for good food. If keeping costs low is vital, buying direct—e.g. from the farm—is usually cheaper. Goods from small independent stores will, sadly, usually be more expensive.

* If you are an older person, without a car, and live in a "food dessert," contact your welfare officer or social worker who will be able to provide you with transport and/or food delivery services.

When to buy food

In order to buy food at its best and keep it in good condition, bear in mind these pointers before shopping:

* Try to do your main regular shopping soon after the major deliveries have taken place, if supermarket shopping. These will tend to be after the weekend rush on a Monday. If you shop Sunday afternoon or

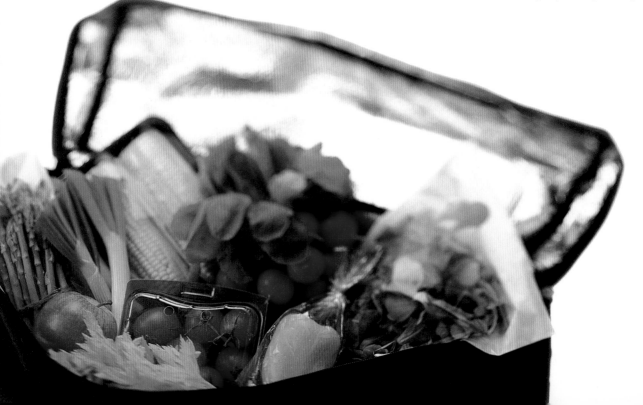

Monday morning you may find stocks—particularly of fresh fruits, vegetables, fish, and meats—are low and what is left is not what you would have ideally chosen.

✱ Don't shop for perishable items if you can't get them back into suitable cool conditions promptly—e.g., if you have to keep them by your side at work all day. This gives bacteria a chance to build up to unacceptable levels and also reduces vitamins B and C in your food.

✱ Don't shop when tired or preoccupied. Your food is important and you need to pay attention to what you are buying, checking sell-by dates, etc.

Menus and lists

Before you do major shopping it is wise to plan out menus for the week ahead, balancing them for health and pleasure. Then write a list. It will help if the list runs in the order in which you will buy.

For safety it is best to purchase chilled and frozen foods last—carried around a warm store while you do other purchasing, they may de-chill or begin to thaw, a possible safety hazard. It is also a good idea to purchase lightweight fruits, salads, etc. after heavy items like cans and bottles, as they may otherwise get crushed, which destroys vitamin C and spoils keeping qualities.

Getting quality in fresh foods

Here are some pointers for choosing the best available food:

✱ Use your eyes. Look for foods that look fresh and "happy." Use your nose, if food isn't in a sealed container. It should smell fresh and sweet.

✱ Meat need not look bright (often a sign it hasn't been aged long enough); it can look dark red (for beef) or pale pink (pork or lamb), but it shouldn't look gray. It shouldn't smell at all, except in the case of some game. In butcher's stores, watch that the butcher doesn't mix serving fresh and cooked meats without washing hands, and make sure he uses separate

utensils and areas of the shop for both.

✱ Fish is often packed for sale atmosphere-controlled (see page 74) so it is hard to evaluate by smell—but fresh fish sold loose should not smell anything other than sweet, fresh, and perhaps vaguely of the ocean. Any ammonia-type smell or anything "fishy" means don't buy it. Shellfish MUST be really fresh both for taste and texture—and to avoid food poisoning. If wild, not farmed, salmon, trout, etc. is on offer, buy it. Go for undyed smoked fish if available.

✱ Buy organic fruit and vegetables whenever you can. Look for fruit and vegetables in season, locally grown fruit and vegetables, and produce that isn't bruised or damaged (this will lose vitamin C and not keep well). A few blemishes are OK. Consider how long you need fruit to keep—ripe fruit will not keep long; unripe fruit can be ripened at home. (Controlled-atmosphere fruit, page 74, may follow its own rules!)

✱ Eggs should be perfect, not cracked or broken. They should be clean. Look for a recent packaging date, and a USDA inspection label.

✱ With all protein foods—meats, fish, eggs—look for quality assurance labels. There are various inspection marks (stamps) used by the USDA, indicating the wholesomeness of these products. Look for descriptions of where or how the animal or fish was raised or in what circumstances hens were kept. With these protein foods, be prepared to pay a little more for quality or organic products; if necessary, forgo the quantity—you only need small portions for good health.

Getting quality in processed foods

As processed foods make up a fair-to-large proportion of most of our diets, it is vital that what we eat is the best we can get. With a little care it is possible to pick products that aren't too high in saturated or trans fats, salt, sugar, etc. It is Read the small print carefully to find out

possible to avoid the less pleasant aspects of processed food, such as mechanically recovered meat (MRM), indiscriminate use of additives, etc.

It is only by buying the quality, healthier options and leaving the garbage on the shelves that we will eventually get the food we want. Here are some pointers for choosing good-quality cans, packages, jars, etc.

Reading the labels

✱ *The name and description*: If you glance at the photographs on some packages, you may find that all is not as it seems. For instance, a UHT (ultrapasteurized) carton or can with a tempting photo of citrus fruits on the front, calling itself "citrus juice drink" may contain as little as 10% real juice, the remainder being made up of water, sugar, colorings, and flavorings. NOT quite so good for you. And this is legal. Strawberry flavor yogurt may never have been near a real strawberry or even real strawberry juice or extract; it will simply use artificial flavoring. This, too, is legal. Meat in inexpensive "pork" sausages and other meat products, such as hamburgers, can include mechanically recovered meat, a kind of slurry removed by machine from a carcass after all the other meat has been removed. "Meat" can also include rind, skin, sinew, and gristle.

Another problem is that the percentage content of what you would consider to be the main ingredients in a product may, in fact, be quite small. For example, you may be getting only a small percentage of meat in a beef burrito. Yet another problem arises for those avoiding ingredients for health or other reasons. Say you're trying to avoid beef products. You may be surprised to find, on reading the ingredients list, that a chicken bouillon cube contains beef extract. Or, you're trying to go vegetarian—only to find that many yogurts contain gelatin, which is often made from beef bone.

FDA GUIDELINES FOR NUTRIENTS CLAIMS (1993)

Fat:
free: ←···0.5 g/serving
low: ←···3 g/serving
reduced: 25% less
less: x% less

Saturates:
free: ←···0.1 g/serving
low: ←···1 g/serving
reduced: 25% less
less: x% less

Sugars:
free: ←···1 g/serving
low: ←···10 g/serving
reduced: 25% less
less: x% less
no added: no sugars, or foods composed mainly of sugars, added to the food or its ingredients

Fiber:
increased: 25% more and ···→ 3 g/100 g serving
more: x% more
source of: ···→3 g/100 g or per serving
high in/rich source of: ···→6 g/100 g or source of per serving

Sodium:
very low: ←···35 mg/serving
low: ←···140 mg/serving
reduced: 25% less
less: x% less
no added: no salt or sodium have been added to the food or its ingredients

Read the small print carefully to find out what you're really buying; even then it may not tell you the whole story; however, the US labeling laws are due to be tightened up and this, it is hoped, will make life simpler for the health-conscious shopper.

∗ *Special health or product claims*: Words like "natural," "traditional," "farm-fresh" have very little meaning when applied to processed foods. For instance, farm-fresh eggs are usually battery eggs. Pictures of country scenes mean nothing. Some manufacturers banner claims such as "free from artificial colorings and preservatives" on their products to distract from the fact that they do contain, say, artificial sweeteners and flavorings. As another example, there is no legal definition of the term "low-sugar" or "reduced-sugar," though maximum 5% by weight is a guideline. "No added sugar" banners may also be misleading as many such products contain high amounts of other, similar, sweeteners, such as syrup, honey, or concentrated fruit juices.

As 70% of the salt that we eat is in processed foods, it is worth seeking out "low in salt" and "reduced-salt" products if you eat them a lot. However, these may be harder to find than "low-fat" or "low-sugar" products—the US food industry is somewhat reluctant to reduce the amount of salt it uses in manufacturing, thus keeping our taste for salty foods high. If the manufacturers won't cut down—perhaps we should cut down on the amount of high-salt processed foods that we put in our basket (a list of high-salt foods appears on page 33). It is called voting with your pocket.

It's also worth reiterating that quite a lot of products that you wouldn't at first think of as having a high salt content, often do; for example, many breakfast cereals do, and many breads do, too. It is currently hard, however, to find out exactly how much salt is in there. Limits for sodium will be phased and foods labeled "healthy" must not provide more than 480 mg of sodium per serving.

The fat content of food is a strong selling point—not only do we have various "low-fat," "90%-fat-free" and so on claims, but now also such things as "high in monounsaturates." The table on the left lists various claims for the major nutrients and what that should mean, according to FDA guidelines set in 1993. However, one omission is that there are none on what constitutes "lean" or "extra-lean."

Another anomaly regarding fat claims is that the percentage of fat content often quoted (e.g., French fries—only 5% fat) is misleading to say the least. By this, the manufacturer means that the fries contain 5% of their total weight as fat—i.e., 5 g fat per 100 g food. This does not mean that the fries only contain 5% of the total calories in the food as fat. All food—including fries, meat, cheese, and so on—contains a high or fairly high percentage of water (e.g. lean meat is 74% water, oven fries are about 60% water, hard cheese is about 36% water) which is calorie-free. So 5% of fat by weight turns out to be a much higher percentage of the total calories. Five grams of fat equals 45 calories, as there are 9 calories per gram of fat. There are about 160 calories in 3½ oz (100 g) of oven fries. So the real amount of fat in the fries is 28%!

A reduced-fat cheese may say something like "only 15% fat" (i.e. 15 g fat per 3½ oz/100 g cheese). Working out the fat content on the only sensible basis—as a percentage of total calories—in fact it contains nearly 52% of its calories as fat. This is the kind of information you really need in order to balance your diet, and yet currently the only way to work out fat content as a percentage of nutrients is to take a calculator with you when you shop! For more on nutrition labeling, see below.

Fiber content can also be a good selling point. To be claimed high in fiber, a food needs to contain at least 6 g of fiber in an average portion. However, sometimes a food is high-fiber because of added bran. High bran intake can inhibit absorption of some minerals such as iron, and it is better to get fiber from natural sources such as legumes, whole grains, fruits, and vegetables.

QUICK GUIDE TO NUTRITION LEVELS ON FOOD LABELS

per serving	A lot	A little
Fat	20 g or more	2 g or less
Saturates	5 g or more	1 g or less
Sugars	10 g or more	2 g or less
Fiber	3 g or more	0.5 g or less
Sodium	0.5 g or more	0.1 g or less

GUIDELINES ON DAILY NUTRIENT INTAKES (FDA)

	2,000 cal	2,500 cal
Total fat maximum	65 g	80 g
Saturated fat maximum	20 g	25 g
Cholesterol	300 mg	300 mg
Fiber minimum	25 g	30 g
Sodium maximum	2.4 g	2.4 g

promotional value—by law, to be a "rich source" of any of these, a product has to contain at least 50% of a day's recommended intake per serving.

Lastly, reduced- or low-calorie content may be a selling point for weight-watchers. A reduced-calorie (energy, joules) product must have 75% or less energy than a similar product for which no energy claim is made, and a low-calorie product must have a maximum of 40 calories per serving.

List of ingredients

So if you can't tell exactly what you are buying from the banner descriptions and illustrations, you check the food label and ingredients list. In the US, the new food label was created to clear this confusion that has prevailed our supermarket shelves and to help us choose healthful diets (e.g., nutrient reference values expressed as % Daily Values are a good tool to see how a food fits into our overall daily diet).

Ingredients are listed in descending order of content by weight, i.e., the ingredient contained in the greatest amount is listed first, and so on, so that the last ingredient listed is the least. Additives must be included in this list, but may be expressed by FD&C number alone, making it hard to detect which you are eating unless you have their names to hand, but additives used in an ingredient (e.g., dried fruits in a fruit cake may have been preserved using sulfur dioxide) needn't be mentioned and neither need flavorings. Sugars, as explained above, come in a variety of

guises, including glucose, dextrose, fructose, corn syrup, lactose, maltose, and treacle. Concentrated fruit juices used as sweeteners, honey, and brown sugar are all similar to basic sucrose and no better for the teeth.

Trans fats (see page 17) will usually appear on the ingredients list as "hydrogenated fats or oils" or "hardened fats." Look out for them in margarines, cakes, cookies, and pastries, though they will be in many more products too. Some ingredients needn't be listed and some foods and alcohol are exempt from having to declare their ingredients.

The new food label

Manufacturers are required by law to provide nutrition information (fat, salt, fiber, cholesterol, etc.) on packaged foods. Historically, food labels were full of figures which were hard to interpret. For example, faty content could be expressed in oz or g per serving or per packet of product. Knowing how much, say, fat there is in 100 g of product when you are not sure of the weight you will be eating is not ideal. Trans fats are not listed (though they will be included in the total fat column). Sodium content is not the same as salt content—for the total salt content you need to multiply sodium content by 2.5.

To help the consumers, the FDA and USDA have created a new food label using Daily Values (DVs). This new dietary reference value helps the consumer use food label information and apply it to their diets. The information provided

shows the percentage of total fat, saturated fat, cholesterol, carbohydrate, and protein, each as a percentage of a 2,000 calorie diet (for labeling purposes 2,000 calories was chosen in part because it is a nice, rounded figure, making it easier for the consumer to calculate their own nutritient needs), and this fits in with the healthy eating guideline pie-chart that appears on page 13. This kind of information is particularly useful in the case of items such as convenience meals and is certainly an eye-opener.

The chart above left offers a simple guide to what is a high content and what is a low content of fat, sugar, fiber, and sodium per serving.The second chart, approved by the FDA, gives total amounts of the major nutrients that you should be eating a day. Take it with you shopping and it is quite easy to see whether a product can fit in with a broadly healthy diet. For example, if a single-serving can of soup contains 2 g sodium you can see that it provides a maximum day's sodium intake for women.

✳ Use-by dates: You should always check the "use-by" dates that are provided on most packaged foods. A "use-by" date means that the food should be eaten by that date at the latest. Sometimes you will find different use-by dates within the same group of foods on the shelf—pick the package with the farthest date. "Best before" dates are for foods with a longer life. The date on these products is a guide only—after that date they may be fine.

Foods at Home

■ Storing foods

* *Fruits, most vegetables, and salad items*: These should ideally be kept in the refrigrator until needed, unless room temperature is needed for ripening. These should be stored in crisper compartments, in ventilated boxes, or plastic bags with holes pierced in them. Mushrooms should be stored in brown paper bags. Bananas are best kept in cool conditions outside the refrigerator. Potatoes should be kept in cool (but not frosted) dark conditions. If fruit and vegetables are stored in warmth and light, they lose their vitamin C quite rapidly. Even in a refrigerator, fruits and vegetables will gradually deteriorate, so use items up on a rotating basis and discard any wrinkled, browned, dry, yellowing, woody, or moldy items.

* *Frozen foods:* These should be transferred immediately to the freezer. Keep different types of frozen food together—e.g., raw meat in one place, frozen desserts and cakes in another. Place raw meats at the bottom of the freezer.

* *Foods to be frozen:* These should be blanched (in the case of vegetables) or otherwise prepared, cooled if necessary, and frozen in containers or heavy-duty plastic bags as soon as possible after purchase (in the case of fruits and vegetables, to retain maximum vitamin C). Fresh foods should be frozen using "fast freeze."

* *Fresh meats, dairy products, and all chilled food:* These should be stored in the refrigerator. Store raw meat, ideally in a covered leakproof container, in the bottom of the refrigerator, well away from cooked meats, to avoid cross-contamination and possible food poisoning.

* *Opened jars:* These should be kept covered and stored in the refrigerator.

* *Opened cans:* These should be decanted into glass or china containers, or at least heavy-duty plastic ones, and the contents used within 24 hours, as chemicals from the insides of cans may leach into the food.

* *High-fat items:* Cheese, butter, pâté, fatty meats shouldn't be wrapped in plastic wrap, as this may contain chemicals that can migrate into them.

* *Cheese:* This should be stored in its own container, which should have airholes. Individual cheeses may be wrapped in greaseproof paper. If bought wrapped in plastic wrap, remove it.

* *Containers:* Once opened, food will NOT keep indefinitely.

■ Preparing food

Careful food preparation can retain water-soluble vitamins B group and C and minimize risk of food poisoning.

* *Avoid* chopping, peeling, or tearing fresh fruits, vegetables, and salads until the last possible minute before cooking or eating, as cut and exposed surfaces lose vitamin C and begin to oxidize.

* *Don't* leave vegetables soaking in water (hot or cold) as this too leaches vitamin C.

* *Cook* vegetables for the minimum amount of time to retain nutrients.

* *Thaw* meats, fish, and meat products' thoroughly before cooking, unless the label advises otherwise. Poultry MUST be thoroughly thawed—feel the cavity to check before cooking and check portions with a sharp knife. Meat that comes out of the refrigerator very cold should also be brought to room temperature before cooking (but don't leave meat for longer than necessary to achieve this). The problem with cooking chicken (etc.) that isn't thoroughly thawed is that the center may remain pink even if the meat looks cooked, meaning bacteria won't have been killed. Don't stuff poultry as the stuffing may also prevent the inside of the bird from thoroughly cooking.

* *Microwave defrosting.* Always make sure that frozen foods thawed in a microwave are turned from time to time for even thawing.

* *When handling raw meat* in the kitchen, use a clean chopping board reserved just for raw meat. A marble board may harbor fewer bacteria than those made from wood or plastic, though some plastic boards now come impregnated with anti-bacterial compound. Chop and put on a plate, and cover if not putting directly into a cooking pan.

Wash hands and utensils plus chopping board thoroughly after use. Steep utensils in boiling water if practical. Dry hands well before handling other foods. Anti-bacterial cleansers may help prevent bacteria build-up. Clean tap handles that may have been touched with infected hands.

* *Keep* all work surfaces, refrigerator, cupboards, food containers, and eating utensils and dishes thoroughly clean.

* *Cook* all meat thoroughly to prevent food poisoning. Ground meat, chicken, sausages, and hamburgers should have no pink left in their centers at all. All microwaved food should be piping hot in the center.

▦ Reheating and leftovers

* If food has to be kept after cooking, allow it to cool and transfer it to a refrigerator (or freezer) as quickly as possible. If hot food is to be kept for, say, less than an hour, cover it and keep at room temperature then reheat to piping hot, or keep in a low oven just simmering. Vitamins B and C group will diminish in food kept warm for long periods. In general, it is better to cool and reheat a meal than keep it hot for long periods. Meals shouldn't be kept at room temperature for any longer than an hour.

* All reheated food should be reheated until piping hot.

* Leftover food, if still in good condition, should be wrapped or put in containers (preferably glass or china), covered and kept in a refrigerator. Use or throw away within 24–48 hours.

* Discard any leftover food that has discolored, has an unusual smell, mold, or white patches appearing on it, a film on top or has dried out, or in any other way doesn't appear fresh and appetizing.

▦ How to avoid food poisoning

Reported cases of food poisoning and deaths from food poisoning are of great concern. In the US, at least 20 million people are poisoned every year. In the UK in 1982 there were only 14,243 reported cases; in 1997, there were over 100,000—a figure which, experts believe, represents one-tenth of the true number of cases, most of which go unreported. No one knows the exact reason for this increase, although as the highest percentage of cases are caused by food "eaten out," the rise in restaurant, café, and take-out eating is an obvious cause. Food eaten in the home accounts for one in six cases and it is thought that demand for a reduction in the amount of preservatives, including sugar, in processed foods, is causing this rise. Another factor is the increased "food miles" raw food travels, and increased number of handlers.

The most common sources of food poisoning are bacteria, although fungi and viruses can also cause it. Worryingly, many cases are caused by bugs virtually unheard of 20 or so years ago. To compound the problem, many food-borne bacteria are resistant to antibiotics, so food poisoning may be hard to treat. Risks can be reduced by following the tips on the right.

* *Campylobacter:* Hardly heard of in the '80s, now responsible for about half of all 1997's reported cases of food poisoning. A recent official survey found the bacteria in 40% of chilled chicken sold in supermarkets. It is also found in meat, unpasteurized milk, and doorstep milk pecked by infected sparrows. It can cause gastroenteritis, paralysis, and death. Chicken and meat should be thoroughly cooked.

* *Salmonella enteriditis:* The second most common cause, accounting for around 40% of cases. There has been little improvement in recent years in the amount of salmonella in eggs, according to the USDA, and research suggests that 36% of chickens in the US are infected. It is also found in poultry meat and other sources. It can cause severe gastric upsets, and even death, especially in the young, ill, pregnant, or elderly. Eggs and poultry should be as fresh as possible when eaten, as bacteria quickly multiply, and they should be thoroughly cooked. Poultry should be thoroughly thawed and stored correctly. Eggs should not be eaten raw. Free-range and organic eggs and poultry have a lower incidence.

* *Salmonella typhimurium:* A newer salmonella strain very resistant to antibiotics and more likely in intensively reared animals. Follow advice for salmonella enteriditis.

* *E.coli 0157:* Another bug that has caused an increasing amount of food poisoning in the last decade. It has a very low infective dose and a common source of infection is meat, which may be contaminated during slaughter and processing. Undercooked meat may then cause food poisoning. Ground meat and under-

cooked hamburgers have been cited as particular risks (the grinding may spread infection through the meat). Dairy products can also be contaminated, and the bacteria can cause severe stomach upsets, even death, especially in vulnerable people.

* *Listeria monocytogenes:* Bacteria found in soft cheeses, such as Brie and Camembert, in pâtés, and chilled convenience meals and deli foods, like pre-packaged salads and hams. The bacteria can thrive at temperatures as low as 41°F (5°C) (many domestic refrigerators function at around this temperature). It is dangerous for pregnant women, young children, and people with weak immune systems.

FOOD SAFETY TIPS

* Buy meat from a reliable butcher who practices high standards of hygiene.

* Never eat meat, fish, poultry, or eggs which is stale or past its use-by date.

* Buy only chilled food that has been stored in cold cabinets under 41°F (5°C) and keep it at this temperature, or lower, at home.

* Transport fresh, chilled, and frozen food home quickly and in cool-bags.

* Store food at home in suitable conditions and don't allow raw meats to drip on other food.

* Cook all meat, fish, poultry, and eggs well. Make sure meat and poultry have lost all traces of pinkness.

* Be extra careful about reheating food and, when using a microwave, make sure the food is piping hot all the way through, turning during cooking.

* Use up leftovers promptly or throw them away.

* Keep all utensils, dishes, pans, and areas of the kitchen very clean.

* Always wash and dry hands after handling raw foods and before handling other foods.

Food Futures

Scientific advances are still being brought to bear on food production, bringing great potential for further improvements and opening new areas for concern.

Genetically engineered (GE) food

Tomatoes that remain ripe without rotting, crops that resist weed-killer, cows that produce human-style milk, and fat-free fats—these are just some of the innovations that the food scientists can offer today. However, can these feats of "biotechnology" really benefit our health? Whatever you want in your food—it seems that the bio-technologists can do it, or will certainly be able to do it soon. They are already promising us cancer-preventing vegetables and red meat low in saturates.

Over thousands of years, crop- and animal-breeders have always tried to improve things like yield, disease-resistance, size, and so on, through selective breeding, but this is a very slow process. Now, there is a much quicker way to alter the characteristics of anything from an apple to a bean to a cow. That way is broadly called genetic engineering or modification, a futuristic technology that appears to have as many detractors as it has enthusiasts.

What is genetic engineering?

Every living organism has a "blueprint" or pattern of genes. Genes contain all the hereditary information that is needed to give a plant, or an animal, or a human, all its special characteristics. Until recently, genes have been passed on through each species via normal sexual reproduction. Now, however, scientists know how to remove genetic material from one living thing and insert it into another, thus giving the second species a new characteristic and bypassing natural evolution.

This "genetic modification" (GM) can not only be done from, say, fruit to fruit, but can also cross the species—for instance, tomatoes have recently been given a gene from fish that helps them to "stay in shape" when frozen, and genetic modification has produced a cow with "human" breast milk, which could in the future be used for healthier formula milk.

So far, genetic engineering has mainly been applied commercially in major world crops, such as soybeans, corn, oilseed rape, cotton, potatoes, and tomatoes. There are, though, test-growing sites all over the world, including the US, for a wide variety of other GM foods.

How much genetically engineered food are we currently eating?

In 1994 the first genetically engineered (GE) food—tomatoes—was introduced into the US market. Today 13–16% of soy crop is GE and GE corn production has increased from 0.6% to 6%. Cheese made using a genetically produced enzyme (instead of rennet) has been widely on sale since the early '90s.

However, up to 60% of the processed food that we eat may contain genetically modified soy, because genetically modified soybeans (engineered to be herbicide-resistant) now comprise at least 30% of the world's soybean crop—the genetically modified soybeans are mixed with traditional soybeans before distribution—and soy is now contained in about two-thirds of all processed foods. Genetically modified corn is also being used in processed foods. In the pipeline are genetically modified potato, chicory—and, no doubt, many more.

What are the advantages of genetic engineering for food consumers?

The companies promoting genetic engineering say that the new technology can have many benefits for the consumer by making food keep fresh for longer,

taste better, and have a healthier profile. For example, scientists in the UK have isolated the gene material in broccoli that contains sulforophane (see page 96), the anti-cancer agent, and are working on implanting it into other vegetables. They also say that if, as a result of genetic engineering, there will be increased yield and less waste—for instance, through production of pest-resistant and weed-killer-resistant grains and vegetables—then there will be more food available, and this should reflect in price control.

What are the drawbacks of genetically engineered food?

Aside from the ethical arguments relating to "tampering" with nature, one of the main problems is that no one knows what the long-term effects of eating genetically modified food may be, nor of their effect on the environment. For instance, much genetic engineering involves using antibiotic "marker" genes, and some experts worry that these will make antibiotic resistance in humans even more widespread and affect our ability to fight disease. It is also thought that genetic engineering may produce new toxins and allergens.

Other experts say that in engineering herbicide- and pesticide-resistant crops, strains of "superweeds" will develop, leading to the need for even stronger herbicides to kill the new weeds. Some people have expressed concern about eating weed-killer-resistant crops sprayed with weed-killer.

How easy is it to avoid genetically engineered foods if we want to?

Unfortunately, it is quite hard. As we have seen, soy products appear in 60% of processed foods, but largely because of resistance from the US soybean producers (who produce much of the world's harvest), genetically modified beans are generally not segregated after harvest but mixed with ordinary beans for distribution (a practice that may change soon due to pressure from retailers and lobbyists); therefore it is impossible to label with any certainty, either. In any case, the FDA states that labeling will only be required if the nutritional composition of the product has changed or if a product contains a food allergen.

For example, the flour and oil from genetically modified soybeans is analytically indistinguishable from that of regular beans, and generally a product is only required to be labeled as containing genetically modified ingredients when the product differs from an equivalent food or food ingredient in either its composition, thus, most foods we eat will not state whether it has been genetically engineered or not.

If you wish to avoid genetically modified soy the only alternatives currently are to read all the labels and avoid all produce containing soy, or choose organically grown soy and soy products, which are guaranteed non-GM. Soy is contained in a wide variety of processed foods, including confectionery, margarines and spreads, mayonnaise, cakes, breads, cookies, gravy, soups, bouillon cubes, meat dishes, and many more.

In Europe, genetically modified tomato paste is labeled on the front of the package as such. Lobbyists are battling to get better regulation for labeling—an urgent priority, as the number of genetically engineered foods for sale will undoubtedly increase rapidly.

▪ What safeguards are there about genetically modified foods?
Currently, the FDA, USDA, and EPA have to give a full safety evaluation to all novel foods before they are allowed on sale. Some genetically modified foods are considered "novel" enough to qualify for a full safety evaluation before being allowed on sale; others may come under a category described as "Substantial

Equivalence" which, briefly, means that they are indistinguishable from the conventional product and therefore have a "fast track" route to approval and need not be labeled. If you are worried about eating genetically engineered foods, labeling of genetically modified foods and how little choice you have in the matter, write to your congressman or congresswoman, or your supermarket.

Other food innovations

Progress—if you like to call it so—is being made in other areas of food research without the application of genetic engineering. For example, plant breeders in Wales are using a variety of rye grass which is very high in the essential fatty acid linolenic acid to feed to cows and thus help promote milk that is lower in saturated fat than normal. Cows at another research station in England are being fed a diet high in heat-treated soy and rape seeds, which also results in milk high in unsaturated fat.

In the US, a device has just been patented which will kill virtually all food poisoning bugs in a millisecond without harming the food, and scientists at the Institute of Food Research in the UK have pinpointed fruits and vegetables which can protect against E. coli.

▪ Functional foods
Functional foods are those that claim enhanced health properties or particular nutritional benefits. Recently launched have been bread containing soy that is said to reduce hot flashes in menopausal women; and a fermented milk drink which claims to increase the "friendly" gut bacteria, i.e. it is pro-biotic (see page 152). Several foods now have added "omega 3 oils" and claim to help reduce heart disease; and in 1997 a cereal-type snack bar said to help prevent cancer because of its added isoflavonoids and

lignans was launched. Hundreds more products like these appear on the market annually.

Nutritionists are often sceptical about these products. They may work, but it is believed that, as with some vitamin and mineral supplements, the "active ingredients" in these foods would be better eaten as part of the food in which they naturally occur. For example, omega-3 fish oils in fish, lignans in natural linseeds, and so on. In other words, the benefits of food are best enjoyed in as natural a way as possible.

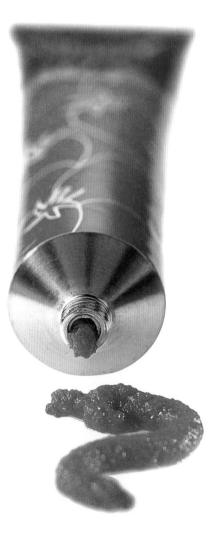

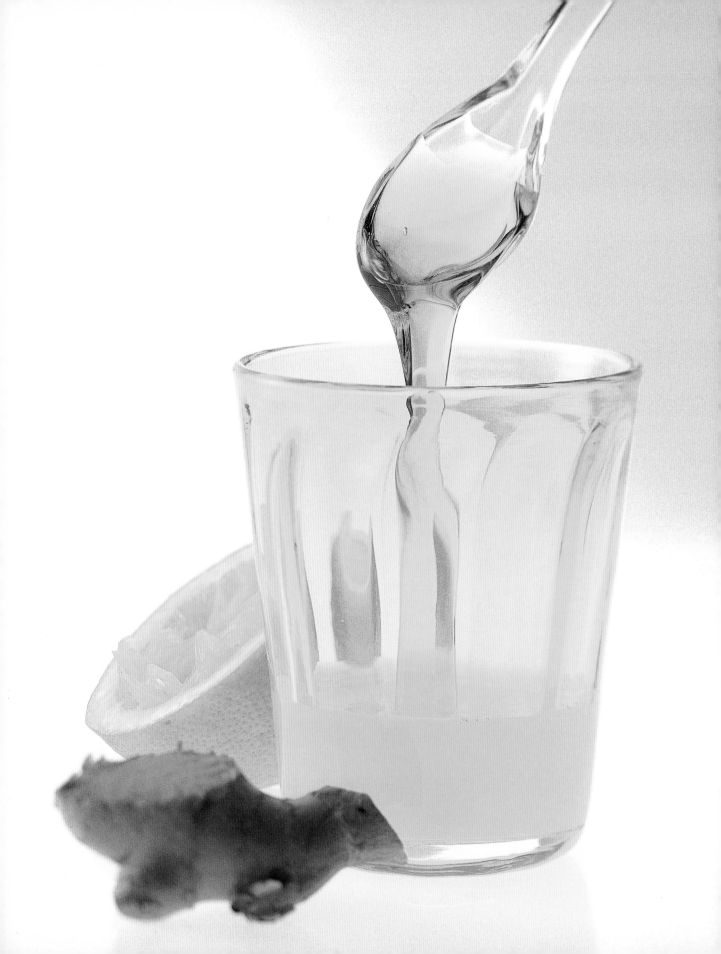

Food as medicine

Twenty—even ten—years ago, who would have believed that we would be being urged to drink up our red wine for a healthy heart, or would be told to eat up our tomato ketchup to help prevent cancer? The last decade has seen a massive increase in interest in the idea of food as medicine—and yet it is nothing new. For thousands of years the medicinal value of plants and food has been appreciated throughout the world. Garlic was first used as a medicine at least four thousand years ago. Five hundred years ago, it was known that fresh fruits and vegetables could cure scurvy. Two hundred years ago, a powerful effect of the foxglove flower (*digitalis*) in helping heart problems was discovered, and 150 years ago salicylic acid (the natural forerunner of today's aspirin) was first isolated from the bark of the willow.

Even as recently as the turn of the century, the largest proportion of medicines was herbal-based. It is only in the mid-to-late twentieth century that Western medicine has become so sceptical of the power of plants—and so reliant upon manmade chemical drugs to effect cures. Now people in their hundreds of thousands—including those in the medical profession and scientific world—are realizing the major drawbacks of a society dependent upon drugs for their health. Drug resistance, drug dependence, and unwanted side effects are three main reasons why alternative, more natural methods of cure and prevention are regaining popularity. Diet is a first choice in this change. We all need to eat—so if what we eat can act like medicine, too, then isn't that a marvelous solution?

Now, with the advantage of modern scientific techniques, we know so much more about food, what is in it, and how it works, that we can fine-tune our diets to suit almost any illness or condition. We are no longer reliant upon the local witch doctor to provide cures without question. We have the greatest minds in the best-funded laboratories in the world, seeking the answers to food as medicine.

ACNE AND PIMPLES

ACNE IS CAUSED by overproduction of sebum—oil—which sits in the pores of the skin, particularly on the face and back. The pores become clogged and are then easily infected. This overproduction of sebum usually occurs in the teenage years, because of increased production of the sex hormones, and is more common in boys than girls. Acne can carry on into the 20s and can also occur in women before menstruation; a mild version may also occur at menopause. Some experts believe that acne is exacerbated by stress, in which case the dietary hints for stress reduction on page 138 may be used in conjunction with these.

SOLUTIONS

All teens should eat a basic healthy diet and follow the particular instructions for them given in Section Three, The Teenage Years (page 167). It is also useful to increase quantities of foods rich in beta-carotene, such as carrots, apricots, sweet potatoes, and broccoli (best sources list on page 23). In the body, beta-carotene converts into vitamin A, which is known to be important in maintaining a healthy skin. Sufferers should eat plenty of zinc-rich foods, such as shellfish, lean meat, and nuts (best sources list on page 31), as acne may be linked with a zinc deficiency. They should also eat vitamin E-rich foods, such as vegetable oils, nuts, and seeds, to aid skin healing (best sources list on page 24). Most experts also agree that a diet high in vitamin C (fresh fruits and vegetables) to fight infection is important. If an acne sufferer refuses to eat a healthy diet such as this, it may be worth considering supplements of vitamins E, C, and zinc.

A diet high in chocolate and saturated fats has often been cited as the cause of acne and pimples, but this has not been proved. Most experts now believe that there is no link, except that if people eat too many sweet, fatty, and "junk" foods, then they will not be getting enough of the nutrients they need. There is some evidence, though, that a high-salt diet may be a contributing factor, so it is worth avoiding salty snacks and foods.

Doctors often prescribe antibiotics for acne, which can help the condition. But if antibiotics are taken for long periods they can upset the gut microflora, which, ironically, may make acne worse! Eat plenty of live yogurt to help avoid this. The acidophilus bacteria in live yogurt may also help acne if applied to the skin at night, rather like a face cream.

AIDS AND HIV

HIV AND AIDS ARE IMMUNE system deficiency diseases in which the body's natural defenses break down and leave the sufferer at much greater risk of infections, such as bronchitis and pneumonia, viruses like herpes and cold sores, and cancer.

SOLUTIONS

There is as yet no cure, but help can be obtained through the right diet, which will help to keep the immune system functioning well. The Immune-Strengthening Diet—rich in vitamins beta-carotene and A, B group, C, and E, as well as zinc—which appears on page 143, is a good basic diet for sufferers, who should, however, show the diet to their physician for approval.

The antioxidant mineral selenium, found in Brazil nuts, lean pork, and fish (best sources list on page 31), for example, may also be lacking in the diet. Research has shown that low selenium levels may be linked with some cancers.

It is important to try to eat enough, as weight loss and malnutrition are common side effects of AIDS. Sufferers should consult a dietitian approved by their physician, for help with their own personal eating plan, depending upon the course their own illness is taking.

ALCOHOL ABUSE

IN OTHER PARTS OF THIS BOOK, the benefits of light to moderate drinking are well documented—for example, in connection with a protective effect against heart disease and Alzheimer's. Safe drinking guidelines for men and women are outlined on page 36, and sensible social drinking and drink/drive limits are discussed on page 66. However, alcohol abuse remains one of the most important causes of ill health throughout the world.

Alcohol is a drug and an intoxicant, and alcohol addiction and dependence is widespread. Experts believe that more than 100,000 premature deaths a year in the US are related to excessive alcohol consumption. Alcohol consumption is linked to half of all murders, accidental deaths, and suicides, one-third of all drowning, boating, and flying deaths, and half of all crimes in the US. About 50% of all fatal car accidents are related to alcohol consumption! The safe drinking guidelines outlined by the USDA (see page 36) are exceeded by approximately 15% of men and 3% of women. The higher above these guidelines your alcohol intake, the more likely it is that you will become dependent and incur a variety of side effects and illnesses.

ALCOHOLISM

A PERSON IS USUALLY described as an "alcoholic" when problem drinking has turned into dependence and full addiction, with bouts of—or chronic—intoxication, cravings for alcohol that can't be controlled, increased tolerance so that more and more alcohol is needed to achieve intoxication, psychological and physical dependence (withdrawal symptoms such as headache, sweating, and tremor), and marked social problems (such as aggression, inability to work, and depression), and lack of concern over appearance.

PROBLEM DRINKING

But how can you tell if your enjoyment of alcohol is turning into abuse? If you find you can tick several of these statements, you are probably becoming a problem drinker, or in danger of becoming one:

* I drink for comfort or confidence.
* I drink when alone.
* I drink every day—or nearly every day—above the USDA guidelines.
* I feel agitated if I can't have a drink when I usually do.

Alcohol dependence—the CAGE questions

Doctors often use the "CAGE" questionnaire when trying to ascertain if a person has become dependent upon alcohol. If the person can answer "yes" to two or more of the four questions, then it is likely that he or she has become dependent upon alcohol:

1 Have you ever felt you should CUT down on your drinking?
2 Have people ANNOYED you by criticizing your drinking?
3 Have you ever felt bad or GUILTY about your drinking?
4 (EYE-OPENER) Have you ever had a drink first thing in the morning to steady your nerves or get rid of a hangover?

■ Alcohol-related problems

People who regularly drink over the safe guidelines, whether or not they are described as alcoholic, will almost inevitably find themselves facing health problems, illnesses, and symptoms associated with alcohol abuse sooner or later, unless they change their drinking habits. (And, even then, for people over 40, some alcohol-induced symptoms may not be reversible.) Here are the main problems the long-term heavy drinker may have to face:

* *Nutritional deficiencies* Alcohol affects the absorption and metabolism of many nutrients, including the vitamin B group and vitamins A and D, the minerals zinc, calcium, and phosphorus, and the essential fatty acids, and may deplete the body of magnesium.

* *Heart and circulatory problems* Heavy drinking—binge drinking or regular intake of four or more alcoholic drinks a day—is associated with abnormal heart rhythms, increased risk of heart attack, high blood pressure, and strokes.

* *Increased risk of some cancers,* particularly cancer of the breast, mouth, larynx, pancreas, esophagus, and liver.

Some studies also link alcohol abuse with colon cancer.

* *Increased risk of digestive tract problems,* including gastritis and duodenal ulcer.

* *Increased risk of gout and diabetes,* and damage to the immune system.

* *Impotence and infertility*

* *Possibly brain and nerve damage* Although a recent large long-term study found no link between cognitive function and heavy drinking, other studies link alcohol abuse with blackouts, fits, confusion, memory loss, hallucinations, etc.

* *Liver damage* Enlarged liver, fatty liver, jaundice, liver cancer, and cirrhosis, which may be more likely if drinks are mixed—e.g., beer and Scotch.

* *Early death*

■ Prevention or cure?

In the light of all this evidence, surely the most sensible solution is to stay within the safe drinking guidelines and enjoy the benefits this will bring. It is much easier to do this than to try to beat dependence later in life. For many people, however, it is too late to do this. Proven methods of

DRINKING AND NUTRITION

As explained, heavy drinking depletes the body of various nutrients. It is, therefore, important either to eat a very healthy diet (which few alcohol-dependent people will do) in an attempt to redress the balance, or to take supplements to avoid deficiencies. Supplements of all the nutrients listed on the previous page may be necessary. Regular moderate-to-heavy drinkers should, as a matter of course, make sure they eat plenty of foods rich in vitamins B and C (best sources lists on pages 26 and 25) and ensure as healthy a diet as possible (see Basic Healthy Diet, page 53), avoiding junk foods, particularly sugary low-nutrient foods like candy, cookies, and sodas, and foods high in saturated fat. This will help to regulate blood sugar levels. Including plenty of essential fatty acids, in the form of fish oils, evening primrose oil, and linseed oil, may help the liver (which has the job of breaking down the alcohol and converting it into harmless components) to cope, and there is some evidence that carrot juice helps, too.

In herbalism, a decoction of dock root is said to aid liver action (see Herbalism). See also Hangover.

cutting down alcohol intake or, perhaps, cutting it out altogether, are by enlisting your doctor's help, attending a "drying out" clinic, joining Alcoholics Anonymous, and, particularly, by also getting help in sorting out any contributory social, emotional, or lifestyle problems.

It also helps to have a strong motivation if you are to succeed in cutting down alcohol—for example, parents may realize that their drinking is affecting their children's emotional and everyday life; an individual may realize that he will ruin his hard-earned career if he doesn't cut his alcohol intake.

ALLERGIES

AN ALLERGY IS an over-aggressive response by the body's immune system to a substance—for example, an airborne pollutant, a chemical, a plant, an animal's fur or feathers—or a food or food additive (though many, many things can be allergens). An allergic reaction can produce a wide variety of symptoms, the most common being skin reactions (eczema, urticaria, for example), digestive reactions (such as vomiting, stomachache, bloating, or diarrhea) or respiratory tract reactions (like wheezing,

runny nose, rhinitis, and other asthma-like symptoms). Other reactions can include headache, flatulence, fatigue, fluid retention, and palpitations.

When an allergic reaction is so severe that it can be life-threatening, this is called anaphylactic shock. The immune system releases a "hit" of histamine within seconds after the allergic individual has come into contact (even slightly) with the allergen; the throat may swell and make breathing difficult, so the sufferer will wheeze, the face may swell, and rashes, stomach cramp, and vomiting may occur. Unless adrenaline treatment is given quickly the sufferer may die.

Diagnosed anaphylactics carry their own emergency kit for treatment. Approximately 1–2% of people in the US are susceptible to anaphylaxis (which usually starts in childhood and is not outgrown), and the most common foods to cause this type of reaction are peanuts, other nuts and seeds, fish and shellfish, and eggs.

The tendency to be allergic (or "atopic") may run in families and may only involve a reaction to one food. However, where there is an adverse reaction to a food, but the traditional allergy tests

are negative, the term "food intolerance" may be used, although it is still possible that immune reactions may be involved.

Intolerance may frequently involve more than one food item and larger quantities may be needed to produce a reaction. However, this term may also be used to describe a specific condition, e.g., lactose intolerance. Normally the digestive enzyme lactase breaks down lactose, the sugar found in milk and dairy products. If this enzyme is deficient, lactose passes into the intestines, resulting in bloating and diarrhea.

Some experts say that over forty million people in the US suffer from allergic reaction to some degree; however, there is evidence that many more people think they are allergic to certain foods, etc., than actually are so the figures could be lower. Some researchers have found as little as 10% of perceived sufferers actually to be allergic to their suspected allergen; their symptoms may be very real, but may be caused by a problem other than food.

There is little doubt, though, that food allergies and intolerances are on the increase and are implicated in a number of other conditions such as arthritis, migraine, irritable bowel syndrome (IBS), PMS, chronic fatigue syndrome (ME, page 125), Crohn's disease, and hyperactivity in children.

There is now a scientific test for true allergic reaction, the RAST test, which measures the amount of immunoglobulin E antibodies (IgE) a person has to a specific substance. There are also "skin prick" tests, in which a tiny amount of the suspected allergen is placed on the arm and a scratch made in the skin, then any reaction (swelling, redness) noted, but this method is more suitable for non-food allergens, such as dust mites, feathers, pollen, etc., and is useless for most food intolerances.

Other tests, such as hair tests by mail or unspecific blood tests offered by alternative practitioners, are probably of little real use in most cases. According to research, some private allergy clinics are notorious for giving out long lists of "problem" foods to people with no known complaints while failing to spot true allergies.

The most reliable test for food sensitivity is the exclusion diet, which should be discussed with your doctor and supervised by a dietitian. This involves a diet usually consisting of a few foods that almost never cause allergic reaction (lamb, bottled water, and rice are prime examples), which is followed for a number of days. Then, if symptoms have improved, one by one, other foods are introduced, at intervals, starting with foods least likely to produce a reaction. If there is no reaction, they can stay in the diet.

Once a particular food triggers a reaction, it should be removed from the diet (possibly for good, although see Living with a Food Allergy or Intolerance overleaf). This method takes a fairly long time as only one new food can be introduced at a time.

A simpler form of exclusion diet involves removing one or two suspect foods from the diet for about 2 weeks; if the condition clears the food is reintroduced. If the symptoms return it is assumed that the reintroduced food is to blame. This type of exclusion diet is only feasible when there is reasonable cause to suspect a certain food or a few foods as being the "culprit(s)" and best attempted with professional advice.

■ **Foods most likely to cause allergy**
Almost any food, additive, or drink can cause allergic reactions, though some, such as rice and lamb, do so less often. Here are the most common food allergens:

* Cows' milk and dairy products See lactose intolerance on page 88. Some people who can't tolerate cows' milk may be able to have goats' milk. Others find that they can drink skim milk and low-fat milk products but not whole milk varieties. Lactose intolerance is one of the most common problems throughout the world.

* Eggs Often egg whites rather than the yolks are the problem. Eggs are an ingredient in many products, so label-reading is crucial. This allergy is most common in young children and, again, may be outgrown.

* Grains Wheat intolerance is common; gluten is not always the "culprit," though it may often be. Any grain can cause allergic reaction, but rice and corn are less likely to do so. Again, grains, particularly wheat and gluten, appear in many products, so vigilance is needed. See Celiac Disease.

* Fish and shellfish Allergic reaction to these is increasing, possibly because of increasingly polluted waters. Most common allergens seem to be shrimp, oysters, crabs, and white fish.

* Nuts and seeds Peanut allergy is quite common, and it is now thought that one in 80 young children are sensitive to nuts. Sufferers may be advised to avoid peanut oil, although a recent study showed that only 10% of peanut-sensitive adults tested were allergic to unrefined peanut oil and none to refined oil. Unrefined oil is more likely to be found in ethnic foods and refined oil can be contaminated if peanuts have been cooked and the oil is re-used.

Other food products may be cross-contaminated with peanut traces. Cosmetics sometimes contain peanut oil. Other common nut allergens are walnuts, brazils, and cashews. There is a growing allergy to sesame seeds—found not only in hummus, tahini, sesame seed bread, and sesame oil, but also often in vegetable burgers, Asian meals, and cakes.

* Fruit Strawberries and oranges are often cited as allergens, as well as other citrus fruits, kiwis, apples, and cherries.

* Soybeans Soybeans and soybean products, such as tofu and soy flour, can cause a reaction, particularly digestive upsets. Soy is found in a multitude of commercial products, and avid label-reading is necessary for those with a soy intolerance.

* Sugar Sugary drinks, candies, and other high-sugar products, including chocolate, may be badly tolerated and can contribute to candida or gut dysbioses, food cravings, and other problems that may have an allergy link.

* Additives Artificial food additives, such as preservatives and colorings, have long been suspected of causing allergic reactions and are especially linked with hyperactivity in children. Likely "culprits" are the azo dyes, such as tartrazine, caramel, benzoates, sulfates, nitrates, glutamates (MSG), and artificial sweeteners such as aspartame.

For more information on additives and health, see page 75.

■ Living with a food allergy or intolerance

Exciting new work has shown that a technique called enzyme-potentiated desensitization (EPD) may be helpful in treating a range of conditions where food allergy or intolerance may play a part, e.g., eczema, arthritis, irritable bowel syndrome, etc. The technique involves injection of tiny doses of the allergens along with a naturally occurring enzyme, producing the desensitizing effect. Doses are given at three-month intervals at the start, and then frequency is gradually reduced.

At the moment, however, this treatment is not widely available and the most obvious course of action for most sufferers is to stick to a diet that excludes the food(s) to which they are allergic or intolerant. As self-diagnosis is often difficult, as has been proven by research, it is unwise to start any limited diet unless the allergy has been confirmed through your physician using one of the techniques described above.

A suitable diet may then be a simple matter to follow (if, for example, you are allergic to oysters only, it won't be too hard for you to follow a diet that doesn't include oysters). If a wider range of foods is involved, however, or if you have an allergy to one of our major foods, such as dairy products or grains or even soy, the diet becomes much more restricted and advice from a dietitian is needed so that you can safely avoid possible nutrient deficiencies.

For example, if you can't tolerate milk products, cheese, or eggs, your diet may fall short in calcium, protein, and several other nutrients, unless you have professional advice to replace those nutrients in your diet by other foods.

The long-term outlook for an allergy sufferer isn't always bleak—sometimes your body will change and tolerate a food that you have had to avoid for a long time. In severe cases, however, returning to a food, particularly for anaphylactics, is a risky business and needs professional supervision if undertaken at all.

ALZHEIMER'S DISEASE

■ ALZHEIMER'S IS THOUGHT of as a disease of the elderly, but it can begin at the age of 50 or even earlier, often with barely noticeable small problems, such as poorer short-term memory, progressing at an unpredictable rate into severe memory loss and confusion. In those with Alzheimer's, plaques and deposits are formed within the brain, but the exact causes of this are still being unraveled.

The first theory in the 1980s was that aluminum intake was a factor, as a core of aluminum was found in these plaques, but now many experts believe that ingestion of aluminum is not a significant factor. Various research programs in the 1990s have, however, uncovered useful data.

Tobacco smoking is now known to increase the risk of Alzheimer's, and the disease has also been linked with the cold sore virus, herpes simplex, with high blood cholesterol, with atherosclerosis, high blood pressure, diabetes, and stroke. There is also a genetic link.

SOLUTIONS

The starting point for everyone should be a basic healthy diet, which can help to prevent or minimize all the conditions above. See entries for each, or follow the Basic Healthy Diet (page 53).

One research program in the US has recently shown that women who take hormone replacement therapy (HRT) could halve their risk of developing Alzheimer's. Another large American study has shown that the antioxidant vitamin E can slow the progress of the disease, and a large French study showed that older people drinking red or white wine was associated with a reduction of up to 75% of the incidence of Alzheimer's. The optimum drinking level in this study was 3–4 glasses of wine a day; 1–2 glasses had little effect and more than 4 glasses actually increased the risk

WHO GETS ALLERGIES?

People who produce too much of the IgE antibody (see page 88) are "atopic" individuals, who are more likely to suffer allergic reactions, and the tendency to this is probably inherited. It may also be that babies are "sensitized" to allergens even before birth by what the mother eats, but this is still the subject of much research. Food allergies do, however, seem more common in childhood. The simple truth is that the experts don't yet have any concrete answer to who will get what allergy, or even when, which means that as yet there is no means of prevention.

of developing Alzheimer's. As usual, moderation seems to be the answer.

Most scientists also believe that a brain "well-used" throughout life is also a factor in avoiding or postponing Alzheimer's, as people who keep mentally active seem to suffer less. In view of this, it may be worth taking the supplement ginkgo biloba, which is said to improve circulation to the brain. There are other as-yet-unproven claims for the benefits of the minerals zinc and selenium in preventing Alzheimer's, as well as the compound co-enzyme Q10, found either in supplements or in a few foods, notably soybeans.

Some experts still stand by the aluminum theory, so it may be worth avoiding cooking foods, especially acidic foods, in aluminum saucepans, as well as avoiding the additive aluminum phosphate, found in some baked goods, and aluminum hydroxide, found in antacids, until further evidence for or against this theory emerges.

Once somebody has Alzheimer's disease, the above dietary measures should still be followed as far as possible, but emphasis should also be placed on providing the sufferer with tempting food that is easy to eat and serve.

ANEMIA

■ ANEMIA IS A CONDITION in which there is a reduction in hemoglobin, the material in the blood's red blood cells that carries oxygen to the tissues in the body. The symptoms of this lack of oxygen can be mild or more severe, including varying degrees of tiredness up to total fatigue, weakness, pallor, breathlessness, dizziness, lack of stamina, and poor concentration.

The most common cause of anemia is iron deficiency, and this can occur for several reasons. Women during their menstruating years are particularly susceptible, especially if periods are heavy, as once iron is lost with the blood it takes a long time to be replenished in the body. Any other form of major blood loss, such as hemorrhage, childbirth, or accident, can also result in anemia.

Pregnant women are also prone to anemia, especially if iron stores are at a low at the start of pregnancy, as there is much more blood circulating in the body than normal and so more iron is needed to go around. To prevent anemia in pregnancy, women are often given supplements of iron with folate, a deficiency of which can also be a factor. Some illnesses can also produce anemia—cancer and leukemia, AIDS, and stomach ulcers, for example. Lastly, a nutritionally poor diet may be to blame.

SOLUTIONS

With iron-deficiency anemia, the solution is to eat a diet containing plenty of iron-rich foods. For a best sources list, see page 30. Your physician will probably also prescribe a course of iron supplements. Animal sources of iron, such as lean red meat, are absorbed more easily than vegetable sources, but absorption of iron in the diet is helped by vitamin C, so eat a C-rich food at the same time as your iron-rich food. Tea, coffee, and cola all hinder absorption, so avoid consuming these drinks within one hour of a meal. Phytates found in bran also affect absorption, but this is not thought to be a significant factor, as the body may adjust to this. Not all anemia is caused by iron deficiency, however, so it is important that you see your physician for a correct diagnosis.

Pernicious anemia is anemia caused by a lack of vitamin B12, or the body's inability to absorb it. Vegans, in particular, may have a B12 deficiency, as it is only found in animal foods or in fortified vegetarian products. B12 supplements suitable for vegans and vegetarians can be obtained from healthfood stores or your physician.

Angina, see Heart Disease and Stroke

Anorexia, see Eating Disorders

ANXIETY

ANXIETY STATES ARE OFTEN a response to an overload of stress in people's lives. When people are under stress, the body's "fight or flight" system pumps adrenaline out in preparation for dealing with a crisis situation, but in modern life the crisis doesn't manifest itself physically—e.g., in a fist-fight or a long run away from danger—and the adrenaline simply stays around, making the person tense, nervous, or anxious. This can be a short-term thing or, in some stressed-out people, an almost permanent state of affairs. Short-term anxiety can also be a perfectly natural response to worrying situations, such as a job interview or an exam.

Anxiety can trigger several other complaints, such as digestive problems, insomnia, muscular pain, skin complaints, palpitations, nausea, and diarrhea. See separate entries for all of these. Acute anxiety can take the form of a panic attack, a severe state of panic that may include palpitations, faintness, dizziness, and fear. Sufferers should see their physician for professional help.

SOLUTIONS

Long term, try to seek out causes of anxiety and think about what changes you can make to your lifestyle to minimize these. Tackle anxiety by mimicking the "fight or flight" response—take some exercise and do some deep breathing. This will help adrenaline to disperse and help you relax. The Bach Flower Rescue Remedy may also help. Other causes of anxious feelings are alcohol abuse or an overload of caffeine drinks and products such as strong coffee, tea, cola, and chocolate. If you are prone to anxiety it would be wise to limit these items severely. Alcohol and, to a lesser extent, caffeine can also disrupt sleep patterns, which may make anxiety worse.

Chronic stress depletes the body of B vitamins, so eating plenty of B-rich foods (see best sources list on page 26) and, perhaps, taking a B-group supplement is a good idea. Eat a good basic healthy diet including lettuce, which is a soporific, and plenty of calcium- and magnesium-rich foods. Herbal remedies for anxiety include valerian, chamomile, passion flower, and lemon balm, all of which can be taken as an infusion or in supplement form. Cloves, rosemary, and lavender are all also said to be calming, and their essential oils are ideal in aromatherapy. Yoga and massage are also worth trying, to alleviate symptoms.

APPETITE, POOR

SEVERAL CONDITIONS CAN BRING about a loss of appetite—anxiety, stress, depression, and shock are four typical situations. Illnesses of many kinds can cause loss of appetite, particularly digestive disorders such as irritable bowel syndrome or peptic ulcer, viral and bacterial illnesses, and food intolerance. Colds, phlegm, and allergic rhinitis can lessen appetite, partly by reducing the sense of smell and taste, as can cigarette smoking. Drugs prescribed for various ailments can cause appetite loss—for example, those the side effects of which may be nausea, or loss of taste or sense of smell. Hormonal changes through the monthly menstrual cycle mean that women's appetites may vary, usually being greater in the week preceding a period and lower in the few days afterward.

Eating disorders such as anorexia nervosa may present themselves as poor appetite, though the sufferer may, in fact, have a normal appetite. Diminished appetite is fairly common in older people (see Section Three, Sixties Plus, page 182); this may be partly due to lessened needs as well as lowered physical activity and a general slowing down of hormone-based responses, of which appetite is but one example.

Poor appetite can also be brought on by a deficiency in certain nutrients—zinc deficiency may contribute to loss of taste and smell and therefore appetite; potassium and magnesium deficiency may also be to blame—likely if the person with a poor appetite has been taking diuretic drugs for fluid retention, as some varieties cause these minerals to be excreted in the urine. Alcohol can reduce the appetite if taken in excess regularly—one drink can, however, be an appetite stimulant. In fact, any kind of drink, including water, sodas, and fruit drinks, can depress hunger signals if taken before meal times. Children with a poor appetite should, in particular, be discouraged from drinking too much before a meal—one study found 15% of preschool-age children took just under 50% of their daily calorie needs in the form of drinks, especially sugary ones.

A short spell of poor appetite in an otherwise healthy person, when the reason is clear, is nothing serious to worry about, and the appetite should return (often with a vengeance!) when the cause is gone. Any chronic loss of appetite should be discussed with your physician.

To tempt a poor appetite, small amounts of tasty and attractive food should be offered frequently. If possible, low-nutrient "junk" foods should be avoided, unless the main consideration is weight gain; meals and snacks should contain plenty of foods rich in vitamins B and C (which are water-soluble and cannot be stored in the body for long), zinc, potassium, and magnesium.

Arrhythmia, see Heart Disease and Stroke

ARTHRITIS

THERE ARE TWO MAIN TYPES of arthritis—osteoarthritis and rheumatoid arthritis, which are dealt with separately here.

Osteoarthritis is a degenerative condition of the joints and is frequently age-related; most elderly people have osteoarthritis to some degree, which is why it is sometimes called "fair wear and tear." A normal healthy joint, such as the knee or hip (two very common sites of osteoarthritis), is covered by a smooth layer of shiny cartilage, which normally allows free gliding movement. With age, or perhaps injury or posture misalignment, the cartilage becomes roughened, resulting in the underlying bone being worn. This is the most common form of arthritis and is more prevalent in women. Symptoms are pain, stiffness, and loss of mobility in the affected joint(s).

Rheumatoid arthritis is determined by blood tests and history, and is most common in adult women. It is a chronic inflammatory condition involving multiple joints and is thought of as having an auto-immune disease component. The immune system, which normally defends us against infection, appears instead to react against some part of the body. Rheumatoid arthritis often starts with pain and weakness in the hands and wrists. Joints may swell and may eventually become deformed. Inflammation may flare up and then disappear again, making it difficult to know exactly what "works" to help. The causes of rheumatoid arthritis aren't fully understood, but there may be an environmental trigger such as a virus or bacterium.

SOLUTIONS

Diet doesn't appear to play a big part in the prevention or management of osteoarthritis in most people, with the main exception being that the symptoms of the condition—and the amount of trouble it causes—will be worse in someone who is very overweight or obese. The "load-bearing" joints, such as the knees and hips, are put under much greater strain if the sufferer is too heavy. So, if you have osteoarthritis and are overweight, lose the excess weight (see Section Four).

However, one recent trial in the US has found that the progress of osteoarthritis can be minimized with high intakes of the antioxidant vitamins C and E, and with vitamin D, found in largest quantities in cod liver oil. More research needs to be done. (Note: Vitamin D can be toxic in excess, but is fine in multivitamin supplements for regular intake up to 10μg.) Some experts in the field of food intolerance feel that an elimination diet may be most helpful for some people, but this is open to debate. Any elimination diet should first be discussed with your physician.

The role of diet and dietary factors in rheumatoid arthritis still remains controversial, but results of a number of trials suggest that diet does have a part to play in managing symptoms. A variety of diets have been reported to be helpful, but, unfortunately, in rheumatoid arthritis, what works for one sufferer may not work for another. Moreover, as explained above, because symptoms often disappear for weeks or longer of their own accord, it is hard to know, when the sufferer suddenly feels better, whether it is diet or a period of remission. However, certain general guidelines seem to achieve best results for many people.

A good starting point is a diet low in saturated fat and high in oily fish (three portions a week at least), fruit, and vegetables, taking on board all the basic healthy eating guidelines. Reduction of saturated fats may work by favoring production in the body of the less anti-inflammatory form of prostaglandins (substances in the body that act in similar ways to hormones). Fish oils may also help reduce inflammation, and fruit and vegetables provide antioxidants, which may be important—one American study showed that people who ate higher levels of vitamin C were three times less likely to have progression of the disease than those eating the lowest; another US study found that low levels of vitamin A and E were linked to the disease's development. Blood tests on people with arthritis have also shown low selenium levels. Recent UK research suggests that the spice turmeric can help relieve inflammation in some people.

There is evidence that a healthy vegetarian or vegan diet can help to prevent rheumatoid arthritis or minimize its symptoms in some people. It may also be helpful to try eliminating from your diet the plants of the nightshade family—potatoes, tomatoes, eggplant, and peppers, which may exacerbate the inflammation of rheumatoid arthritis. Do not eat them for a period of eight weeks; if, by then, the symptoms are improved, you may want to avoid those foods in future. Tobacco is also a member of the nightshade family, so smoking should be avoided if you seem to have rheumatoid arthritis that is triggered by the nightshade family.

Many other foods are reported as "triggers" for attacks of rheumatoid arthritis. Dairy foods and grains, especially wheat and corn, are the most common triggers mentioned. Coffee, nuts, and fruits with seeds have also been cited, as well as red wine and citrus fruits. However, because these vary so much and because some, such as dairy foods and grains, form such an important part of many people's diets, and eliminating them without proper dietary advice could cause nutrient and energy deficiency, it is important to be medically supervised if you want to attempt to pinpoint a particular trigger.

Recent studies using supplements of evening primrose oil and fish oil in cases of rheumatoid arthritis have shown encouraging results, but response takes time—up to three months. Linseed oil—like fish oils, rich in omega-3 fatty acids—may have a similar effect. Some experts believe that supplements of vitamin E, C, zinc, and selenium may help, but this is still debated. Various other supplements—including nettle tea, green-lipped mussel extract, glucosamine, and cider vinegar—are said to help some people, but the evidence for their usefulness is much more anecdotal than scientific.

People who are on anti-inflammatory drugs for their arthritis may become anemic and should therefore be sure to eat plenty of iron-rich foods. People who are on steroids should take plenty of calcium-rich foods. See also Gout.

ASTHMA

THE INCIDENCE OF ASTHMA is increasing rapidly in the Western world. This may be due to a number of factors, including air and chemical pollution. The symptoms of asthma are wheezing, cough, tight chest, and difficulty in breathing, due to the air passages in the lungs narrowing. Asthma is the most common long-term disease in the West—one in seven children and 4% of adults are thought to suffer.

There may be a genetic connection. Asthma may be triggered by many things, including house mites, cigarette smoke, household sprays, cold air, exercise, pollen, animals, and, less commonly, by some foods (often dairy products and fish) and food additives. Generally, when foods are involved, they may sensitize the air passages and result in some other trigger causing an attack.

It is hard to find the food link in such cases, but certain items are known to be more sensitizing than others. The food additives containing sulfites are common triggers and are most likely to be found in wine, beer, hard cider, vinegar, dried fruits, quick frozen shellfish, and some ready-prepared salads—read the labels to check—as are the azo dyes such as tartrazine found in fruit drinks, candy, and other commercial products. Some asthmatics are allergic to the salicylates in aspirin.

An asthmatic reaction is possible in anyone with a true food allergy or intolerance. However, asthmatics should only carry out food avoidance or elimination diets under medical supervision, as serious reactions may be experienced.

For more information about allergies and food intolerance, see page 88.

SOLUTIONS
Asthmatics can follow some dietary precautions to help minimize attacks even if a food intolerance isn't the problem. A low-salt diet is a good idea, because salt can increase the reactivity of the airways (for a list of high-salt foods to avoid, see page 33). A diet high in the mineral magnesium may help, because magnesium reduces the reactivity of the muscles in the airways and of certain allergy cells (MAST cells)—for best sources list, see page 32. A diet rich in antioxidants—selenium and vitamins C, E, and the carotenoids (for best sources list of all these, see pages 22–33)—can help boost the body's defense mechanisms against attack.

Asthma can begin at any age, so it is important to try to protect yourself against it. Research shows that people who eat a poor diet, low in fruits and vegetables, and therefore antioxidants, are more likely to develop asthma than people who eat healthy diets. A recent lung study in the UK found lung function better in children who ate fruit every day compared with those who didn't.

A new system called enzyme-potentiated desensitization (EPD) is showing promising results in helping to control asthma, where minute doses of allergens are injected up to four times a year.

See also Allergies and Hay Fever.

Atherosclerosis, see Heart Disease and Stroke

Bad Breath, see Halitosis

BLOOD PRESSURE

■ HYPERTENSION (HIGH BLOOD PRESSURE) is an extremely common disorder, affecting approximately one-fifth of adults in Western countries. If left untreated, it can cause strokes, heart attacks, and kidney disease, and yet symptoms are not easy to spot.

Some people have a hereditary predisposition to it; short people in particular are susceptible; the middle-aged and elderly are more prone to it than young people; and men are more often affected than women (although incidence rises among women during pregnancy). People who smoke are also more likely to have high blood pressure, as are women on the Pill and people under stress.

SOLUTIONS

Medication can help to reduce hypertension, but there are also various nutritional methods of helping to prevent or control high blood pressure. One of the major factors is body weight—overweight and obese people are much more likely to have raised blood pressure than slim people; so, if you have hypertension—or risk factors as described above—and are overweight, follow a sensible dieting plan such as that in Section Five and get down to a reasonable weight slowly. Yo-yo dieting is very negative and may actually make hypertension worse.

Alcohol is another factor—high alcohol intake may result in raised blood pressure levels, so if you drink more than the safe guidelines (see Alcohol Abuse, and Social Drinking, pages 86 and 66) you should cut down.

People who have hypertension often find that a reduction in their sodium intake helps to reduce blood pressure—try to limit salt intake to no more than 4 g a day, equivalent to 1.6 g of sodium, which is within the US DRV guidelines of no more than 2.4 g of sodium a day, or take advice for your own case from your physician. A list of the major sources of salt in the diet appears on page 33. Other tips for cutting salt intake are to stop adding salt to cooking vegetables and to food at the table, and to eat a diet as high in natural produce as possible, because it is highly processed foods that tend to contain most salt.

There are salt substitutes available, which you may find helpful, and there are many commercial foods that are "reduced salt." It is also quite easy to wean yourself away from a taste for salty foods—cutting down gradually is the best method; after one month the transformation should be complete. Additional herbs and spices in the diet may help to perk up taste buds used to a lot of salt.

While cutting salt, increase your intake of foods rich in potassium (see page 32), such as dried apricots, legumes, and nuts, because research shows that high potassium intake can help lower blood pressure. NOTE: Do not eat a high-potassium diet if you have any sort of kidney disorder or are on certain medications (consult your doctor).

Two other minerals, calcium and magnesium, have also been shown to lower blood pressure (see their respective best source lists on pages 29 and 32), as have omega-3 essential fatty acids in the form of oily fish and linseed, garlic, fruits high in soluble fiber (see the Food Charts), and moderate alcohol consumption (one or two drinks a day).

Data from the UK Vegetarian Society shows that vegetarians have less incidence of hypertension than meat-eaters, but this could be for a variety of reasons. However, many vegetables are good sources of potassium, calcium, and magnesium, and, in China, celery has long been a widespread remedy for hypertension. Ginger and the herb rosemary are also traditional herbal remedies for raised blood pressure.

BRONCHITIS AND COUGHS

■ BRONCHITIS is an acute or chronic inflammation of the bronchial tubes—the airways that lead to the lungs. There will often be an underlying infection. Bronchitis is accompanied by a mucus-producing cough and often a raised temperature. The most common cause of bronchitis is smoking, but it can also be caused by infection or viruses, pollution, or an allergic reaction to, say, dust or airborne fumes.

SOLUTIONS

Avoidance of tobacco and known allergens is the obvious starting point in avoiding bronchitis. People who are prone to chest infections should also build up their immune system with a diet rich in antioxidants, zinc, and other known immune builders (see Immune-Strengthening Diet, page 143). Some nutritionists advocate avoidance of "mucus-forming" foods, such as dairy products, saturated fats, and white bread, although this theory has never been proved.

Once bronchitis has taken hold it is important to take action quickly to minimize its duration and severity. Take plenty of fresh garlic—one of its active compounds, allicin, is a powerful antibiotic. To a lesser extent, onions and leeks are effective, too. Increase your intake of vitamin C, with plenty of fresh fruits and salads. Honey is a useful antiseptic and expectorant, and can be taken twice daily as a drink with fresh lemon juice and a little warm water.

The herbs hyssop, eucalyptus, and thyme are antiseptic and can be taken as an infusion daily (see Herbs for Health, page 154). It is also useful to inhale their oils in recently boiled water. Bronchial and other coughs and sore throat can be soothed with licorice and with the honey drink mentioned left. A honey and cider vinegar gargle and zinc lozenges can also be effective in some cases.

Bulimia, see Eating Disorders

CANCER

■ A QUARTER OF all deaths in the industrialized world are due to cancers. One in three Americans is at risk of contracting cancer, and approximately 560,000 a year die of the disease—a figure that is rising. There are over 100 different types of cancer, and it is now believed that the causes and triggers may be almost as diverse. However, the consensus of opinion is that 60–70% of all cancers could be prevented by doing just two things—eating the suggested healthy diet and giving up smoking.

The latest report from the World Cancer Research Fund (WCRF) estimates that up to 40% of cancers—that's four million cases throughout the world—could be avoided through a good diet and maintaining correct body weight. Both the WCRF and the American Institute for Cancer Research (AICR) have similar dietary recommendations for cancer prevention. These recommendations, in most points, are similar to the recommendations of many international cancer societies. Let's look at these recommendations one by one:

Increase intake of a wide variety of fruits and vegetables

It seems that in the fight against cancers, fruit and vegetables may hold the most vital key. Increased intake is linked with, for instance, a decreased incidence of cancers of the colon, stomach, lung, breast, mouth, pancreas, and bladder. In one study, cancer deaths in vegetarians were found to be 39% lower than in others. Not only do fruits and vegetables contain fiber, vitamins, and minerals needed for health, but scientists are now discovering the wealth of "hidden" compounds they contain. These are the biologically active non-nutrients in food called phytochemicals.

Under that umbrella term there are many different groups of phytochemicals, such as flavonoids, indoles, and phenols, and within each group are yet more specific compounds, each with its own function(s). It seems that many of these phytochemicals are marvelous at helping to prevent, block, or suppress carcinogens or tumors. Here are some examples:

* **Tomatoes** contain the carotenoid lycopene, one of the phenol group, which protects against cancer-causing pollutants. One trial found that men eating ten servings of tomato a week were 45% less likely to get prostate cancer (one of the leading causes of death in US men).

* **Broccoli** and other cruciferous vegetables contain indoles, a group of cancer-fighting agents. Broccoli contains glucosinolates, which break down in the body to form sulforophanes that fight cancers of the lung and colon in particular.

* **Brussels sprouts** contain another glucosinolate, sinigrin, a compound that suppresses pre-cancerous activity.

* **Watercress** is rich in phenethyl isothiocyanate, which is particularly good at helping to prevent lung cancer.

* **Carrots, broccoli,** and other dark green, red, orange, and yellow vegetables contain carotenoids, which help to protect the immune system and may help fight lung cancer.

* **Yams** are high in phytoestrogens, which may help to protect against breast cancer and other similar hormone-driven cancers.

NUTRITION AGAINST CANCER

* Increase intake of a wide variety of fruits and vegetables. Five portions a day are recommended as a minimum, and total weight should be around 1 lb (450 g).
* Increase intake of starchy plant foods in general, including wholegrain cereals and legumes, and a total weight around 20 oz (600 g) minimum.
* Increase intake of dietary fibre (NSP), see page 14, from a variety of sources (the first two points would achieve this). Intakes of up to ¾ oz (24 g) a day from natural sources is a healthy average.
* Reduce intake of saturated fats and meat. The World Cancer Research Foundation recommends reducing meat intake to less than 2 ¾ oz (80 g) a day.
* Reduce total fat intake to approximately 30% of total calorie intake.
* Maintain a healthy weight and be physically active. Avoid obesity—keep to a reasonable body weight throughout adult life.
* Limit consumption of alcohol to within recommended safe drinking guidelines (see page 36).
* Limit consumption of salt-cured, pickled, char-grilled, and smoked foods.
* Do not smoke or use any tobacco products.

* **Asian mushrooms** such as shiitake contain lentinan, which strengthens the immune system and helps fight cancer.

* **Grape skins** and many other fruit skins are rich in resveratrol, a compound that inhibits cancer development. It is also found in red burgundy wines. Grapes also contain ellagic acid (found in cherries and strawberries, too), another cancer blocker.

* **Citrus fruits** such as oranges, are high in antioxidant flavonoids and the phenol lutein.

And so on! For more information on the phytochemicals and their powers, see pages 34–5. Many fruits and vegetables also contain rich levels of the important antioxidants, vitamins C, E, and beta-carotene, which also offer considerable protection against cancer.

Increase intake of starchy plant foods
Starchy, "complex carbohydrate" foods, such as wholegrain cereals, rice, pasta, oats, legumes, and potatoes, are high in fiber (NSP), see page 14, and high intakes are linked to low levels of bowel cancer as well as of cancers of the prostate and breast. Experts believe that a high-fiber diet can reduce colon cancer by speeding

the passage of waste through the large intestine so that potential carcinogens have less contact time with the intestine wall. New research also suggests that a substance called butyrate, produced by fermentation of complex carbohydrate in the bowel, is essential for colon mucosal health. It helps prevent conditions that promote cancer and increases the rate of death of cancer cells.

Whole grains are high in lignan, a compound similar to fiber, which is a phytoestrogen. This seems to reduce the risk of hormone-dependent cancers, such as breast cancer. Soybeans are high in isoflavones, another phytoestrogen linked with a reduced risk of hormone-dependent cancers.

Reduce intake of saturated fats and meat
High-fat diets, and particularly those high in saturated fat, have long been linked with increased incidence of cancers of the colon (more marked in males). A high-fat diet also seems to increase risk of cancer of the prostate, ovary, and breast. Although the link isn't scientifically proved, the cause is thought to be that a high-fat diet increases estrogen production. High-fat foods, such as whole-

OTHER NOTES ON CANCER AND DIET

* Garlic contains anti-cancer compounds. In animal studies, the phytochemical diallyl sulfide helps to prevent and suppress tumors by up to 60%. Raw garlic is the best medicine— its compounds appear to be much less effective if taken cooked or in dried form.

* Green and black tea contain antioxidants that help protect against cancers.

* The mineral selenium is an antioxidant and is powerful in fighting the free radicals that are thought to increase risk of cancer. Brazil nuts and tuna fish are two good sources of the mineral. For best sources list, see page 31.

* Aspirin appears to be anti-cancer: 300 mg a day may reduce the risk of cancer of the colon and rectum.

* Nitrate fertilizers, used by commercial growers to fertilize vegetables such as lettuce and greens, are no longer thought to be cancer-causing. In fact, there is evidence that they turn into nitric oxide in the body and offer health benefits.

* Supplements of beta-carotene appear to be ineffectual in cancer protection. One trial found that smokers who took supplements of the antioxidant actually had more incidence of lung cancer. However, vitamin E supplements may reduce risk of prostate cancer in men.

* Polyunsaturated cooking oils can oxidize if heated too many times or kept too long and may be carcinogenic. Oils should be stored in a cool, dark place, and discarded after use.

* Smoked and cured foods, such as smoked salmon and bacon, are carcinogenic and should be eaten in moderate amounts.

milk dairy products, fatty cuts of meat, and high-fat convenience foods, should be limited to reduce saturated fat intake.

Several studies have also concluded that a diet high in meat predisposes to certain cancers, e.g., colon and prostate, hence the new recommendations from the WCRF. This is still a subject of debate, but it makes sense to cut down on meat intake in any case, in order to make room in the diet for increased levels of the recommended food groups and in order to help reduce saturated fat levels.

One reason that meat-eating may be linked with cancer could be that meat increases levels of nitrosamines in the body. These are chemicals known to be cancer-inducing: one UK study showed that people who eat large amounts of meat had three times the levels of nitrosamines in their urine. The eating of overcooked meats and char-grilled meats has also been linked with increased incidence of cancer— probably because the high cooking temperature creates carcinogens.

Reduce total fat intake
By following all the above guidelines, our total fat intake should automatically be reduced to within recommended levels (most cancer research agencies agree that this is a maximum of 30% of total calo-ries). A high-fat diet is linked to several types of cancer (see above) and is a major cause of obesity and overweight (see next paragraph). However, some types of fat are necessary in the diet and probably have a role to play in cancer prevention. Adequate amounts of omega-3 fatty acids appear to protect against cancer of the prostate, breast, and bowel, probably by having a "calming" effect on the inflammatory prostaglandins in the system. Omega-3s are found in oily fish and linseed (flax) oil. It is, therefore, a good idea to replace some of the meat meals in the diet with oily fish meals as well as plant-based meals. According to latest research, there is also a link between high olive oil intake and lower cancer risk.

Avoid obesity and overweight
Overweight is linked to breast cancer, which is one and a half times more likely in overweight post-menopausal women. There is a less obvious link between being cervical cancer and overweight, and cancer of the gallbladder in women and prostate in men. By following the advice given above, a weight within the body mass index guidelines (see page 188) should be fairly easy to maintain for everyone.

Limit consumption of alcohol
Excessive alcohol intake increases the risk of several cancers, including those of the mouth, pharynx, larynx, esophagus, breast, and liver. It may also increase risk of rectal cancers. Beer can be a major source of nitrosamines, which are carcinogenic, and heavy beer drinkers appear to be more at risk from pancreatic cancer.

Alcohol drinking should therefore be kept within safe guidelines (see page 36). A protective effect against cancer has been shown in red wine, which contains resveratrol, also found in grape skins, but moderate intake guidelines should still be observed.

See the Anti-Cancer Diet on page 140.

■ THERE ARE SUGGESTIONS THAT a yeast— Candida albicans—may be involved in causing a range of symptoms that are attributed to food sensitivity. However, this is highly controversial, as there is no scientific proof that this is the organism that causes the problems that may lead to such a "Candida" diagnosis. It may be that the balance of microorganisms in the gut is disturbed, with the beneficial bacteria being reduced, allowing other bacteria— or possibly yeasts—to establish them-

CANDIDA

selves. This may particularly be the case where antibiotics are taken (which kill off the "friendly" gut flora), or after severe stomach infections. It has also been suggested that this perhaps should be called Gut Dysbiosis.

The most frequently seen symptoms are irritable bowel, wind and bloating, constant fatigue, mild depression, muscle or joint pains, headaches, vaginal yeast infection, a craving for sweet foods, and an intolerance of alcohol. Other problems may include a sensitivity to foods containing yeasts and molds, and even sensitivity to musty or moldy atmospheres and damp weather. Foods containing sugar, in particular those high in sugar, are commonly reported as causing symptoms. This could be due to the troublesome bacteria and yeasts that feed on sugar.

Candida-type infections can also occur in people whose immune systems are not functioning well, perhaps after a long illness or long period of stress. Longterm use of steroids, for conditions such as asthma, can make people more susceptible and deficiencies of vitamins and minerals can affect the immune system.

SOLUTIONS

The nutritional treatment of dysfunctional gut is three-sided:

1: Follow a special diet, which may discourage the growth of the offending organisms. This can be achieved by avoiding foods containing sugars, and also yeasts and molds (to which there appears to be some form of sensitivity). There is also some evidence that a diet high in garlic may help.

2: Take a course of prescribed antifungal medication from your doctor.

3: Re-colonize the gut with friendly bacteria. This can be achieved by taking a pre-biotic supplement known as fructo-oligosaccharides (FOS), which feeds the beneficial bacteria, together with a probiotic supplement containing lactobacillus acidophilus and bifidobacteria. These are also present in reasonable quantities in some live yogurts.

There are many different "anti-candida" diets being offered by private nutritional therapists and doctors. Some are unnecessarily strict—for example, forbidding all grains or dairy products. Some patients respond to these diets because, in fact, their symptoms were not of candida-type infections at all, but, instead, a grain or dairy allergy. Other "therapists" recommend avoidance of all fruit—a tactic that is neither necessary nor wise. The avoidance list that appears on page 141 (with the Anti-Candida Diet) is the one that many experts now agree achieves results, without being too strict.

Longterm, people who have had candida-like infections may, after treatment, be able to tolerate some or all of the "forbidden" foods again. However, a healthy lifestyle and a good immune system (see the Immune-Strengthening Diet on page 143) are the best ways to fight the condition. Turn to page 141 for the Anti-Candida Diet and food avoidance list.

Cataracts, see Eye Problems

Catarrh, see Colds and Flu

CELIAC DISEASE

AN INFLAMMATORY CONDITION of the gastrointestinal tract, celiac disease is caused by intolerance of the protein gluten, which is found in wheat and rye, and similar proteins in barley and oats. The gluten damages the intestinal lining, thus reducing the sufferer's ability to absorb nutrients. This can then result in conditions such as malnutrition, anemia, osteoporosis, and other problems.

First symptoms may appear when gluten is introduced into the diet of susceptible children after weaning, but the disease can also present symptoms at any age. Adults may have only mild symptoms or, in some cases, none at all. One in 2,500 of the US population suffers from celiac disease, and the average is higher in insulin-dependent diabetics and with some other auto-immune conditions.

Symptoms can vary enormously, but in children they commonly include poor weight- and height-gain, crying and general miserableness, diarrhea, bloating, and vomiting. In adults, there may be weight loss, diarrhea or constipation, anemia, tiredness, lethargy, flatulence, mouth ulcers and sore tongue, painful joints, depression, amenorrhea or infertility.

SOLUTIONS

If you suspect celiac disease see your physician, who will make arrangements for diagnosis to be made.

Once celiac disease is diagnosed, management involves avoiding all foods containing gluten, wheat, rye, barley, or oats. These include ordinary breads, biscuits, pasta, cakes, cookies, many breakfast cereals, and pastry and pies. A recent study produced evidence that oats may not be harmful in adults; however, until there is further evidence, oats should still be avoided.

The avoidance list may sound fairly daunting at first, but specially produced gluten-free foods are available, e.g., breads, cookies, and pasta, where the gluten is removed from the wheat, leaving gluten-free wheat starch. There are also those versions of such foods made from grains such as corn and rice, which are naturally gluten-free.

A small proportion of celiacs may also need to avoid wheat starch if they do not improve, and an even smaller proportion still may be helped by a diet that is also milk-free.

Some special products are available on prescription. Specific dietary advice for celiac sufferers should be obtained from a dietitian and, once diagnosed, the diet needs to be life-long. In proven cases of nutritional deficiency, e.g., anemia, appropriate supplements will be needed. A general multivitamin/mineral may be helpful for the first few months after diagnosis, but this should be discussed with your physician first.

The American Celiac Society has annual lists of manufactured foods that are guaranteed to be gluten-free. (See Appendix on page 320.)

Chicken Pox, see Herpes Simplex 1

CHILBLAINS

■ Chilblains, which usually appear on the hands or feet, are painful swellings that may itch and burst like blisters. They are an extreme reaction to cold, caused by poor circulation to the extremities, and are therefore more common in cold weather.

SOLUTIONS

Smoking is a contraindication and should be avoided if you suffer from chilblains. Aerobic exercise, which helps maintain good circulation, is the main prevention—chilblains are more common in people who take little exercise, and in the elderly, although young children also seem to be prone to them. For other advice on improving circulation, see Circulation, Poor.

Food methods of increasing blood-flow to hands and feet include regular consumption of ginger, chili peppers, and mustard. External remedies include potato poultices, mustard baths, and bathing in carrot juice—none of which is proved but won't do you any harm, so may well be worth a try. Lastly, keep hands and feet warm in winter, with good socks, gloves, etc., and have a warm foot bath every day.

Chronic Fatigue Syndrome, see ME

CIRCULATION, POOR

■ PEOPLE WITH POOR CIRCULATION often feel cold when others don't and may look a little pale, with pale hands and feet. Their metabolism may be slower and they may suffer from related problems, such as chilblains, a sluggish digestive system, including constipation, problems waking up in the morning, and a general feeling of lethargy. When blood is circulated, the heart pumps it through the arteries to all parts of the body. The blood is then returned with the help of muscular activity through the veins. Poor circulation can then be caused either by a weak heart muscle, or by the hardening of the arteries (atherosclerosis), when the blood is not easily able to move through the arteries because build-up of deposits such as cholesterol on the arterial walls has narrowed them.

For more details of both these problems, see the Heart Disease entry on pages 118–120.

SOLUTIONS

A major factor in good circulation is regular aerobic exercise, such as walking, jogging, or cycling, during which blood is naturally pumped faster. Also, exercise encourages the muscles to remain fit and strong and in "good working order"—in other words, more efficient in helping the circulatory system.

Garlic, ginger, buckwheat, and the supplement ginkgo biloba are all aids to circulation, and may be used as part of a healthy diet. Vitamin E and omega-3 fatty acids, such as fish oils and linseed oil, also help to "thin" the blood and aid its flow through the circulatory system.

Cirrhosis, see Alcohol Abuse

COLDS AND FLU

A COLD—symptomized by sneezing, blocked-up nose, perhaps cough, and body temperature changes—is a viral infection, as is flu. Although colds and flu are "caught" from an infected person, in the air or by touch, you are more likely to get a cold or the flu if you have a weak immune system—perhaps through long periods of stress or other chronic illness, or through poor diet.

SOLUTIONS

The Immune-Strengthening Diet on page 143 will help to prevent colds and flu. This includes plenty of foods rich in vitamin C and zinc. It has been suggested that mega-doses of vitamin C—up to 5 g a day—help prevent colds, but this has never been proved in scientifically conducted tests. High doses of vitamin C

taken for more than a few days can cause stomach upsets, diarrhea, kidney stones, and other problems. If you feel a cold coming on, however, its severity and duration may be lessened by immediately increasing your daily intake of vitamin C to 500 mg a day, and continuing at that level for as long as the cold lasts. It is hard to get 500 mg of vitamin C a day in your normal diet, so a supplement will be necessary—try a chewable one with added bioflavonoids, and add to this a one-a-day zinc supplement.

Cold Sores, see Herpes Simplex 1

COLITIS

THIS IS A GENERALIZED TERM for inflammation of the colon. Several conditions can be grouped under the name, including ulcerative colitis, Crohn's disease, and irritable bowel syndrome (this last one is dealt with in a separate entry).

Ulcerative colitis is ulceration of the lining of the colon; symptoms include watery stools, which may contain mucus and/or pus, abdominal pain, tenderness, colic, and intermittent or irregular fevers. It is unclear how the condition is actually caused, although there may be an irregularity in circulating antioxidants, i.e., vitamins A, C, and E and the minerals selenium and zinc.

Crohn's disease is inflammation that can attack any section of the gut, from the mouth to the anus. Symptoms may be diarrhea, abdominal pain that can be mistaken for appendicitis, fever, loss of appetite, weight loss, and a bloated feeling. Again, it is not clear why Crohn's disease starts, but some trials have shown that there could be a food intolerance link, and that avoiding the problem foods significantly reduces the time before the disease recurs. Foods primarily found to be a problem include milk, grains, dairy products, and yeast.

SOME OTHER IDEAS FOR MINIMIZING YOUR COLD

* Garlic and onions—anti-bacterial and decongestant. Include plenty of the fresh product in your diet and take garlic oil supplement.
* Oils of thyme and eucalyptus may help to clear congestion. Use a few drops in boiling water as an inhalant and use plenty of fresh thyme in your cooking.
* Ginger and chili peppers are stimulating spices, said to help fight off the viruses, and are decongestant. Use plenty fresh in your cooking.
* Echinacea, which stimulates the immune system.
* Drink plenty of fluids throughout your cold, preferably citrus-based.
* It may also help to avoid dairy products, chocolate, and all foods high in saturated fat throughout your cold. These are said to be mucus-forming and may encourage your cold to develop into sinusitis or catarrh.

SOLUTIONS

Constipation may bring on an attack of ulcerative colitis, in which case a high-fiber diet will help, such as that outlined on page 14, avoiding too many refined and low-nutrient foods. A basic healthy diet, including plenty of vitamin C-rich foods, will help to minimize symptoms. Research shows that, during an attack, 20% of patients have benefited from a milk-free diet.

Antioxidant supplements may be useful, and fish oil supplements may help to speed up the pace of recovery and reduce the number of subsequent attacks—probably because the omega-3 oils from oily fish have anti-inflammatory properties.

Some sufferers of Crohn's disease do best on a low-fiber diet, avoiding certain fruit and vegetables, which could result in nutrient deficiencies (a dietitian's advice will be needed on supplementation), while in others a high-fiber diet may reduce the recurrence of the disease. Again, supplements of antioxidants and fish oils may help in either case. If food intolerance is suspected, it is important not to self-treat, but to seek professional help from a dietitian (via your physician).

With both ulcerative colitis and Crohn's, some research suggests that certain natural chemicals in foods can act as irritants, and citrus fruits, pineapples, bananas, cheese, coffee, and milk are often implicated.

Compulsive Eating, see Eating Disorders

Conjunctivitis, see Eye Problems

CONSTIPATION

■ CONSTIPATION—the infrequent passing of stools—is one of the most common physical complaints in the Western world. More than just an uncomfortable problem, if left untreated it can cause or contribute toward diverticular disease, and the occurrence of hemorrhoids, and may even put the sufferer at greater risk of bowel cancer. Largely, it is our Western diet that is to blame, although lack of physical activity undoubtedly makes the problem worse. Sometimes other factors can cause sudden constipation, especially stress or a change in daily routine (as when you are on vacation).

To function correctly and regularly (which may be less or more than the "once a day" people usually regard as normal), our bowels need high-fiber foods and plenty of fluids to help bulk up the stools and make them easy to pass—about 4 pints (1.75 liters) of water a day is ideal.

Health experts recommend we intake a minimum of 20 to 30 g of fiber a day, but some people may need much more than this in order to maintain a regular bowel, particularly if constipation is or has been a major problem in the past and if their general levels of physical activity are low.

SOLUTIONS

To get this amount of fiber you need to make a real effort to include some high-fiber foods at every meal. Prunes and rhubarb are also known to contain further special compounds that also produce a laxative effect, but they should not be relied on to the exclusion of a varied high-fiber diet. The food charts on pages 260–317 list the fiber content of over 300 foods, and the best sources of fiber are listed on page 14.

Fiber is found in all fruits and vegetables, grains, nuts, seeds, and legumes, but not in animal products, so the best diet to prevent constipation is one that contains lots of natural unrefined plant foods. Refined products such as sugar, white breads, white rice, manufactured cakes and cookies, refined breakfast cereals, and white pasta, contain much less fiber than their natural, unrefined counterparts.

Some people add a spoonful or two of bran to their daily diet to help keep them "regular." While true bran is a very good source of insoluble fiber, many experts believe it is better to get fiber as a natural part of your foods, because bran in this form can hinder absorption of some minerals.

If stress rather than a low-fiber diet is causing your constipation, then a mild herbal relaxant taken for a few days should help the problem—try chamomile tea twice a day or the supplement kava kava—and see what lifestyle changes you can make. Exercise not only helps regulate bowel movement, but also helps you relax.

Millions of people rely on daily doses of branded laxatives to try to cure their constipation. However, these are generally best avoided except for really very occasional use, because long term they can make the problem much worse—your colon comes to rely on them instead of trying to work for itself. So when you stop taking them your constipation is likely to become much worse than before. It is best to cure constipation slowly, through appropriate diet, exercise, and lifestyle modifications.

NATURAL REMEDIES FOR CONSTIPATION

Various other foods and herbal remedies are recommended for constipation. Some of the herbs, such as senna, are strong purgatives, and the same applies to them as to over-the-counter laxatives (see right). More gentle remedies include rose hip syrup, olive oil, honey, licorice, blackstrap molasses, and psyllium seeds infused in water. Strong spices, such as curry powder, ginger, and chili, have a laxative effect.

CHD (Coronary heart disease), see Heart Disease and Stroke

Coughs, see Bronchitis and Coughs

CRAMP

■ EVERYONE HAS A MUSCLE CRAMP now and again and it is unmistakable—an extremely painful, and sometimes prolonged, powerful contraction of a muscle, often in the leg, usually sudden. Cramp may be due to over-exercise, perhaps without sufficient prior warming-up of the muscles involved, and may be exacerbated by insufficient fluids and minerals before or during prolonged exercise.

SOLUTIONS

A range of minerals is involved in muscle contraction and relaxation. It makes sense to have adequate amounts of salt in the diet if you exercise a lot, particularly in hot conditions when you will lose salt in the sweat. However, salt intake should still not exceed healthy eating guidelines (see page 33). Adequate calcium intake is important, too, as is magnesium, which works with calcium in the body (best sources lists, page 29 and 32).

Drink plenty of fluids when exercising, and see Circulation, Poor, for further information about nutritional deficiencies that may result in poor circulation. Cramp may also occur at other times—for example, in bed at night—and this is likely to be a circulatory problem.

Once a cramp has begun, the best way to relieve it is to massage the affected area and, if possible, stretch it out. Try to relax and breathe calmly.

Crohn's disease, see Colitis

Cuts and Grazes, see Wounds, Cuts and Grazes

CYSTITIS

■ CYSTITIS is a bladder infection, the main symptoms of which are a need to urinate very frequently, but then finding that you can only pass a few drops, a burning sensation when you do pass urine, and, if the attack is left untreated, pain in the kidneys (felt in the center of the back). Urine may be cloudy, or even red, through traces of blood, and you may feel generally unwell.

SOLUTIONS

Some research seems to show that regularly drinking cranberry juice can help to prevent cystitis and may lessen the severity of an attack. At the onset of an attack it is essential to cut out tea, coffee, and alcohol, and to drink plenty of water, which helps to dilute the urine and so makes it less painful to pass as well as reducing infecting bacteria. Sufferers should also obtain sachets of potassium citrate, available from a pharmacy, which neutralizes the urine, and should see their physician. A basic healthy diet, low in refined sugar and low-nutrient foods, will help to prevent infection.

DEPRESSION

■ DEPRESSION is usually treated medically with a variety of drugs that enhance mood, but, unfortunately, few are free from side effects. However, with dietary alterations and other natural methods, many cases of depression can be helped or even cured. Symptoms of depression can be severe or mild, short term or long term. Cause is often difficult to pinpoint, but symptoms may often include a general "slowing down" both physically and mentally; inability to concentrate; loss of self-esteem; loss of libido; insomnia; deep feelings of unhappiness and/or worthlessness; fear of life in general and withdrawal from social life; and feeling at odds with the world.

SEASONAL AFFECTIVE DISORDER

One common form of depression is SAD (Seasonal Affective Disorder), which is the term used to describe the depression that many people in northern latitudes feel throughout the long, dark winter months and thought to be the result of the lack of light, which in turn results in low levels of serotonin in the brain. This can be alleviated using all the methods outlined below, and it has been found that regular light therapy works well in the winter months.

See also: Menopause (page 178); Menstrual Problems (126); ME (chronic fatigue syndrome, page 125); Fatigue (page 111), and Anxiety (page 92).

Depressives sometimes lose their appetite, possibly because of a knock-on effect from the "slowing down" syndrome that is so symptomatic of depression, and possibly because the will to "look after yourself" goes. Poor or meager eating habits will result in nutrient deficiencies, which can also contribute to depression.

Other depressed people frequently turn to food for comfort, perhaps bingeing on lots of high-carbohydrate foods, such as cakes, candy, and cookies. This is a downward spiral, because comfort eating inevitably results in weight gain and even lower self-esteem.

SOLUTIONS

Interestingly, there is probably a genuine reason why so many people crave sweet foods when they are feeling miserable. There is evidence that high-carbohydrate, low-protein meals help in the metabolism of tryptophan. Due to the action of insulin, after such a meal, tryptophan is free to enter the brain for conversion to serotonin, a compound that enhances mood. (Incidentally, many of the new wave of antidepressant drugs, including Prozac, also work by increasing available serotonin.) However, healthier carbohydrate foods, such as bread and fresh and dried fruits, may help mild depression.

It is vital for any depressed person to be encouraged to eat a basic healthy diet. This will include regular portions of the protein foods such as lean meat, low

fat-milk, cheese, and eggs, which are rich in the amino acid tryptophan. Recent research in the UK showed that women deprived of tryptophan showed symptoms of depression within hours.

American researchers have found a link between a high intake of omega-3 fatty acids, such as those found in oily fish, and low levels of depression. As omega-3s are healthy anyway, it is worth including plenty of oily fish or a supplement in the diet. The basic healthy diet should also include plenty of foods rich in the vitamin B group (for best sources lists, see page 26), which keeps the nervous system healthy. Research has shown that people who follow a diet low in B vitamins suffer from more mood swings and are less happy than others. Vitamin C is depleted more easily in the body when it is under stress (which includes depression), so plenty of C-rich foods should be included. If the depressed person isn't eating properly, then daily supplements of B group and C are indicated.

Alcohol should be avoided—in very small doses it has a stimulant effect, but after the first drink or two it is a depressant and particularly likely to have an adverse effect on a person who is prone to depression anyway. Alcohol also robs the body of the B group vitamins and C. Caffeine can make depression worse, so tea, coffee, cola, and chocolate, are best kept to a minimum.

It is important to take as much regular aerobic exercise as possible when depressed—there is much research to

show that mood is enhanced by exercise because it releases endorphins into the body. A daily brisk walk would be good, as fresh air also has a stimulating effect and can help to banish that "what's the point" feeling, which is so consistent with depression. Taking that first step is all that is needed.

Herbalists will recommend the herb hypericum (St. John's Wort) for depression. Tests show that it is, indeed, effective as a mild antidepressant, with few, if any, side effects and can be taken for periods of several weeks (in dosage as specified). Hypericum can be bought as dried leaf from some specialist stores and healthfood stores or as tablets called Kira, now fairly widely available.

DIABETES

■ THERE ARE approximately 10.3 million diagnosed diabetics—and perhaps six million undiagnosed diabetics—in the US alone and the figure is increasing. Diabetes mellitus is caused by lack of the hormone insulin, which is responsible for regulating levels of sugar in the blood and its utilization by tissues. Without insulin, the level of sugar in the blood rises.

The first signs of diabetes are increased thirst, frequent urination, weight loss, excessive tiredness, and, perhaps, skin and fungal infections and blurred vision. If diabetes is not treated it can damage the heart, kidneys, eyes, and other organs. Urine and blood tests can diagnose diabetes, which can be either Type 1, insulin-dependent diabetes (IDDM), or Type 2, non-insulin-dependent diabetes (NIDDM). Diabetics of both types are at greater risk than normal of cardiovascular disease, kidney disease, eyesight problems, and infections.

NOTE: Anyone with diabetes should be regularly monitored and counseled individually by their physician/consultant and dietitian. The notes below are for general guidance only. Any diabetic who wishes to follow any of the diets or diet tips recommended below should get professional approval.

■ Insulin-dependent diabetes

People with this type of diabetes don't produce any insulin themselves and need to have regular daily injections of insulin coupled with correct diet (see below) in order to control the diabetes.

Who gets it?

About 25% of diabetics are insulin-dependent. This type of diabetes is more common in children and young adults, and it is thought that about 10% of cases are found in people with one or other parents also IDDs. There is some evidence of a link between a virus that attacks the pancreas, where insulin is normally produced, and the onset of diabetes. Sudden shock also seems to precipitate the start of diabetes. At the moment, however, there is no proven cause and no cure.

■ Non-insulin-dependent diabetes

People with this type of diabetes either produce a little—but not enough—insulin, or there is a defect in its use. However, the diabetes can be controlled either simply by modifications in diet (and weight) or, in addition, with the help of tablets.

Who gets it? This is the most common form of diabetes, accounting for about 90% of all cases. It is also most common in people aged from 40 upward, which is why it was often called "mid-life onset diabetes." More women suffer than men. Insulin production doesn't appear to decrease with age, but increased age may produce a resistance to insulin's action, probably because of weight gain and lack of physical activity.

Many people with Type-2 diabetes are overweight. A recent large trial, over fifteen years, of men in middle age found that a body mass index (see page 188) of over 26 more than trebled the risk of diabetes, and a BMI of 30 or over increased the risk ninefold. Losing surplus weight means less insulin is needed.

Type-2 diabetes may also be triggered by steroid medication or other factors, and up to a third of Type-2 diabetics have other family members who are also diabetic. Diabetes occurs more frequently in people of Asian, Jewish, Mexican American, or Afro-Caribbean descent.

Coping with diabetes through lifestyle

The three best things a diabetic can do to help the condition are to keep to a reasonable body weight (losing weight through a sensible gradual diet, if necessary), eat a healthy diet, and take regular moderate exercise.

Type-2 diabetes can often be controlled by modifications in diet (and weight if necessary) alone. If the diabetic is overweight, he or she should follow a sensible diet plan such as that in Section Five until the body mass index is down to the ideal range of 20–25. (For middle-aged people who have been severely overweight, a target of no less than 22 is probably realistic and sensible.) The American Diabetes Association no longer endorses any one single meal plan, however, many diabetics are prescribed specific meal plans which are similar to the healthy eating recommendations we should all follow.

This diet should be low in saturated fat (and overall fat intake to be kept to around 30% or less of total calories) and low in simple sugars, such as sugar itself and candies, which cause sharp rises in blood sugar levels, and low-nutrient, highly processed "junk" foods. It should include plenty of complex carbohydrates, fiber, fruit, and vegetables, and adequate protein and essential fatty acids. Salt and alcohol intake should be moderate, and alcohol should be taken only with meals.

To help keep blood sugar levels from fluctuating too much, for many diabetics it helps to have regular small to medium-sized meals and snacks, including plenty of low-to-moderate glycemic index foods (see page 195), especially legumes, oats, and fruits, which are high in soluble fiber. These also have the benefit of lowering blood cholesterol levels, which are often high in diabetics. (However, individual needs vary and a dietitian's advice is needed.)

The nutritional requirements of a diabetic can be met by following the basic healthy diet in Section One, or the Healthy Heart Diet on page 142. Or, female diabetics may prefer to try the PMS and Diuretic Diet on page 145.

Plenty of water and fluids should be taken to help keep the kidneys working well, and a diet high in antioxidants, zinc, and garlic will help to protect against infections. If you would like the odd sweet treat, chocolate, or dessert, eat it with a main meal to help keep blood sugar levels constant.

New research also indicates that a diet high in both vitamin E and fish oils (which can be taken by eating more oily fish or in the form of a supplement) is particularly beneficial for diabetics, offering protection against cardiovascular disease—the leading cause of ill health and death, because of the diabetic's increased levels of cholesterol and fat in the blood. A diet that is high in fruit and vegetables, and low in salts, may also help to reduce high blood pressure.

Exercise

Some regular moderate exercise, such as walking, will help to get or keep surplus weight off and strengthen the circulatory and immune systems, as well as lower blood pressure and blood cholesterol. However, exercise "uses up" blood sugars for energy, and the insulin-dependent diabetic should take care to eat sufficient carbohydrate before exercise to avoid hypoglycemia (a "hypo"), when too much insulin is present and blood sugar levels crash. If this should happen, blood sugar needs to be raised quickly with glucose tablets or similar. After exercising, it is a good idea to have a healthy snack containing carbohydrate and a little protein, such as a banana and yogurt.

DIARRHEA

■ DIARRHEA can be a symptom of several different illnesses or disorders. An acute (short-term) attack of diarrhea is often related to food poisoning, when bacteria such as salmonella or E. coli are present in foods and have not been killed by appropriate cooking. It is also frequently experienced by travelers who may drink contaminated local water or eat new foods. When out of the US on long-distance travel, it is sensible to drink only bottled water and stick with foods that have been well cooked.

Food allergy or intolerance is another common cause; for example, diarrhea is a symptom of lactose (milk sugars) intolerance and celiac disease, which is caused by intolerance to the gluten in wheat and other products. Diarrhea can also be the result of eating too much food that has a laxative effect—for example, rhubarb or oranges. Many infections and illnesses may result in diarrhea, particularly in small children.

SOLUTIONS

Sufferers from an acute attack should drink plenty of bottled water to which is added a little salt and sugar for rehydration, and eat no solids for 24 hours. When able to eat a little again, eat bland, easily digested, energy-rich, low-fat foods, such as potatoes, rice, white bread, and bananas. Also get plenty of potassium-rich foods, such as bananas, potatoes, seeds, lentils, and nuts, into your diet as soon as possible, as diarrhea depletes the body's potassium levels, and potassium is particularly important in stabilizing your body's fluid levels after a bout of diarrhea.

Get back to a basic healthy diet when you can, paying particular attention to foods rich in B-group and C vitamins—water-soluble vitamins that will also have been depleted by the condition. Live yogurt will help to restore the digestive system to normal by restoring its healthy bacteria levels.

Attempts should always be made to ascertain the cause of an attack of diarrhea, and suitable precautions should be taken so that the problem doesn't recur. Diarrhea that lasts longer than 48 hours, or recurring bouts, for which you can find no simple explanation, need investigating by a physician. The cause could be irritable bowel syndrome, colitis, or other

---

"DIABETIC" FOODS—WORTH THE EXPENSE?

There is a huge range of commercial foods available, produced especially for diabetics and often sold in pharmacies or healthfood stores. These are items, such as diabetic jams, confectionery, cookies, and so on, and they are usually more expensive than ordinary products. Although they are often as high in fat and nearly as high in calories as their ordinary counterparts, they usually contain fructose (fruit sugar) or another sweetener, sorbitol, instead of sucrose. Many experts feel that these products are unnecessary.

These days, supermarkets carry a very good range of products low in fat and sugar which are equally suitable for diabetics. There is not really any such thing as a "diabetic food" and, in any case, high intake of fructose and sorbitol can cause problems—such as diarrhea or other digestive upsets. A diabetic should discuss the whole topic of how sweet foods can be included in the diet with their own dietitian.

more serious problems.

See also entries on Allergies, Celiac Disease, Colitis and Irritable Bowel Syndrome, and Safe Food on page 81.

Digestive Disorders, see Heartburn and Indigestion

DIVERTICULAR DISEASE

■ DIVERTICULAR DISEASE is a common problem in older people, when small pockets or sacs form in weakened areas of the wall of the colon. Half or more of the population over 60 may have diverticular disease, but only 25% or less will have the symptoms—abdominal pain, particularly in the lower left-hand side above the groin, and a change in bowel habits, e.g., alternating diarrhea and constipation. If the pockets (diverticuli) become clogged with waste matter and infected, symptoms may also include fever and bleeding, and hospital treatment will be needed. The cause of diverticular disease is probably our highly refined Western diet, with inadequate amounts of fiber, particularly soluble fiber. This can easily lead to constipation, and the diverticuli may form when straining to pass hard stools.

SOLUTIONS

To prevent diverticulitis, follow the Basic Healthy Diet (page 53), or, if prone to constipation, a high-fiber diet. Follow all the tips in the separate entry for Constipation, paying particular attention to getting enough cereal fiber and soluble fiber in the diet, found in excellent quantities in legumes, fruits, and oats. The Food Charts on pages 260–317 list the soluble fiber content of all common foods. On average we need 18 g of fiber a day, of which at least 6–8 g should be soluble.

Also make sure to get enough fluid in your diet—insoluble fiber needs fluid to form stools that are easy to pass. If upping your fiber intake, you should drink plenty of water—at least eight 8 fl oz (225 ml) glasses a day. Fiber is best obtained through a natural high-fiber diet—avoid sprinkling raw bran on foods, as it may irritate the colon.

Duodenal Ulcer, see Peptic Ulcer

EATING DISORDERS

■ ANOREXIA NERVOSA, BULIMIA NERVOSA, AND COMPULSIVE EATING are the three main categories of eating disorder, which most experts agree are an outward expression of psychological conflict rather than simply a problem with food and body image. In practice, it is sometimes not simple to categorize a sufferer as being precisely one or another of the three. For example, anorexics may later become bulimic; compulsive eaters may from time to time be bulimic, and so on. However, there are distinct differences between the disorders and their effects, described here in more detail.

■ Anorexia nervosa

The term means "loss of appetite due to nervous reasons" but, in fact—at least in the early stages of the disease—most anorexics do generally feel hungry and do want to eat, but they don't allow themselves to do so. Later, appetite may indeed disappear and, even though the anorexic may want to be cured, she or he may find that that decision is no longer within her or his grasp (ironically, because anorexics frequently fear being out of control).

Neither is anorexia simply an obsession with becoming slim (although thinness is outwardly one of the anorexic's main goals), or a disease brought about by modern society's increasing accent on

ZINC AND ANOREXIA

There has been some evidence that supplements of the mineral zinc can help anorexics to regain their appetite and taste-buds, and may help the depression from which many anorexics suffer. It has also been suggested that a zinc deficiency may also be one of the factors in the development of anorexia, although this is yet to be proved.

good looks—anorexia was recognized as long ago as the Middle Ages, and given its name nearly 130 years ago. Some cases, certainly, may be triggered by a need to have a particular body image (which is why the incidence of anorexia, and bulimia, is high among people like dancers, models, and actors, many of whom have the "anorexic personality type" described below).

Anorexia nervosa is thought not to have just one cause, but several, although many sufferers do tend to have certain things in common. The disease is ten times more prevalent in females than males, and is thought to affect up to one in two hundred women, and up to one in a hundred girls in their late teens, although it can also effect older people (including menopausal women).

Many experts believe that there can be a genetic tendency toward anorexia, with extra factors acting as triggers. Sufferers tend to be high achievers and often from families where academic achievement is important. Many anorexics appear to be confident and efficient and perfectionist, wanting to be good at all they do (though some may be introverted and shy), but underneath may have a constant feeling of not being good enough, and of, literally, being "anxious" to please, particularly peers (including parents). They may feel that the parents don't care about the person so much as what is achieved.

Experts say that the two most common traits in the anorexic personality are perfectionism and obsessionality. It is thought that giving up food may be a way of exercising control over life, over

others, and over oneself. Anorexia may be a solution to this personality type, whereas others may turn to alcohol, drugs, or crime, for example.

The symptoms of anorexia are a preoccupation with weight and weight loss, and, perhaps, with eating only foods perceived to be low in calories, such as lettuce or celery. The anorexic's goal is to lose weight, and she or he is terrified of being fat, with a distorted image of her or his own body size. Anorexics may go to great lengths to avoid eating food, and become adept at making excuses for missing meals. Often, though, they will enjoy preparing and serving delicious meals for the rest of the family.

Weight loss is the obvious first physical sign, although many anorexics disguise this well with big and baggy clothes. Anorexics are often restless and hyperactive, and may be obsessional about exercise and orderliness. In women, periods will cease. As the anorexia progresses, the sufferer will face severe constipation and malnutrition, will feel very cold all the time, and may grow hair on the body while hair on the head may be thin. As time goes on, anorexics will tend to eat less and less, until eventually their diet may consist of a lettuce leaf and some water every day. Unless the anorexic is treated, death through starvation or related causes, such as heart failure, will occur.

The sooner the anorexic can be persuaded to accept treatment, the greater the chance of recovery. Treatment often consists of a stay in the hospital, where the patient is fed until sufficient weight

is gained, coupled with psychological and practical counseling. It has been found that unless the underlying causes of the original anorexia are addressed, the anorexic will often quickly lose weight again. Recovery often takes several years. About half of diagnosed and treated anorexics recover completely, while others remain ill long term, and about 5% die.

It is very hard for an anorexic to make a recovery without the support and help of other people, as many refuse to admit that they have a problem. Various private clinics and residential homes now exist where the anorexic can be helped to work through problems and be taught to eat again. Overeaters Anonymous has a network of support and self-help groups, which also have a high degree of success.

Some nutritionists who specialize in eating disorders have a program that helps sufferers to eat normally again, through a process of teaching them the real value of food and why the nutrients it contains are important for a healthy body; by suggesting several small meals a day, beginning with foods the anorexic feels she or he can manage to eat, and learning to accept that the taste and texture of food is something to enjoy not fear; and then gradually reintroducing other healthy foods.

■ Bulimia nervosa

It is thought that bulimia nervosa— when the sufferer binges on, sometimes huge, amounts of food and then purges through vomiting, diuretics, or laxatives—is much, much more common in the Western world than is anorexia, but because most bulimics feel shame at what they do and follow the binge/purge cycle in secret, many cases go undetected. Bulimia also affects predominately young women, though more and more young men and older people seem to be becoming sufferers.

The causes of bulimia may often be very similar to those of anorexia, but, whereas the anorexic uses not eating as the "answer" to her or his problems, the bulimic uses secret binges as a way to help them alleviate stress, loneliness, anxiety, or depression, feelings that she or he doesn't feel able to share with anyone else, as it is very important for her or him to appear successful and self-contained.

This desire to binge is usually overwhelming in the bulimic, who seems to have no control over the binge sessions. Once a binge is over, the sufferer regains control by purging, vowing never to binge again—but sooner or later is compelled to do so. Some bulimics begin purging themselves after fairly normal-sized meals, as a way of controlling their weight without conventional dieting, and then find it difficult to stop.

Typical binge foods are refined carbohydrates, such as cakes, cookies, bread, chocolate, and pastry. Cheese, butter, ice cream, and other fatty foods are also common binge components. However, some bulimics gorge on meat, and even fruits and vegetables.

Symptoms of bulimia in others are often hard to spot, particularly if the bulimic is of normal weight (as is often the case), appears to eat normal meals, and may seem perfectly happy. Drastic fluctuations in weight may be an indication, however, and many bulimics do have long or short periods of semi-starvation before a binge. Also, in order to buy the quantities of food needed for a binge, some bulimics may resort to stealing money, or shoplifting.

Physical signs of bulimia will not, however, take long to appear. If vomiting is the main way of purging, the bulimic's teeth will quickly be affected. The acid in the vomit erodes tooth enamel and severe tooth decay follows. The bulimic may also face digestive disorders, including severe irritation of the lining of the intestines, severe chronic sore throat, gum disease, hair loss, general fatigue and depression, as well as malnutrition, imbalance in tissue salts in the body, and, finally, possible kidney failure, even heart failure and death.

Sufferers of bulimia can be helped with the aid of counseling and advice on diet. The compulsive binges that bulimia sufferers experience are, at least in part, brought on by the periods of starvation and the imbalance in blood sugar levels these cause. The binge is the body's way of telling the sufferer that food is needed.

It is now known that female bulimics tend to binge more in the week preceding a period (when hormonal changes cause most women to eat more) than at any other time. Explanation of this and help with a suitable premenstrual diet, as well as any other medical treatment as necessary, are all important.

One leading expert in bulimia advocates the "little and often" theory for bulimics—several small meals a day, avoiding refined carbohydrates, but including protein and fresh fruit. Most of all, bulimics need to be shown how to be around food in a normal manner again, to re-learn eating for the right reasons and eating a healthy diet without guilt; if slimness was their main goal, they need to be shown what constitutes a sensible body weight for them, achievable without starvation or purging. As with anorexia, they also need to be helped to deal with any underlying psychological problems.

■ **Compulsive eating**
The third, and possibly largest, group of people with an eating disorder are the compulsive eaters—people who regularly eat very much more food than is necessary, often in the form of bingeing as bulimics do, but without purging. The result is that, inevitably, they gain weight, and many compulsive eaters

become chronically or morbidly (life-threateningly) obese. This overeating and bingeing often begins when the sufferer faces particular major problems in life—divorce, redundancy, a death, etc.—and the food is used as a comfort.

However, compulsive eating is more than the kind of "comfort eating" that most people indulge in now and then. Vast quantities of food can be eaten over long periods of time, or sometimes in a short space of time. The sufferer is almost like an alcoholic—he or she needs his or her fix of food. Soon the initial reason for bingeing is forgotten, as compulsive eating becomes a habit and an important part of the sufferer's life.

Compulsive eating may also be interspersed with periods of semi-starvation—a state that may begin as the typical "yo-yo dieting" of someone trying too hard to lose weight, and then giving in and bingeing. A sufferer of this type of alternate binge/starve compulsive eating may either fluctuate in weight or be a fairly average weight, as the periods of starvation cancel out the effects of the binges.

If the sufferer is obese (with a BMI of over 30, see page 188), he or she should see a physician and begin a weight reduction program, as obesity can cause many physical problems and illnesses, including heart disease. This may require close monitoring. Counseling or a self-help groups such as Overeaters Anonymous local groups are usually vital if the sufferer is to overcome compulsive eating long term.

Binge/starve compulsive eaters will benefit from similar practical counseling to that for bulimia sufferers. A new idea is that a lack of essential fatty acids in the diet may result in food cravings, but this has yet to be proved.

See also Section Four, Food for Weight Control, and the Teenage Section in Section Three.

ECZEMA

■ SOMETIMES CALLED DERMATITIS, eczema is an allergic inflammation of the skin, with a red, itchy rash that may form small bubbles under the skin. If scratched, these may burst and infection may occur. There may be dry and flaky skin otherwise. Eczema is a common disease in childhood, with 50% of cases starting before six months of age, but it may start at any time. The severity may change with time, and could resolve as the child gets older.

SOLUTIONS

Contact allergy—e.g. to house dust mites, washing powders, clothing, nickel, rubber, or pets—is a common cause. These possible allergens should be investigated before dietary intervention.

UK trials have shown that Chinese herbal medicine can have beneficial results with standardized preparations; with impure herbs, however, side effects (including problems with liver and kidney function) may occur, so it is important to work only with an experienced herbal practitioner.

Several studies have shown that foods can provoke symptoms, and up to 40% of sufferers could benefit from exclusion diets as explained in the Allergy entry. However, it is often hard to predict which foods may provoke a response, although if increase in itch is noted after eating a certain food, this may indicate it is worth a trial. One or two (or, very occasionally, several) foods may be "culprit" foods. Any exclusion diet should only be carried out under experienced medical supervision. If any foods are permanently excluded, the nutritional adequacy of the remaining diet needs to be checked.

In breast-fed babies, there may be food from the mother's diet aggravating the symptoms, which may also appear when weaning begins or a switch to cows' milk is made. You should see your dietician for advice. See also Allergies.

FOODS THAT CAUSE ECZEMA

Foods commonly reported to cause problems are milk, cheese, and eggs, citrus fruits, food colorings and preservatives, nuts, fish, and tomatoes. Eczema sufferers often find that inflammation is reduced if they follow a diet low in saturated fats and high in essential fatty acids.

Evening primrose oil has, in trials, been shown to be effective for eczema. Some anecdotal evidence exists that fish oil and zinc supplements may also help.

Energy, Lack of, see Fatigue

EYE PROBLEMS

■ GRANNY WAS RIGHT—good eye health really is a lot to do with eating up your carrots. She didn't know why, but we do now— the extremely high beta-carotene content of carrots, which converts to vitamin A in the body—is essential for good eyesight and healthy eye tissue. Beta-carotene is an antioxidant, and, for general eye health, it is essential that you get enough of all the main antioxidants in your diet—the carotenoids, vitamin C, and vitamin E. Below specific problems and solutions are dealt with in more detail.

* *Night blindness* is nearly always due to lack of vitamin A in the diet. Around 2–3 carrots a day, lightly cooked, should help ease the problem.

* *Blepharitis* (red-rimmed eyes), bloodshot eyes, dull eyes, corner cracks, and sties are often a sign of vitamin B2 (riboflavin) deficiency. Take a daily vitamin B-group supplement and eat plenty of variety meats, nuts, seeds, and legumes, as well as antioxidant-rich foods and plenty of zinc for the immune system, as persistent eye problems are often a sign

of being run down. Get adequate sleep. Bathe the eyes in an infusion of eyebright herb (1 teaspoon to 1 cup boiling water).

* Conjunctivitis can be caused by an infection or allergy, and produces red, sore, painful eyes. Eat a basic healthy diet high in garlic and onions, which fight infection, and take a daily tincture of echinacea to help quickly boost your immune system. Eyebright bath may also be soothing and helpful.

* Dry eyes, gritty eyes are often a problem with contact lens wearers, but can be triggered by dry atmospheres, lack of sleep, or lack of essential fatty acids in the diet. Eat plenty of oily fish for omega-3s, and try a daily spoonful of linseed (flax) oil, another source of omega-3s. Evening primrose oil is also useful. All the antioxidant vitamins are important, especially vitamin E, so eat plenty of avocados and walnuts, and other E-rich foods. Try eyebright solution as above.

* Puffy or baggy eyelids are often caused by fluid retention (see entry). Follow the PMS and Diuretic Diet on page 145. Lie with cucumber or potato slices or chamomile tea bags (used and cooled) over each eye for 10 minutes each morning.

* Cataracts are very common as people age, but their development can be slowed by a diet rich in antioxidants, especially vitamin C sources rich in flavonoids, such as oranges and black currants; rich in quercetin-containing foods, such as tea, onions, and red wine, as well as vitamin B2 (best sources list, page 26), and a general basic healthy diet.

FATIGUE

FATIGUE IS A SYMPTOM with many possible causes. Short-term bouts of fatigue may be due to illness or overwork/stress or simply lack of sleep, and the tiredness is the body's way of asking for more rest. In these cases the answer is usually sleep and rest, plus a healthy diet, until the fatigue has passed. See also Insomnia and Stress.

Chronic fatigue, sometimes called the "TATT" or "tired all the time" syndrome, may be due to an underlying physical cause—for instance, food allergies, anemia (more common in women), ME (or chronic fatigue syndrome, which often occurs after a viral illness such as glandular fever and can last for a year or more), or possibly even more serious problems such as heart disease or cancer.

It may also be, at least partly, psychologically based, for example linked with chronic stress, depression, or boredom. Chronic fatigue should always be investigated by a physician. More detailed advice on dealing with these ailments nutritionally appears under each of the separate headings.

In women, many cases of fatigue are linked to the monthly menstrual cycle. Tiredness that occurs regularly in the premenstrual week or few days and then disappears on day one or two of the period is almost certainly linked to hormonal changes.

Diet itself can cause or exacerbate fatigue. Too much alcohol or caffeine on a regular basis can cause long-term fatigue. A diet that is regularly high in refined carbohydrates, such as sugar, cakes, and cookies, can contribute toward low blood sugar levels, a symptom of which is fatigue.

Crash-type weight-loss diets, where inadequate calories are consumed, can cause tiredness, as can irregular meals (low blood sugar again) or eating only once a day. Occasionally, vegan and vegetarian diets can cause fatigue through being too low in iron and perhaps the B group vitamins.

SOLUTIONS
To help beat tiredness you should follow a good healthy, varied diet, rich in whole foods, complex carbohydrates, and a

wide range of nutrients, particularly vitamin B12 (which has been shown in trials to alleviate fatigue when injected), folate and iron, which are responsible for maintaining healthy red blood cells, antioxidant vitamins C and E, the minerals zinc and magnesium, and the essential fatty acids. For best sources of all of these, see Section One. The herbal supplement ginseng helps some people feel more energetic when taken as a four- to six-week course at 500 mg a day. Avoid consumption of caffeine while taking ginseng.

You should also take regular exercise (if your health allows), preferably in the fresh air, because tiredness is made worse by a sedentary lifestyle and worse again by stuffy offices and homes that don't get enough air-flow through them. Our bodies need oxygen to function properly; oxygen is supplied in fresh air via our lungs and circulatory systems. These work most efficiently in a fit and exercised body.

Studies have shown that just a 15-minute walk in fresh air can revitalize and refresh, and may be exactly what is needed rather than going back to bed. Deep breathing exercises by an open window (in good weather) are also useful for helping to oxygenate the body and clear a fuzzy brain.

FEVER

FEVER—raised temperature (normally considered 102.2°F/39°C plus), usually accompanied by sweating, shivering, aches and pains, and sometimes bouts of nausea or diarrhea—is normally a symptom of some sort of infection, which should be treated according to the advice on page 122.

Most of the symptoms of the fever can be improved with aspirin. Herbal methods of bringing down a high temperature include use of garlic, ginger, and chili, all of which promote sweating (the body's own natural method of cool-

SIX TIPS TO MINIMIZE FLATULENCE

1 Cook food well, particularly legumes, which helps to remove the problem. Canned beans may be tolerated better than dried ones. Soak all dried beans well and discard soaking water before cooking thoroughly.
2 Purée foods before eating, e.g., as a side dish or in a soup.
3 Chop food small.
4 Chew food thoroughly, and relax and enjoy your food.
5 Eat slowly and keep the mouth shut. Some excess wind is caused by swallowing air as you eat.
6 Get used to new foods slowly, e.g., if you are beginning to eat more healthily, all the extra fiber in your diet may be too much for you.

ing the skin and bringing fever down).

Garlic is also a strong antibiotic. A chamomile infusion is also useful for controlling the symptoms of fever, and a supplement of borage oil (starflower oil), which is a cooling herb and an infection fighter, may also help.

Prolonged sweating means that the body will quite soon become dehydrated, so anyone with a fever should drink plenty of fluids, preferably diluted lemon or orange juice, perhaps with a spoonful of honey added. If the feverish person has lost his or her appetite and is not eating, which quite often happens, the fluids should also contain a little salt—approximately 1 teaspoon for every 1 quart/1 liter.

The appetite of the feverish person may be whetted by easy-to-eat, tasty, or cooling foods, such as ice cream, stewed fruits, berry fruits, small peanut butter sandwiches on white bread, poached egg on mashed potato, and mashed bananas with honey. On the other hand, if the feverish person is feeling chilled and shivery, a little mug of hot soup may be a good idea.

As soon as the patient is eating well again, ensure he or she gets plenty of foods rich in vitamins C and B, which will have been depleted by the illness, as part of the basic healthy diet.

See also Diarrhea, Infections, and Nausea.

FLATULENCE

EXCESS WIND in the digestive system can be both uncomfortable and unsightly—causing a bloated feeling and distension—as well as being noisy and embarrassing. This excess wind, called flatulence, often occurs when gases are formed as the bacteria in the intestines feed on food. Certain foods seem to cause more problems with wind than others. The resistant starches in some high-fiber foods seem to be the worst culprits of all: the leguminous peas, beans, and lentils, and under-ripe bananas, for example. Bran, dried fruits such as prunes, and cruciferous vegetables—particularly Brussels sprouts and cabbage—are also foods that cause overproduction of wind for many people. As these foods are all healthy and provide us with much-needed fiber and nutrients, they are best incorporated in the diet using the tips above.

There may be other causes of excess wind. Caffeine, beer, sodas, high-fat foods, such as cream and pastry, and fresh bread are all known to be culprits.

There may also be an underlying disorder or illness causing the problem. A food intolerance or allergy is likely, or lactose intolerance or celiac or Crohn's disease. Candida is a fairly common cause, and so is irritable bowel syndrome. These should be investigated by your physician.

For everyday flatulence, relief can be

obtained with an infusion of one of the following herbs: peppermint, chamomile, dill, lemon balm, basil, or fennel leaves. Or, a decoction can be made with fresh chopped ginger or fennel seeds. The condition may also be helped with regular servings of live yogurt, as long as lactose intolerance has been discounted.

See also Heartburn and Indigestion.

Flu, see Colds and Flu

FLUID RETENTION

SURPLUS FLUID IN THE BODY is often mistaken for surplus fat or wind and can result in weight gain of many pounds. The symptoms are a bloated and puffy feeling and visible swelling, especially of the stomach, breasts, face, hands, ankles, and feet. Fluid retention is caused by a variety of different things.

Women frequently suffer during times of hormonal change—with PMS, during pregnancy, when on the Pill, or at the menopause. Before a period, a woman can put on 6–9lb (3–4 kg), much of which will be fluid. The Pill may add this much, too, and the extra fluid tends to stay until the woman comes off that form of contraception. For more detailed advice on fluid retention in pregnancy and the menopause, see pages 172 and 178.

Another common cause is a high-salt diet—experts say that up to 4 lb (1.8kg) of surplus fluid may be retained in the body through a typical Western diet high in commercial foods with lots of added salt and salty snacks. Refined carbohydrates such as cakes, cookies, and low-cost white bread may also contribute to fluid retention, so it is wise to cut intake of these right down, especially, if female, at vulnerable times such as before a period.

Allergies are another common cause (see Allergies entry). Certain health problems predispose toward fluid retention—heart disease and kidney disorders being the most common—as do certain drugs. In these cases, talk to a physician.

SOLUTIONS

Most cases of fluid retention can be helped by an appropriate diet, such as the PMS and Diuretic Diet on page 145. Salt intake should be kept to a minimum (see list of high-salt foods on page 33) and so should refined starches as above. It is important to drink plenty of plain water, as, contrary to popular belief, this doesn't make fluid retention worse, but, in fact, allows salt to be excreted more easily.

You should also eat a diet high in potassium-rich foods, such as bananas, tomatoes, and whole grains. Potassium works with sodium in the body to balance fluids properly, and a high potassium intake is a natural way to help flush out surplus salt.

Some experts also believe that a lack of essential fatty acids in the diet may contribute toward sluggish elimination of fluids, so it is worth eating plenty of oily fish and pure vegetable oils, and perhaps taking a supplement of evening primrose oil for 2–3 months.

Exercise is important in helping to flush surplus fluid out of the body—a swimming session is ideal, or a brisk walk. If you are retaining fluid you will notice that as soon as you have finished the exercise you need to go. Certain types of body massage are also effective.

Avoid anything more than very occasional use of over-the-counter diuretic pills. Misuse of these can affect the correct balance of body fluids and minerals, and will eventually make the problem worse. Natural diuretic foods can be incorporated into your diet though—these are most fruits, especially melon and citrus fruits, carrots, salad vegetables, including tomatoes, celery, lettuce, watercress, sweet peppers, and cucumber, and infusions of dandelion, parsley, lovage, nettle, or rosemary.

Food Intolerance, see Allergies

Food Poisoning, see Diarrhea, Infections, Nausea and Travel Sickness, and Stomachache

GALLSTONES

MANY PEOPLE HAVE GALLSTONES—some reports put the figure as high as one in three of all women (men are much less likely than women to suffer)—but only a minority of those will ever experience problems because of the stones. Pain in the upper right-hand side of the abdomen, which comes on several hours after eating, may be due to stones, which are generally caused by an excess of bile (which helps in the digestion of fats) and cholesterol in the gallbladder that can build up, particularly when the sufferer eats a high-fat diet. Inflammation or pain can occur if the stone tries to leave the gallbladder and becomes lodged in the bile duct. Pain can spread to the back and right shoulder. Flatulence is another common symptom.

SOLUTIONS

Gallstones are less common in vegetarians and in people who eat a basic healthy diet of small regular meals, low in saturated fats and sugars and high in fiber, fruit, vegetables, oily fish, folate, magnesium, and vitamin C. A diet high in fat, sugar, and junk foods and low in water and fiber may predispose to gallstones. One study has shown that gallbladder pain can be overcome by testing for food allergies on an elimination diet. When foods were reintroduced, the foods that most often triggered symptoms were eggs, pork, and onions.

Gastric Ulcer, see Peptic Ulcer

GLANDULAR FEVER

CAUSED BY THE EPSTEIN-BARR VIRUS, glandular fever is a fairly common illness of the teens and twenties, after which it becomes quite rare. Symptoms are enlarged lymph glands (e.g., in the neck and armpits), muscular aches and pains, fever, headache and tonsillitis, tiredness and weakness. Glandular fever usually lasts at least two weeks, but can carry on, with recurring bouts of the symptoms, for a year or more. Some people diagnosed with glandular fever go on to suffer from ME (chronic fatigue syndrome).

SOLUTIONS

To help shorten the duration of glandular fever you need to build up your immune system by, for instance, following the Immune-Strengthening Diet on page 143. There is evidence that a diet rich in essential fatty acids can also help, and a daily supplement of tincture of echinacea, 10 drops in 7 fl oz (200 ml) warm water, is a good idea. If the illness has reduced appetite, daily supplements of vitamin B group and vitamin C, both of which are important for the immune system and which are quickly depleted in the body, may be useful. Sensible diet, plenty of rest, and gradually building up to a little regular exercise will help to ensure that glandular fever doesn't develop into ME. See also ME.

GOUT

A FORM OF ARTHRITIS, gout is caused by the build up of uric acid, a metabolic waste product, in the blood. Gout affects single joints, usually the big toe, and happens when not enough uric acid is passed in the urine, or too much is produced. When the urate level increases, uric acid crystals form, and deposit in the cartilage or joint space, causing inflammation and pain, which can be very severe.

SOLUTIONS

Treatment is usually by drugs, but the right diet can be helpful. The sufferer should drink plenty of non-alcoholic fluids and avoid becoming overweight. If already too heavy, a sensible weight-loss plan (such as that on page 192) should be followed. However, crash diets and fasting should be completely avoided as these could precipitate an attack. A diet rich in vegetables and low in fatty foods has been shown to be helpful.

Foods high in purines, which may lead to increased uric acid, should be avoided. These are variety meats, shellfish, sardines, mackerel, whitebait, herrings, anchovies, fish roe, and game. As fish oils are healthy and particularly useful in helping to prevent heart disease, supplements of linseed oil can be used to replace oily fish in the diet. Individual tolerance varies, but alcohol often makes gout worse. Drinking should be well within healthy guidelines (see page 36).

Some food supplements, such as vitamin A and niacin, may be harmful. Vitamin C is often quoted a being helpful, but should only be used under medical supervision. See also the Arthritis entry.

GUM DISEASE

IF YOUR GUMS, OR ANY PART OF THEM, ARE SORE, puffed up, red and inflamed, painful or bleeding (or any of those symptoms), you need to visit a dentist and get the condition rectified. If you leave the condition untreated it will probably get worse and eventually result in loss of teeth. The most common gum disease is gingivitis, which is mostly caused by insufficient oral hygiene and is often characterized by halitosis and the symptoms described above.

If teeth and gums aren't brushed and flossed at least twice a day, layers of plaque (sticky, opaque residues that are a mixture of food particles and the bacteria contained in the mouth saliva)

SIX STEPS TO AVOIDING GUM DISEASE

1 Regular dental check-ups and scaling.
2 Twice daily thorough oral hygiene, including flossing.
3 Healthy diet rich in fruit, vegetables, vitamin C, and zinc.
4 Avoid long periods of chewing on sweet food, such as caramels.
5 Always brush teeth as soon after a meal or snack as possible.
6 Avoid lots of sweet, sticky, or starchy snacks.

are left and build up on your teeth and gum margins. If left longer, these gradually harden into tartar, which it is not possible to remove without going to the dentist. If the tartar isn't removed, infection in the gum margins can set in and gingivitis results.

People who eat a healthy diet, high in fruit and vegetables and wholefoods, and low in sugary and refined foods, may build up less plaque, but this isn't necessarily always the case. Some people seem more prone to plaque production, whatever their dietary habits. Nevertheless, a healthy wholefood diet provides the mouth, teeth, and gums with a good workout and may help to keep them in good condition.

However healthy the diet, it is important to brush and floss regularly, making sure to brush the gums as well as the teeth. Very occasionally, bleeding gums may be caused by a vitamin C deficiency. A diet very low in fruit and vegetables and all the other C-rich foods (see list), compounded, for instance, by smoking and drinking alcohol, both of which deplete the body's vitamin C, or maybe another vitamin C "robber," such as stress or illness, may possibly result in such a deficiency. Bleeding gums are also quite common in pregnancy.

See also the Tooth Decay entry.

HAIRLOSS

WHEN HAIR SUDDENLY BEGINS FALLING OUT, hormonal changes are often to blame. After childbirth, during the menopause, and the "male menopause," hair loss is common. In most cases this isn't totally preventable. Other causes of hair loss are hypothyroidism (a medical condition), stress, long-term illness, and large doses of vitamin A. It is also possible that poor circulation in the scalp may affect the hair follicles from which the hair grows. Stress will make this worse by tightening the scalp.

SOLUTIONS

Exercise, relaxation techniques, and scalp massage may all help. See Stress and Circulation, Poor for more information. Once hair is lost in male-pattern baldness or menopause, little can be done nutritionally, but a basic healthy diet will help anyone keep their remaining hair in good condition. Hair lost after childbirth or through illness will usually be replaced quite naturally, but, again, a healthy diet will help to ensure this. Adequate iron and zinc intake, and vitamins B group and C are particularly associated with good hair.

HALITOSIS

BAD BREATH—OR HALITOSIS—has various causes, and successful treatment relies on making the right diagnosis of the cause and then eliminating it. Here we run through the most common causes and suggest appropriate action:

* **Oral infection** Gum disease or tooth decay can cause bad breath. Get the problem sorted out by your dentist and help any necessary healing with plenty of zinc and vitamin C.

* **Poor oral hygiene** Insufficient brushing and flossing will leave particles of food between the teeth and around the mouth, which can smell bad when they decay. Brush and floss at least twice a day, three minutes a time on both.

* Type of food eaten Everyone knows how pungent raw garlic is on the breath. The odor of curried food, alcohol, tobacco, and some other foods can so linger on the breath. Odors like this can be masked by chewing parsley or mint and, when caused by foods eaten, should disappear within hours.

* Food allergy or intolerance These can cause bad breath. If you have accompanying symptoms, e.g., bloated stomach, feeling "off color," headaches, get your physician to check you over to see if an allergy may be the cause. The solution then is to avoid the item(s) that produce the allergy symptoms. For more detailed advice on allergies and food intolerances see appropriate entry.

* Throat or mouth infection Tonsillitis, sore throat, and oral thrush (sore mouth) are often accompanied by halitosis. In most cases, when the infection clears up so will the bad breath. Meanwhile, drink plenty of water.

* Sinusitis and phlegm Nasal blockages may cause you to breathe through your mouth and/or to leave your mouth open most of the time. This encourages bad breath by drying out the mouth and lowering levels of saliva, which contains oxygen to keep the mouth fresh. Try a dairy-free diet for 2–4 weeks and see if your sinusitis or phlegm improves. See also Colds and Flu.

* Sleeping with mouth open If your bad breath is worst in the morning, it could be that you are sleeping with your mouth open, which encourages bad breath (see previous paragraph). If a nasal problem is causing you to breathe through your mouth, get it sorted out by the physician. Also try avoiding dairy products in the evening (see the previous paragraph on Phlegm).

* Constipation If you are constipated you may have bad breath, probably because the stored-up waste in the bowel is causing back production of gases, which are being eliminated via the breath. If you are constipated, switch gradually to a high-fiber diet, take lots of exercise, and drink plenty of water, which will also help to keep the mouth moist.

* Medication Some drugs can cause bad breath. If you are taking any medications and can find no other reason for your halitosis, check with your physician and see if perhaps another similar medication could be used instead (if the drug you are taking is long term). If short term, it is probably best to live with the problem for just a few days, and chew parsley or mint to sweeten the breath.

* Predisposition to halitosis According to some experts, some people have higher than normal concentrations of the bacteria that can cause bad breath in the back of their throat and mouth. However careful they are, they may still have bad breath.

Best help is to scrape the area regularly with special tongue scrapers. Mouthwashes are not a good idea, as, although they work short term, long term they make the mouth drier and encourage the halitosis.

HANGOVER

IF YOU ARE GOING OUT for the evening and know you are likely to be drinking more than usual, you can do a lot toward preventing a hangover the next morning by taking one or two precautions beforehand.

First, eat a meal and drink some milk. This helps to slow the absorption of alcohol (some of which is absorbed straight through the stomach lining without waiting to go the route of other things that you eat and drink—which explains why we can begin to feel "tipsy" in a very short time after taking our first drink).

Then drink a glass or two of water, and continue drinking water throughout the evening in between alcohol. This not only helps you to drink less alcohol, but helps to stop you dehydrating. Dehydration is the major cause of hangover. Alcohol is a diuretic, which means that you will pass more urine than usual during and after drinking, and become dehydrated. When body fluids are too low, we get the classic hangover symptoms of headache, throbbing head, and so on.

When you get home you can do yet more to help prevent that hangover. If you can face it, drink a mug of warm milk, the calcium in which will help you sleep. Alcohol, while probably sending you to sleep well at first, disrupts REM sleep (the deep sleep that we all need in order to feel refreshed) and may cause wakefulness from the early hours. Drink more water before you go to bed—preferably with a soluble vitamin C tablet in it—and keep water by the bed for sipping if you wake in the night.

In the morning, if, despite everything, you do have a hangover, continue drinking plenty of fluid, preferably water or diluted fruit juice. If you feel queasy, skim milk is a good idea. Avoid coffee, particularly strong black coffee, and tea, both of which are also diuretics and will compound the problem. If your hangover has left you feeling a bit jittery and jumpy, the caffeine they contain will make you feel worse.

You should eat something as soon as you feel up to it—if you can't face anything bigger, a banana is a good idea. This will help boost your blood sugar levels. Low blood sugar is another cause of some of the symptoms of hangover, such as irritability, dizziness, and tiredness. "Hair of the dog"—i.e., another alcoholic drink—is absolutely not a good idea, whatever you have been told. A drink may make you feel temporarily better, but will just compound the problem long term. It is also the road to addiction. Proprietary preparations for hangover usually contain high levels of alcohol; avoid these too (check the label).

You can try non-alcoholic herbal remedies, such as an infusion of rosmary (a couple of sprigs infused in a teacup of boiling water for 5 minutes, then strained).

Some freshly juiced carrot or mixed vegetables may help your liver (which has to process all the alcohol that you drink) to recover. As soon as possible, eat a nutritious meal and then get back to bed for some REM sleep. If hangovers are a common occurrence for you, read the entry on Alcohol Abuse (page 86) and consider ways to cut down your drinking.

KNOW YOUR POISON

Choose your alcoholic drinks very carefully. Some drinks are much more likely to cause hangovers than others because of the congeners—the additives—that they contain. Many alcoholic drinks contain a great deal of additives. The additives that give alcohol color seem to be the worst culprits in producing a hangover. So stick to pale-colored or colorless drinks—vodka is best, followed by gin and white wine. Then follows, in best-to-worst order: lager, beer, hard cider, Scotch, rum, sherry, stout, brandy, red wine, and port.

HAY FEVER

SEASONAL ALLERGIC RHINITIS, or hay fever, is an extremely common allergic reaction to airborne pollens from grass, trees, and/or fungi, usually characterized by several of the following symptoms: inflammation of the nasal passages; itching in mouth, nose, throat, and eyes; streaming eyes and nose; sore throat, mouth, eyes, and nose; sneezing; blocked-up nose; disturbed sleep; and head-, face-, and/or earache.

Diet is not thought normally to play a part in this, but, in a minority of people, some foods may cause a problem. These foods contain substances that are similar to the pollen allergen, which the body may recognize, and a reaction will be set up—e.g., birch pollen cross-reacts with a number of fruits and vegetables, including apples, raw carrots, and peaches. People with hay fever may be more susceptible to food allergies or intolerances, and there are anecdotal reports that people who sort out their food intolerances that may cause other symptoms—e.g., irritable bowel syndrome—find that their hay fever may reduce in severity or disappear. See Allergies.

Headaches, see Migraine and Headaches

HEARTBURN AND INDIGESTION

HEARTBURN, which can cause sharp and even severe chest pains, is the result of too much acid in the stomach when a meal is being digested. The excess acid spurts back up into the esophagus, which connects the stomach and mouth, and the acid causes pain and discomfort, often known simply as indigestion. Heartburn is also a symptom of hiatus hernia, which is more common in people who are very overweight, and may also be a common problem in late pregnancy, when the expanding uterus can literally "squash" the digestive system.

SOLUTIONS

Whatever the cause, a few simple dietary guidelines can help minimize occurrence and the discomfort caused by heartburn and indigestion. Certain foods are more likely to cause an attack. Both acidic foods, like pickles, sauces, and vinegars, and fatty foods, such as fries and pastries, are the most common culprits. Both stimulate the output of acid in the digestive system. Raw vegetables, such as onions, bell peppers, and radishes, curries, chili peppers, and unripe fruit, are also best avoided, as are alcohol, strong coffee and tea, sodas, all of which can cause irritation.

How you eat is also important. Have several small meals rather than one or two large ones; the digestive system will find this easier to handle. Chew food thoroughly, eat slowly, and try to relax while eating. After you have eaten, an infusion of fennel, dill, or apple mint leaves will help to prevent heartburn.

If heartburn or indigestion occur frequently and these tips don't work, it is important to have a check-up with your physician, as there may be an underlying problem that needs attention. If you are overweight, follow a sensible weight-loss diet (such as that in Section Four).

HEART DISEASE AND STROKE

CORONARY HEART DISEASE (CHD) is the number one cause of death in the US and the greatest single cause of premature death in men. It develops when the coronary arteries, which supply blood to the heart, become narrowed by a build-up of plaque (cholesterol and other deposits). This is called atherosclerosis. Blood supply to the heart is reduced and there may be chest pain (angina) and/or irregular heart beat (arrhythmia). In time the arteries may become completely blocked, either by more build-up of plaque and/or by a blood clot (thrombosis), supply of blood to parts of the heart will be blocked, and a heart attack will occur. Similarly, a blocked artery that supplies blood to the brain may lead to a stroke.

There are several internationally recognized risk factors for heart disease: old age (most CHD occurs in people aged 70 plus), hereditary factors, diabetes, smoking, heavy drinking, stress, lack of exercise, obesity, high blood pressure, and high blood cholesterol levels. Also, men are more likely to get CHD than women, until after menopause when women appear to lose their hormonal protection and the risk becomes equal. The more of the risk factors that you have, the higher the likelihood of your developing CHD.

There is also much recent research into other possible risk factors for CHD. For instance, there is now growing evidence that CHD may also be linked with bacterial infections, particularly those that cause chest infections and gum disease, all of which may be controlled with antibiotics. To reduce risk of contracting infections, see advice on page 122, and follow the Immune-Strengthening Diet on page 143. See also Gum Disease, Tooth Decay, and Bronchitis and Coughs.

There is also strong evidence that a diet lacking in adequate fruits and vegetables and other plant foods is a risk factor in itself, probably because these foods contain the vitamin antioxidants E and C and beta-carotene, the phytochemicals such as flavonoids, and B vitamins, particularly folate and B6, which all now appear to have an important role to play in lowering risk of CHD. A diet high in red meat may also be an important risk factor. A recent study by the Imperial Cancer Research Fund in the UK found that vegetarians have a 24–45% decreased risk of dying from CHD.

Preliminary measures to help reduce your risk of CHD are to give up smoking; keep alcohol consumption to a minimum (see page 36); seek ways to reduce high stress levels (see page 134); and take regular exercise (latest research says that 11 minutes of aerobic exercise a day will cut the risk by nearly a half).

If diabetic, sensible management of the condition (see page 105) will help reduce risk of CHD. High blood pressure puts extra strain on the heart and blood vessels, especially if atherosclerosis is present, so should be regularly checked and controlled with the help of your physician and lifestyle and dietary advice.

Obesity can increase risk of heart disease (one large study showed it doubled), because it is associated with raised blood pressure and cholesterol and tryglyceride levels. If you are overweight, with a BMI of 26 or more (see page 188), and partic-

ularly if your waist-to-height ratio (see page 188) is high, you should lose weight.

Cholesterol and heart disease

Cholesterol is a soft, waxy substance that is manufactured mainly in the liver and then circulated in the blood, and is necessary for the smooth running of a variety of bodily functions. The amount of cholesterol that the liver makes may be due to hereditary factors and/or related to the amount of fat, particularly saturated fat, eaten. Cholesterol production and action is also affected by a variety of factors. Some of these seem to involve various aspects of diet, which are discussed below.

There are two major types of cholesterol—low-density lipoprotein (LDL) and high-density lipoprotein (HDL). A surplus of LDL in the blood is a major factor in the "furring" of arteries and formation of the plaques that lead to atherosclerosis, heart disease, and stroke; whereas HDL—often called "good" cholesterol—actually helps to remove cholesterol from the tissues and delivers it to the liver for excretion. There are various things you can do, nutritionally, to help lower LDL levels, in conjunction with any medical treatments your physician may suggest.

1: You can reduce intake of the types of foods that cause the liver to manufacture more LDL. These are foods high in saturated fats, such as full-fat dairy products and fatty meat, and those high in trans fats, such as many commercial margarines and ready-made products. Cholesterol is also found in some foods, particularly liver, eggs, shellfish, meat, and dairy products (see page 19). Intake of high-cholesterol foods may have a small relationship to blood cholesterol levels, but is less important than saturated fat intake. For more information about saturated and trans fats, see Section One.

2: You can reduce intake of foods that lower HDL levels in the blood, thereby lowering the amount available to transport the surplus cholesterol away.

Recent research has shown that trans fats can reduce the amount of HDL by up to 20%. So trans fats get the "thumbs down" on two counts, and seem to be worse for your blood cholesterol levels than butter. Very high intakes of polyunsaturated fats will also lower HDL levels, so, in their case, "enough" is good, "too much" is bad. (See page 16 for more information on polyunsaturated fats.)

3: You can eat more of the foods that seem to lower production of LDL, or increase production of HDL and therefore encourage its excretion. The foods that appear to achieve this are:

* ***Unsaturated fats*** When replacing saturated fats in the diet, polyunsaturated fats—particularly those high in linoleic acid, such as corn oil and sunflower oil—and monounsaturated fats help lower LDL levels. Monounsaturates, found in greatest quantities in olive and canola oils, do not lower HDL levels, so it may be a good idea to eat more monos than polys, as the latter can lower HDL if taken in excess.

* ***Garlic*** Its phytochemicals, including allicin, help lower LDL cholesterol.

* ***Soybeans and soy milk*** Some research has shown that regular intakes of soy equivalent to about 2½ cups/600 ml of soy milk per day can lower LDL by up to 25%.

* ***Soluble fiber*** Found in greatest quantities in oats, legumes, and many fruits and vegetables, fiber can help lower LDL.

* ***Beer and wine*** There is some evidence that a glass of beer or wine most nights of the week may increase HDL.

Lastly, your diet can also help to prevent cholesterol from forming the artery-narrowing plaques, and it can help to prevent blood clots from forming. To do this your diet should be rich in:

* ***Oily fish*** The omega-3 fatty acids in oily fish, such as salmon and mackerel, will "thin" the blood and help prevent blood clots. Fish oils also have the effect of lowering blood triglycerides (see below) and slightly lowering blood cholesterol levels. If taking fish oil supplements, an evening primrose oil supplement taken at the same time will ensure correct metabolism of the N6 fatty acids (see page 16), which can be inhibited by supplements high in omega-3s.

■ Heart disease and antioxidants

Although, as we've seen, antioxidants aren't found solely in fruits and vegetables, experts now believe that a diet rich in fruits and vegetables may reduce heart disease by up to 20%, five varied portions a day being the minimum recommended by the American Heart Association. One recent large trial of middle-aged men found that those who had a vitamin C deficiency had a three and a half times greater risk of heart attack.

■ Heart disease and homocysteine

Recent research has found a strong link between raised blood levels of plasma homocysteine and increased incidence of CHD and strokes. More research needs to be done, but it appears clear that low levels of the B vitamin folate predispose to this condition. Other B vitamins, particularly B6, may be involved in homocysteine metabolism, and a B-group-rich diet may help to protect against, or reverse, this condition. Legumes and green vegetables are rich sources of folate and other B vitamins (for best sources list, see page 26).

■ Heart disease and triglycerides

Triglycerides are another type of fat found in the blood, and evidence suggests that higher than normal levels can contribute to increased risk of heart disease, particularly in women, diabetics, and older people. Your physician can test your blood for high triglyceride levels. Levels can be reduced by eating small, regular, high-fiber meals not too high in fat, by eating oily fish or fish oils, and by restricting intake of alcohol and sugar.

WHAT ARE ANTIOXIDANTS?

Antioxidants are vitamins, minerals, and phytochemicals that help prevent fat from oxidizing. They can prevent the oxidization of food in the pantry (for example, when added to fatty foods such as margarine, they can help prevent it from going rancid) and they have a similar role to play in the body. The importance of this is that surplus LDL blood cholesterol needs to be oxidized before it can form the plaques, and so a diet rich in antioxidants can help prevent the furring up of the arteries that leads to atherosclerosis.

The chief antioxidants are vitamins C, E, and beta-carotene, the mineral selenium, and various and numerous phytochemicals, such as flavonoids (found in citrus fruits and other fruits), lycopene (found in tomatoes, ruby grapefruits, and watermelon), quercetin (found in tea, onions, apples, and red wine), and the glucosinolates (found in broccoli and kale). Olive oil also seems to make LDL cholesterol more resistant to oxidation, and garlic, too, is an antioxidant.

■ Heart disease and supplements

Several large trials have been carried out to see if dietary supplementation, primarily with the antioxidant vitamins C, E, and beta-carotene, can help reduce incidence of and deaths from CHD. Results have been varied (indeed one major review for the World Health Organization found that mortality from heart disease increased in smokers who took beta-carotene supplements), and the message from experts is that it is better to get adequate nutrients from a varied diet high in fruits and vegetables than to rely on supplementation. One reason is that eating natural foods minimizes the risk of "overdosing" on one particular nutrient; another is that it may be an array of different elements that offer protection (phytochemicals working together, for example), rather than just one.

One problem is that there is no definitive amount of any vitamin, nutrient, or phytochemical that is known to offer protection, because there are so many variables: for example, other risk factors for CHD (e.g., smoking increases the need for antioxidants), diet (e.g., high intakes of polyunsaturated fats such as sunflower oil increase the need for vitamin E). However some experts think that the current RDIs of various nutrients may be too low for optimum protection from diseases such as CHD, and others say that it is hard to get adequate amounts of vitamin E from a normal diet.

For more information on antioxidants see page 24, and for more information on supplements see page 146. The Healthy Heart Diet appears on page 142.

HEMORRHOIDS

■ THESE ARE VARICOSE-VEIN-LIKE SWELLINGS of the blood vessels in the wall of the anus, and are usually a result of prolonged constipation, or occasionally chronic diarrhea or IBS, which may irritate the veins. Straining to pass stools disrupts the support around the tissue, which becomes displaced and congested. Hemorrhoids are not caused by sitting on cold seats or hot radiators! The pressure that builds up can cause the swellings to prolapse or protrude from the anus, when they are known as external (rather than internal) hemorrhoids.

They often occur in people in middle and old age, and may also occur in pregnancy, when blood flow in the lower abdomen may alter, and constipation can be a problem. Hemorrhoids may be painful, and a common symptom is bright red blood in the toilet after passing stools. Once symptoms are noticed, you should see a physician to check that your problem is caused by hemorrhoids.

SOLUTIONS

Dietary prevention is similar to that of constipation, with plenty of high-fiber foods, water, and fresh fruit, and vegetables. A mash of linseeds, available from the healthfood store, may be helpful.

HERPES SIMPLEX 1

■ COLD SORES are caused by the herpes 1 virus, which is related to the other herpes viruses: genital herpes (simplex 2) and chicken pox (herpes zoster), which may cause shingles later in life. It is not thought that having one form of the virus can make you more likely to get the others. Herpes 1 virus usually produces an initial attack, which can make the sufferer quite ill—a cold sore appears, usually around the mouth, and there may be fever, headache, aches and pains, and lethargy. The attack can last a week, and the sore take up to two weeks to go. The virus then lies dormant in the body and may produce other cold sores in the future (usually with less severe side effects), particularly if you are run down or stressed, or when your immune system has been weakened for any reason.

SOLUTIONS

By keeping the immune system as strong as possible, the likelihood of frequent recurrence of cold sores is reduced. If they do appear, they will be milder and of shorter duration. Correct diet is important in achieving this—you should regularly eat foods that are rich in immune-boosting nutrients zinc, vitamins C, A, and E, and essential fatty acids found in oily fish and olive and sunflower oils. Best sources of vitamin C are those rich in flavonoids, such as citrus fruit and black currants. Other "best sources" lists appear in Section One.

You should also take plenty of garlic, onions, ginger, and thyme. Black and green tea are useful for the quercetin and catechins they contain, which have been shown to be antiviral. Iron deficiency may be linked to cold sores as well; best sources of iron are listed on page 30. There is some evidence that the protein amino acid lysine helps block the herpes virus. Lysine-rich foods are lamb, fish, chicken, and milk.

The herb echinacea is a powerful immune strengthener. If you feel a cold sore attack is imminent (usually a tingling around the mouth will tell you), take 8–10 drops in warm water twice a day for a week. Also, dab a little tea tree oil onto the tingling area. The Immune-Strengthening Diet on page 143 is ideal to help prevent cold sores or to reduce their duration if one appears.

HIV, see AIDS and HIV

■ ALSO KNOWN AS "attention deficit hyperactivity disorder," this is a condition that effects up to one in ten children (though most will have only mild or moderate symptoms) and can continue on into adolescence, or even begin then. Its symptoms are disturbed behavior, such as overactivity and fidgeting, distractibility, impulsiveness, inability to concentrate, and aggressiveness.

For the one in two hundred children who do have severe symptoms, life for everyone involved, at home, at school, and socially, can be difficult.

SOLUTIONS

Diet is thought by some experts to play a large part in causing hyperactivity. Diet from weaning onward should be low in processed and highly refined foods, particularly those containing artificial additives, and drinks high in caffeine and additives, such as cola. Other foods that often seem to cause hyperactivity are

chocolate and fresh orange or apple juice. In some cases, further food intolerances may be involved, and a carefully supervised elimination diet may be indicated.

The diet should contain adequate amounts of all the necessary nutrients, by ensuring the child receives three good meals a day with plenty of fresh and home-cooked ingredients. Each hyperactive child should receive personal dietary advice and nutrient supplementation given as necessary.

Supplements found to be effective include zinc taken as a liquid supplement, magnesium, vitamin B complex, and the essential fatty acids DHA, GLA, and vitamin E. For more information on children's healthy diet and feeding problems, see Section Three.

Hypertension, see Blood Pressure

■ HYPOGLYCEMIA is commonly known as "low blood sugar." Hypoglycemic symptoms include feeling dizzy and/or weak, palpitations and tremor, feeling "spaced out," and often hungry. Hypoglycemia can be a problem for diabetes sufferers when the level of insulin in the body isn't matched by correct food intake. Prolonged or extreme physical effort (such as marathon running) without adequate intake of carbohydrate can also result in low blood sugar. To avoid this, runners take sugary drinks along the route, and other athletes, like professional tennis players, take drinks and eat bananas (a quickly digested source of starch and sugars that will rapidly provide a source of blood glucose).

Poor dietary habits can also result in hypoglycemia for ordinary people. If meals are skipped, blood sugar levels can dip. This will be compounded if a meal

HYPERACTIVITY

HYPOGLYCEMIA

is then eaten that is high in refined carbohydrate, such as sugars and snack foods, which is absorbed rapidly into the bloodstream. The body releases an overabundance of insulin to cope with this sudden influx, and within an hour or more hypoglycemic symptoms may begin again. Alcohol has a similar effect to sugary foods.

Some people seem more prone to fluctuating blood sugar levels than others. Women may find they suffer more before a period (see Menstrual Problems); caffeine and cigarette smoking may exacerbate the problem.

There is also some evidence that a chromium deficiency may be a cause of low blood sugar levels, but chromium is best taken naturally in chromium-rich foods, such as shellfish, cheese, whole grains, and legumes.

SOLUTIONS

Hypoglycemia can be controlled by a sensible and healthy diet (see Basic Healthy Diet, page 53) and by eating "little and often." The diet should contain plenty of wholefoods and enough protein, which will release their energy slowly into the bloodstream and thus keep blood sugar levels on a more even keel.

Sugary snacks when you are hungry should be avoided. Ideal between-meal snacks are small pieces of low-fat cheese with a rice cake, or an apple and some low-fat yogurt.

For more information on foods for maintaining even blood sugar levels, see Glycemic Index in Section Four. See also Diabetes.

IMPOTENCE

■ DIET DOESN'T APPEAR TO PLAY a large part in preventing or curing male impotence (failure to get or maintain an erection), but there are some dietary tips that may help the problem, the most important of which is to eat a diet rich in the mineral zinc. Some research shows that zinc deficiency is linked with a lack of the male sex hormone testosterone, and trials have shown a return to potency for men with low zinc levels after supplementation. For a list of the best sources of zinc in the diet, turn to page 31. Zinc supplements are available over the counter and are best taken with vitamin C. It is also wise to avoid caffeine, which can affect absorption of zinc. However, if a male is not deficient in zinc, taking extra is unlikely to be of any benefit.

One alcoholic drink may help relaxation and enhance libido that way, but too much alcohol is associated with loss of libido (by reducing the long-term production of male hormones) and loss of sensitivity in the sexual organs. Long term, a healthy diet low in saturated fats and cholesterol and high in antioxidants and fruit and vegetables (such as the Basic Healthy Diet, page 53) will help maintain potency, as tests have shown that a cause of impotency is blocked arteries to the penis.

A diet rich in garlic will also help to thin the blood and maintain good circulation. Stress is frequently a cause of impotence, and in such cases relaxation techniques and the anti-stress diet hints on page 138 may help.

INFECTIONS

■ AS BACTERIA ARE BECOMING more and more resistant to our usual antibiotic drugs, and viruses are rarely killed by antibiotics in any case, it is important to find natural ways to fight infection. We now know that several foods and herbs do have strong antiviral, antibacterial, and antifungal effects, and it is likely that in the next few years many more important discoveries will be made in this field.

To ward off infections of the respiratory system, digestive and urinary system, and the skin and eyes, and to help minimize the effects of bacterial problems such as food poisoning, a general healthy diet (Basic Healthy Diet, page 53) should be followed. Or, at times of particular stress or vulnerability, the Immune-Strengthening Diet (page 143) can be followed.

Once an infection has set in, try the following:

* **Garlic** and its less powerful but still effective relatives, onion and leek, have been used as an infection-fighter for thousands of years all over the world. Scientists are now beginning to discover not only that garlic does work, but how it works. Fresh raw garlic can not only kill bugs, such as listeria and salmonella, but will also kill the new "superbugs" that antibiotics don't work on any more. Its main active ingredient is allicin, which, sadly, becomes much less potent when the garlic is crushed and then stored before using, or when cooked. Garlic is an expectorant and can help ease symptoms of coughs and colds. Raw garlic can be eaten in salads or dressings, such as pesto and salsa. Or, high-quality garlic capsules can be taken.

* **Honey** is very useful for skin infections, and rubbed on wounds and burns, it has been shown to heal the skin, leaving minimal scarring. It can also be used to treat mouth ulcers, the fungal infection athlete's foot, and the eye infection conjunctivitis. Internally, honey will help ease coughs and sore throat.

HERBS TO FIGHT INFECTION

Several herbs have antibacterial effects. Thyme is one of the most powerful of the herbal antiseptics. Others are sage and rosemary, which, along with thyme, are best used fresh in cooking and in salads or as an infusion to drink, or can be gargled if sore throat is a problem. Infused mustard seeds also make a good gargle for tonsillitis and throat infections. Oils of peppermint, eucalyptus, lavender, and thyme can be used in solution for skin infections.

* Green tea has been shown to help kill bacteria when taken as an infusion, and can also be used as a bathing fluid for skin infections.

* Ginger Fresh gingerroot is thought to be a mild antibacterial food, which will also help to clear up chesty coughs and colds. Use it grated in cooking, or infuse for a drink with honey and lemon.

* Lemon An antioxidant and antiseptic, lemon is, of course, rich in vitamin C (see next paragraph). Taken as juice, with ginger and honey, it is an ideal drink for sufferers of coughs, colds, bronchial problems, and flu.

* Vitamin C Long talked about as a "cure" for colds, it is now recognized that lack of C-rich foods can be a factor. For best sources, see page 25. A daily supplement of up to 500 mg with added bioflavonoids (phytochemicals that help the vitamin be effective) may shorten length and severity of an infection.

See also entries for Colds, Bronchitis and Coughs, etc.

INFERTILITY

FEMALE INFERTILITY—inability to conceive—may be due to several different medical or physical problems, but diet does play an important role. Regular menstruation and a reasonable body weight are both linked to ease of conception. Women who over-exercise and/or who follow over-restricted diets, which contain neither enough calories nor enough nutrients, may cease menstruating and, therefore, at least temporarily, fail to ovulate. A certain amount of body fat, which helps regulate hormone levels, and a Body Mass Index (page 188) between 20 and 25 are important factors in conception. Anorexics and people who exercise a great deal professionally, such as sportswomen and dancers, are frequently unable to conceive; if a sensible diet is followed and less exercise taken, however, periods can

usually be restored to normal. Recent studies show that women who are trying to conceive should not drink alcohol.

Obesity can also cause infertility, probably by hampering ovulation, so a BMI over 30 should indicate a weight-loss diet. A general basic healthy diet, containing all the nutrients for good health, will help to facilitate conception. New evidence shows that the polyphenols in tea may increase fertility. For more information on pre-conceptual care and on eating for a pregnancy, see Section Three.

Male fertility can be boosted with an adequate intake of zinc-rich foods (see best sources list on page 31) and with a diet high in vitamin C, essential fatty acids, and selenium. All males intending to father a baby should eat a general basic healthy diet—preferably organic, as chemical residues may reduce fertility—cut down on alcohol, caffeine, and smoking, and get plenty of exercise.

INSOMNIA

INSOMNIA—the inability to "get a good night's sleep"—is frequently related to psychological symptoms such as stress, anxiety, and depression. For more information on these conditions, see the appropriate separate entry. Prescription sleeping pills can be an occasional effective remedy, but, used too frequently, the body adapts to them so that they work less well. When you try to do without them, insomnia can be even worse than before. Therefore, natural remedies—of which there are plenty—are a more sensible idea.

SOLUTIONS

Regular exercise is an important factor in good sleep—according to research, a daily walk or other activity in fresh air produces a 50% improvement in sleep patterns. Before bed, a warm bath sprinkled with some calming essential oils, such as lavender or ylang ylang, aids relaxation.

The right diet can do much to help you get a good night's sleep. In general, avoid both overeating in the evening (which can cause sleeplessness through indigestion) and going to bed hungry, which will keep you awake. The ideal pattern of eating in the evening is to have a medium-sized meal no later than three hours before bedtime, consisting mainly of complex carbohydrates, such as pasta, rice, or potatoes, and vegetables, with a small amount of low- or medium-fat protein, such as fish or chicken, eggs, lean meat, or low-fat cheese.

Research shows that carbohydrate foods have a calming effect upon the brain, probably because they stimulate the production of a chemical called serotonin, sometimes referred to as the "happy" chemical, because of its ability to produce a good mood. A low-carbohydrate, high-protein supper, such as a steak and green salad, tends to have a "stimulating" effect. However, small amounts of protein are important in your evening meal, as they help to provide the amino acid tryptophan, which, in turn, converts to serotonin as discussed above.

People who sleep badly in winter, but not in summer, may be suffering from low serotonin production, as production naturally decreases in winter. This can be increased with light therapy—or a winter vacation in the sun! Before bedtime it is a good idea to have a small snack or drink rich in both carbohydrate and tryptophan-containing proteins, such as hot milk and a graham cracker, a banana, a rice cake, and a little low-fat cheese (unless cheese disagrees with you if eaten later in the evening, see above), or peanut butter on bread.

A drink is most easily digested—and milk really is the perfect bedtime drink, because not only does it contain tryptophan in the milk protein, it also contains carbohydrate in the form of the milk sugar lactose, and is an excellent source of the mineral calcium, which is some-

FOODS AND DRINKS TO AVOID FOR INSOMNIA

* Caffeine-rich strong coffee and cola drinks
Cocoa contains caffeine, so a malted drink is better if you prefer that to plain milk. Caffeine is a stimulant and will help to keep you awake.

* Alcohol
One drink may help you to get to sleep, but too much alcohol effects REM sleep and blood sugar levels, which may be an important cause of waking in the middle of the night. Beer contains hops, which are a known sedative.

* "Bad dream" foods
Some foods, such as cheese and red meat, seem to spark off bad dreams and nightmares in some people. If you think this may be a problem, try eliminating these foods from your diet in the evening.

times called "nature's tranquilizer." Insomniacs should ensure they get adequate calcium in their diet (see best sources list on page 29, plus RDI) and also magnesium, which may also be a calming mineral.

There are several herbs that are natural tranquilizers and sleep-inducers. Chamomile, lettuce, passion flower, valerian, and lemon balm all have a reported effect.

IRRITABLE BOWEL SYNDROME

■ ONE IN FIVE OF THE US POPULATION is said to suffer from IBS, and it affects twice as many women as men. Sometimes called spastic colon, symptoms are abdominal pain, which is related to bowel function, with either constipation or diarrhea present, and perhaps nausea, wind, bloated stomach, an urgent need to empty the bowels, a feeling of incomplete emptying, passage of mucus, and sharp pains in the rectum. These may often be accompanied by depression, fatigue, backache, and other symptoms.

The cause of IBS is not certain, One major study found that 10% of cases develop after an acute bout of diarrhea. Another possible cause is food intolerance, and wheat and dairy products appear to be two foods strongly associated with IBS. Others are coffee, potatoes, corn, onion, beef, oats, cheese, and white wine. A low-sugar and low-yeast diet may also help. However, virtually any food or drink may provoke an individual response. Intolerances should be investigated with the help of a dietitian. See Allergies, page 88.

There is also an association between IBS and psychological factors. One study reported that two-thirds of IBS sufferers have experienced severe stress before onset of symptoms, and stress may significantly or certainly worsen symptoms for some (see page 134).

SOLUTIONS

During an attack, it is wise to avoid high intakes of tea, coffee, cola, sodas, and alcohol (although some people report that alcohol helps), and excessive intake of wheat bran, wind-forming vegetables, such as cabbage and Brussels sprouts, and under-ripe fruit (see Flatulence).

Aloe vera, slippery elm, and evening primrose oil have all been used successfully in some cases. Peppermint tea is antispasmodic, and fresh ginger tea will help nausea. Long term, a basic healthy diet, with regular relaxed meals eaten slowly and thoroughly chewed, will help. For IBS with constipation, a high-fiber diet is helpful, but raw bran should be avoided. Soluble fiber—found in greatest quantities in fruits, oats, legumes, and linseed—may help (for a best sources list, see page 14). Fluid intake of 4 pints (1.75 liters) a day is recommended.

See also the Colitis entry.

KIDNEY STONES

KIDNEY STONES are usually made predominantly of calcium (and this is the type we discuss here), which is why it has always been presumed that a low-calcium diet would help to prevent them. This now appears not to be the case. Men are three times as likely to get kidney stones as women, and it now seems likely that, in fact, a calcium-rich diet can help to prevent the stones, which may be formed when oxalate-rich foods, such as rhubarb, tea, beets, spinach, peanuts, and chocolate, are eaten. Calcium may interfere with the absorption of the oxalates. It has also been shown that a basic healthy diet—rich in fruits and vegetables and high-potassium foods, such as bananas and dried apricots, high in fluids and with not too much meat protein—helps to prevent stones from forming in the first place.

Mastalgia, see Menstrual Problems

ME

MYALGIC ENCEPHALOMYELITIS, also known as ME, chronic fatigue syndrome, and post-viral fatigue syndrome, is said to affect 4–10 people per 100,000 adults and about 80% of those affected are women. It is often described as feeling like a severe hangover or influenza with muscle pain and deep exhaustion (as if having run a marathon) all at the same time.

The effects of the syndrome can last for months or even years, and is highly disabling—sufferers frequently have to give up work or school. The diagnosis is often not accepted or recognized by the medical profession.

The name myalgic encephalomyelitis is probably a misnomer, as it implies chronic inflammation of the brain and spinal cord, and there is no evidence of this in sufferers.

Other symptoms can include sore throat, tender lymph glands, feverishness, poor memory and concentration, abnormal sleep patterns, depression, mood changes, and bowel problems, e.g., IBS. Symptoms can vary from day to day, or within the day, and are often worse after exertion.

ME may result from an infection, but sometimes seems to come on for no real apparent reason. It may develop in the wake of a stressful event, or there may be gradual onset.

SOLUTIONS
The Immune-Strengthening Diet (page 143) may be useful in helping to prevent ME. Otherwise, follow a basic healthy diet, including plenty of fresh fruits and vegetables, oily fish, and whole grains. Foods rich in potassium may be helpful (see page 32).

Known food intolerances should be avoided. For people with irritable bowel syndrome or other symptoms that may be caused by allergy or intolerance, sufferers may like to try an elimination diet as explained in Allergies, with the help and guidance of an experienced dietitian.

For some, various dietary supplements seem to help. One trial showed quite significant improvement in symptoms with a regular combination of evening primrose oil and fish oils. Another showed that a course of magnesium injections helped—oral magnesium may also be helpful. Other suggestions have included supplements of multivitamins/ minerals, vitamin E, zinc, C, and co-enzyme Q10.

See also the Fatigue entry.

MEMORY, POOR

SLIGHT LOSS OF MEMORY is quite common as we age, and this isn't necessarily a sign of the beginnings of Alzheimer's Disease, although loss of memory, particularly short-term memory, is a symptom of that. Many women report a deterioration in their memory at the time of the menopause, and others find their memory is worse in the few days before a period, both of which are probably connected to changing hormone levels.

The disorder hypothyroidism also produces loss of memory as one of its early symptoms. If you also have problems with tiredness and constipation, and tend to feel cold all the time, it may be worth seeing your doctor to have him check out your thyroid function.

SOLUTIONS
Help your memory to stay in top condition throughout your life with a basic healthy diet rich in the antioxidant vitamins A, C, and (especially) E; and eat plenty of foods rich in B-group vitamins, especially B1.

A recent study showed that people deficient in B1 had poor memories, which were improved with supplementation. (However don't take supplements of B1 alone; you should take the B group together.)

Include in your diet plenty of essential fatty acids, found in oily fish, vegetable oils, olive oil, evening primrose oil, and linseed oil.

BRAIN BOOSTERS

Supplements of ginkgo biloba are claimed to increase brain capacity and memory, and Siberian ginseng is said to have a similar effect. Excess intake of alcohol will impair short-term memory, and may impair long-term memory, too, although studies on this are divided.

MENSTRUAL PROBLEMS

PROBABLY THE MOST COMMON COMPLAINT associated with periods is premenstrual syndrome, or PMS, the various symptoms of which—such as weight gain, fluid retention, bloating, food cravings, breast pain, tiredness, and depression—appear in the 4–10 days before a woman's period begins and disappear a day or two after it has started. These symptoms are caused by changing levels of the hormones progesterone and estrogen, and all can be helped with dietary intervention and/or supplements.

Heavy bleeding, or menorrhagia, can be a problem from time to time, particularly in the teens and when women near the menopause. If you regularly suffer from heavy periods, you should get checked by your physician, who may diagnose an under-active thyroid, often present when there is also weight gain, dry skin, and lethargy. Iron supplements, taken with plenty of vitamin C, may be needed to correct iron-deficiency anemia.

Painful periods (dysmenorrhea), with or without heavy bleeding, can be eased through exercise, such as walking and yoga, extra EFAs, and supplements of calcium and magnesium. The herb meadowsweet is a natural analgesic, and foods high in tryptophan may help pain by producing a calmer mood.

Absence of periods (amenorrhea) is usually a sign of pregnancy, which is the first option to have checked. Other reasons are stress, over-exercise, and under-eating. Any woman who loses a lot of weight quickly, goes on a crash diet, or, for any other reason, doesn't eat enough, risks amenorrhea. Prolonged amenorrhea can result in osteoporosis and possible infertility. Periods will usually return if lifestyle and eating habits return to normal. Periods can also cease due to the effects of diabetes or an over-active thyroid.

SOLUTIONS
The basic healthy diet is a good starting point for eating on most days of the month. It contains all the nutrients you need for healthy periods. These are: enough calories to maintain a reasonable body weight; and enough essential fatty acids, B and E vitamins, iron, zinc, calcium, and magnesium to keep the female hormone system functioning well.

However, to alleviate—or even prevent—the PMS symptoms, or whichever ones you may get, a little further dietary help may be necessary.

* **Watch the salt.** Fluid retention is a natural occurrence before a period, accounting for up to 7 lb (3.25 kg) of extra weight, but if you watch your intake of salt (see high-salt foods list on page 33) and refined carbohydrates, such as white bread, cakes, and cookies, fluid retention will be kept to a minimum, and stomach bloating and breast tenderness will also be helped. You should also eat plenty of potassium-rich foods, which have a role in fluid elimination. See also Fluid Retention, page 113.

* **Eat extra vitamin B-rich foods** including yeast extract, whole grains, and dark green leafy vegetables. The vitamin B group is important for healthy nerve functioning and is depleted when we are under stress. Vitamin B6, in particular, has been found to be important in minimizing PMS, because it helps to break down estrogens, and high doses up to 200 mg have been used by therapists with success. However, latest UK government recommendations suggest that vitamin B supplements available over the counter should contain no more than 10 mg B6 per day's intake because, they say, large doses can cause nerve damage. Many nutritionists disagree with this. Women wishing to increase their B6 intake through food should eat wheat germ, legumes, whole grains, oily fish, bananas, and poultry (see the best sources list, page 26).

* **Eat more essential fatty acids,** found in vegetable oils, fish oils, nuts and seeds, and in supplements of evening primrose oil, linseed oil, and starflower oil. The EFAs are particularly useful in helping to prevent breast tenderness (mastalgia). One research study showed that two-thirds of women with premenstrual breast pain had lower levels of EFAs than other women. Mastalgia is caused by increasing levels of estrogen, and the link is probably that EFAs somehow reduce the sensitivity to this hormone. Vitamin E appears to have a similar effect.

* **There is some research** to show that extra calcium and magnesium in the diet can help ease PMS—up to 1 g of calcium and 200–300 mg of magnesium a day may be the optimum level.

* **Food cravings** in the week before a period can be controlled by following the tips in the Hypoglycemia (low blood sugar) entry and by avoiding alcohol. Low moods and depression can be alleviated by a diet high in complex carbohydrates, such as whole grains and legumes, and by eating tryptophan-rich foods (see Insomnia), which produce the mood-lifting chemical serotonin. Bananas are a particularly ideal food before a period, as they are high in serotonin, potassium, vitamin B6, and carbohydrate.

* **Constipation** can be a problem before a period—follow all the advice under the separate entry.

* **For undue tiredness,** see separate entry on Fatigue; however, tiredness will be reduced to a minimum in most cases with the other tips in this entry.

* **Iron deficiency** could also be a problem if periods are heavy (see page 126).

* **Drink plenty of fluids**, preferably natural water, before a period (this will not make fluid retention worse), and cut down on consumption of both caffeine and alcohol.

* **PMS** is often helped by solving any food allergy or intolerance problems; for some, an "anti-candida" diet may help.

See the PMS and Diuretic Diet on page 145.

MIGRAINE AND HEADACHES

■ COMMON MIGRAINE—a severe throbbing headache, which is often one-sided and may be associated with nausea, vomiting, and aversion to bright lights or noise—affects one in ten of the population and is twice as frequent in women. First attacks usually occur between childhood and early adulthood, with 90% first occurring before the age of 40, although menopausal women sometimes experience a first attack at this time, probably because of reducing levels of the hormone estrogen. In women, attacks may also occur more frequently pre-menstruation and less frequently during pregnancy, again no doubt due to the changing estrogen levels.

Classic migraine, which affects 20% of sufferers, includes all the above symptoms, but also aura, which may include flashing lights, split- or half-vision, blind spots, and mood changes before the attack begins. Migraine can last from a few hours to three days, and can occur rarely or as frequently as 2–3 times a week.

Research indicates that there are very many triggers for migraine, several of which are dietary. In general, skipping meals and any crash or severe diets are to be avoided as they can cause hypoglycemia (low blood sugar), which may precipitate an attack. Regular meals, adequate fluid intake, and plenty of foods rich in magnesium (see best sources list on page 32) and oily fish are all thought to help prevent migraine.

Individual foods can also trigger an attack. Cheese and chocolate contain amines called tyramine and phenylethylamine, which may trigger an attack. Caffeine over-consumption, or even withdrawal, may well set off a reaction. Red wine contains phenolic flavonoids, which can cause migraine in some people. Many other foods can start a migraine and this is thought to be due to allergy or food intolerance. The mechanism by which a particular food triggers a migraine is not yet fully understood, but published trials have shown that up to 70% of migraines in adults may be caused by various foods. Another trial in children has shown that, if the trigger foods can be avoided, other known triggers for migraine, such as perfume and cigarette smoke, no longer provoke a migraine. In view of these results, if other typical allergic symptoms are present, such as urticaria or irritable bowel syndrome, then an elimination diet as explained on page 89 in the Allergy entry may be a good idea.

■ Other headaches

Headaches can be caused by many factors, including eye problems, hangover, allergy, catarrh, infection, high blood pressure, stress, and hypoglycemia. Check the different entries for all these. Other causes can be poor posture, dehydration, and a diet that is high in protein and low in carbohydrate. See the Basic Healthy Diet on page 53 for information on improving the balance of your diet. Persistent headache or migraine should be checked by your physician.

MOUTH ULCERS

■ SMALL PAINFUL ULCERS inside the mouth, also called canker sores, are a common occurrence, and it is often not at all easy to pinpoint the exact reason for a flare-up. However, certain food intolerances may cause them, and they can be a symptom of celiac disease—see Allergies. Dairy products, wheat, strawberries, yeast extract products, tomatoes, and even oranges may be to blame.

NATURAL REMEDIES FOR MOUTH ULCERS

✳ Eat some plain yogurt, high in acidophilus bacteria, every day. Keep it in the mouth as long as you can—these "healthy" bacteria may clear the ulcer up more quickly.

✳ Put honey (set, not clear) on the ulcer—honey is antiseptic, soothing, and healing, and will stay in place for longer than most of the gels that are sold for mouth ulcers.

✳ Eat plenty of garlic, also an antiseptic. Try opening a garlic capsule and dabbing the contents on the ulcer.

✳ Sage leaves are said to heal mouth ulcers—crush a leaf lightly and dab it onto the ulcer directly, or make a strong infusion and, when cool, use as a mouthwash.

✳ The herb echinacea is said to help—use tincture of echinacea to dab on the ulcer, or dilute in warm water and use as a mouthwash.

SOLUTIONS

If you think a particular food may be the problem, you could try excluding that food from your diet. If ulcers recur, you will know that food wasn't to blame and you could try eliminating another one. However, this type of exclusion diet needs to be carried out prudently, eliminating only one food at a time, otherwise nutritional deficiencies can occur. For example, dairy products are an important source of calcium and protein.

People who are run-down or recovering from illness, or under great stress, may be more likely to get mouth ulcers. Try the Immune-Strengthening Diet or the anti-stress diet hints, pages 143 and 138. A diet low in vitamins, minerals, and other nutrients, and high in junk foods, may also be a factor. Follow the Basic Healthy Diet on page 53 and include plenty of vitamin B-rich foods and iron (for best

sources lists, see pages 26 and 30).

Acid foods in general will be painful to eat while you have a mouth ulcer—avoid ketchup, vinegar, vinaigrette dressing, citrus fruits, tomatoes, and so on, until the ulcer has gone.

MUSCULAR PAIN AND RHEUMATISM

■ MUSCULAR PAIN can be caused by any activity you are not used to—e.g., a bicycle ride, if you haven't cycled for years, will cause a build-up of lactic acid in the used muscles and result in them aching, a result that can be minimized by doing stretching exercises on the used muscles immediately before and after the activity. Another prevalent muscular pain is cramp, and a further common cause of aching muscles, particularly in the neck, shoulders, and back, is stress anxiety or tension.

Muscular pain can also be associated with various other conditions, or called by various other names, and sometimes this involves what people often term "rheumatism." Rheumatism isn't, in fact, a real medical condition, but a blanket term used to cover all kinds of aches and pains in the joints, muscles, ligaments, and tissue. There may be local tender spots or pain, inflammation, "shooting" pains up limbs, stiffness, and, perhaps, swelling and general discomfort. Associated syndromes are polymyalgia, fibrositis, repetitive strain injury, tendonitis, ankylosing spondylitis, housemaid's knee, tennis elbow, and so on! Aches and pains associated with tiredness, fever, and weakness, and a general feeling of being unwell may, in fact, be rheumatoid arthritis. Joint pains may be osteoarthritis. See also the Arthritis entry.

SOLUTIONS

There is no guaranteed diet that you can follow to prevent muscular aches and rheumaticky problems, but the Basic Healthy Diet on page 53 is a good starting point, including plenty of essential fatty acids, which are known to help inflammation. Selenium, vitamin E, evening primrose oil, and cod liver oil may also be of help. Take extra selenium in the form of foods rich in the mineral (see best sources list on page 31); vitamin E, evening primrose oil, and cod liver oil may be taken as daily supplements. Any chronic or acute joint or related pain with no obvious cause should be discussed with your physician.

NAUSEA AND TRAVEL SICKNESS ■

NAUSEA, a feeling of queasiness or sickness that may or may not result in vomiting, can have various causes. A food allergy could be the cause (see Allergies). Frequent bouts of nausea that don't seem to have a cause may be a food intolerance (see also Allergies). In women, nausea is a fairly common side effect of PMS and can often be relieved by a small, low-fat, high-protein snack such as a spoonful of cottage cheese. It is also common in pregnancy; see the Pregnancy feature in Section Three (page 172).

If the problem is food poisoning, nausea will soon be followed by vomiting and diarrhea. Drink plenty of orange juice diluted with water and avoid food until the vomiting is over. Another likely cause of nausea, especially in children, is the onset of an infection. Again, plenty of fluids should be taken and food ignored until the child feels like eating again. Stress and worry can cause feelings of nausea, often associated with appetite loss. Eat small meals or take nutritious drinks until appetite returns; also see page 175.

Travel sickness is a type of nausea that happens because of the motion of traveling. One of the best cures for this is fresh ginger—some tests have shown it to be more effective than travel sickness pills from the pharmacy. Try an infusion of grated gingerroot half an hour before traveling, and eat a little crystallized ginger as you travel. To settle the stomach before bed after a day of traveling, a small glass of ginger ale may be a good idea. Peppermint alleviates nausea—a few peppermint candies will help, or peppermint tea.

Any unexplained nausea lasting more than a day should be discussed with your physician.

Nervousness, see Anxiety

Nettle Rash, see Urticaria

NEURALGIA ■

NEURALGIA is a blanket term for nerve-related pain in any part of the body, and can include pain from trapped or compressed nerves, as in a slipped disk or, sometimes, in late pregnancy; damaged nerves due to illness such as Multiple Sclerosis or viruses such as shingles; and the long-term pain that can carry on after the acute stage of shingles.

SOLUTIONS

The health of the body's nervous system is dependent, at least in part, upon a healthy diet, containing adequate supplies of all the nutrients, particularly the B vitamin group and vitamin E. Check out the best sources for these on pages 22–33, and follow the Basic Healthy Diet on page 53, including plenty of essential fatty acids. In one trial, high doses of vitamin E cured post-shingles nerve pain in almost three-quarters of sufferers. The herbs meadowsweet and chamomile are said to ease the pain of neuralgia. Meadowsweet is called "nature's aspirin." Both can be taken as an infusion. Elderberries are also said to be a good remedy for the pain.

Night Blindness, see Eye Problems

■ NOSEBLEED may be a symptom of high blood pressure—if you have a nosebleed it is wise to see your physician, to have this possibility investigated. Dietary advice similar to that for people with high blood pressure may be of use in preventing recurrence. The tannin in tea is said to help prevent nosebleed. Tea can be used as a drink, and cold tea bags or absorbent cotton soaked in tea can be used as a poultice over the nose to help stop bleeding. Nettle tea may have a similar effect.

Osteoarthritis, see Arthritis

■ OSTEOPOROSIS causes over 1.5 million bone fractures a year in the US. It affects approximately 75 million people in North America, Europe, and Japan, including one in three women aged 50 plus, and one in 12 men. It can effect all ages, but is most common in postmenopausal women, due to reduced levels of estrogen in the body after the menopause, which causes acceleration of loss of calcium and other minerals from the bones.

Osteoporosis is sometimes called "brittle bone disease," but that really is a misnomer—the condition happens when skeletal bone loses its substance and density, becoming thinner, more fragile, more porous, and therefore much more at risk of fracturing. People with the condition are sometimes unaware that they have low bone density until they suffer a fracture, which is why osteoporosis is often referred to as "the silent disease."

Areas commonly affected are the hips, spine, and wrists, and it can cause severe backache, pain, and disability, as well as loss of height—up to 5 in (12.5 cm)—and may cause spinal curvature, known as "dowager's hump." Once bone density is lost, as yet there is no complete cure, although progress is being made—for example, the drug alendronate sodium is claimed to rebuild bone at all affected sites and reduce the risk of fracture.

Still, the best method of dealing with osteoporosis is in prevention—particularly by building strong, large bones. The human skeleton is a dynamic structure that is constantly changing. A child's skeleton is totally rebuilt every two years, and an adult's every 7–10 years. When the bones stop growing in length (which happens by the late teens in most people), they still increase in density until about 30–35, when "peak bone mass" is reached. After this time, bone mass should be maintained by sensible precautions, including correct diet.

Maximizing the amount of bone in your body may mean that in later life, even if bone thinning occurs, enough bone density may be retained to prevent fractures. After the early thirties, there is a natural slow reduction of bone density in most people—approximately half a percent per year in both sexes, caused when the body loses more bone than it can replace. At menopause, and for the next five or so years after, there is a marked increase in the rate of bone loss (without intervention, see below), estimated at an average total loss of 15%. After this, loss slows down again.

■ **Factors that will help to achieve and maintain your peak bone mass are as follows:**

Calcium intake
Calcium is the major component of bone, and adequate amounts in the diet from birth are vital in order to reach peak bone density in adulthood. However, there is considerable debate over the optimum level to prevent osteoporosis. In the US, the National Institute of Health (1994) recommends higher levels of calcium intake than the RDI amounts (see page 28). The suggestions are 1,200–1500 mg for those aged 11–24, 1,000 mg for those between 25–50, and 1,500 mg for women over 51, unless on ERT/HRT, and for all over 65. But heredity, lifestyle, and other dietary factors, such as those discussed later in this entry, will affect everybody's personal optimum amount in any case. Best sources of calcium are listed on page 29.

Vitamin D intake
Adequate vitamin D is needed in order for calcium to be absorbed from foods. Vitamin D is obtained by the action of sunlight on the skin and from certain foods (for best sources list, see page 23).

Magnesium intake
Calcium and magnesium "work together" in the body, and magnesium is involved in a number of reactions in the formation of bone, which is why some experts believe that adequate magnesium intake is as important as calcium intake. For best sources list and RDIs, see page 32.

Essential fatty acid intake
The EFAs—found in fish oils, vegetable oils, and evening primrose oil, for example—are now thought to be important in helping to build and maintain bone mass by helping calcium absorption and delivery of calcium to the bones.

Intake of other nutrients
Bone health and maintenance may also be affected by a range of other nutrients, including vitamin K, zinc, folic acid, B6, vitamin C, and potassium (plus other trace elements that are rarely lacking in the diet). There is some evidence that the mineral boron may reduce loss of calcium and magnesium and increase estrogen and testosterone in the body, but more research needs to be done.

Maintenance of reasonable body weight

Thin people are more prone to osteoporosis than people with a sensible body mass index (or, indeed, than overweight people, although excess weight is not a sensible way to prevent osteoporosis, as it involves so many other health risks). This is because thin people may have lower levels of the hormone estrogen, which helps to prevent bone loss, and because they have less weight to carry around, thus minimizing the beneficial effects of weight-bearing exercise (see below).

Also, if diet is seriously inadequate, menstrual periods may become infrequent, or cease completely, and this will have a similar effect to early menopause (see below).

Weight-bearing exercise

Regular exercise that involves using the body's own resistance or weight (or any other type of weight) is an important factor in building and maintaining bone. Walking, dancing, or step exercising is weight-bearing exercise for the legs (but not the arms); tennis is a weight-bearing exercise for the racket-holding arm (in tests, players' playing arms have significantly more bone than the non-playing arms). Swimming is a non-weight-bearing exercise.

Weight-bearing exercise should be carried out regularly in moderate amounts, as excessive exercise may actually make osteoporosis more likely, not less (see Anorexia, Menstrual Problems).

Hormone replacement therapy

One of the major benefits of HRT for women of menopausal age is that the accelerated bone loss at this time, due to marked decrease in the body of the hormone estrogen, can be largely prevented. Estrogen replacement can reduce bone loss to premenopausal levels and therefore reduce fracture rates. Any woman considering HRT should see her physician to discuss the possibilities.

Soy-rich diet

Soybeans, and foods made from them, contain phytoestrogens (sometimes called isoflavones), which are natural substances that appear to mimic the body's estrogen hormones. In one study, postmenopausal women who took soy, to the equivalent of 2 glasses of soy milk a day, experienced no accelerated loss of bone density. Replacing some, or all, of your cows' milk daily allowance with soy milk may, therefore, be a good idea. However, soy milk is naturally much lower in calcium than cows' milk, and this is also important for healthy bones as we've seen, so it is best to choose a calcium-enriched soy milk. See also Menopause in Section Three, page 178.

■ Factors that may have a detrimental effect on your peak bone mass:

Inadequate intake

Inadequate intake of all the correct nutrients and/or calories (see above).

Sedentary lifestyle

Osteoporosis is on the increase worldwide, not only because the numbers of older people are increasing, but because of our sedentary lifestyles. Look at ways to build more mobility into your life, particularly weight-bearing exercise (above).

High-salt diet

A diet high in sodium causes increased excretion of calcium in the urine, and the higher the salt intake the greater the rate.

Alcohol intake

Heavy drinkers and alcoholics often suffer from low bone density. This may be because alcohol reduces absorption of calcium, a direct effect of alcohol on the bone, or through general malnutrition. However, one study has shown that moderate consumption of alcohol has no detrimental effect and may even have a beneficial effect on bone density.

It is possible to find out your risk of osteoporosis and fracture with a simple low-dose x-ray to measure your bone density. This is called a DXA scan and is becoming more widely available.

Cigarette smoking
Heavy smokers are more at risk of osteoporosis than other people. The longer you smoke, and the more you smoke, the higher the amount and rate of bone loss. The WHO cites double the risk.

Excess protein
Too much protein—particularly animal protein—in the diet can cause increased excretion of calcium in the urine. However, one study showed that in a high-protein diet more calcium is absorbed to "make up for" the extra calcium excreted, so perhaps excess protein may only be a problem if overall calcium intake is low. Therefore, it is wise to limit protein intake to no more than the recommended levels listed on page 20, unless advised otherwise by your dietitian or physician. Milk is an interesting food in this debate—it is one of the best sources of calcium, but is also a good source of protein. However, the lactose (milk sugars) it contains help the calcium to be absorbed and so, despite its protein content, it still is an excellent source of easily absorbed calcium.

Caffeine intake
Caffeine—found in coffee, tea, chocolate, cocoa, and cola drinks, as well as some food supplements such as guarana—increases calcium excretion in the urine; therefore, it is wise to limit intake of these, especially for individuals who may be at high risk of osteoporosis (see below). One major Norwegian study found that drinking more than nine cups of coffee a day almost doubled the risk of hip fracture in women—but, interestingly, not in men.

Intake of foods high in phytates and oxalates
Raw wheat bran, spinach, rhubarb, chocolate, and tea should be limited, because the phytates or oxalates they contain hinder calcium absorption.

High phosphate intake
Diets high in phosphate-containing items, such as sodas and processed foods, will limit calcium absorption.

Other factors, which may be unavoidable, can effect bone density and the likelihood of developing osteoporosis. These are: early menopause, early hysterectomy, long-term use of cortisteroids, irregular or infrequent periods (see Menstrual Problems, Anorexia), low body weight due to natural tendency, lack of sunshine and therefore of vitamin D, diseases such as hyperthyroidism and celiac disease (gluten intolerance), race (Caucasians and Asians have much greater risk of osteoporosis than black people), and genetic tendency—i.e., a family history of osteoporosis.

Calcium—to supplement or not?
As we've seen, an adequate intake of calcium is vital, especially in childhood and youth, in order to reach "peak bone mass." Yet, according to the WHO, data appears to show that optimum levels are not being met. In two separate trials, youngsters who received calcium supplementation achieved greater gain of bone mass than those who received no supplementation, and the WHO report suggests that intake of 1,000–1,600 mg a day appears to be optimal for children and young adults between the ages of 2 and 30. Many international experts suggest that calcium intake should be higher than the levels recommended. Levels such as this may not be easy to obtain through diet without consuming too many calories, so supplementation with calcium tablets may be advisable, especially if several of the risk factors are present. However, exactly what level of supplementation is necessary, and for how long, will continue to be debated.

Little data is available on the effects of supplementation for premenopausal adult women or males, but several studies have been carried out on the effects of extra calcium for postmenopausal women. Calcium supplementation has been shown to reduce bone loss and fracture, but the benefits appear to be greatest after the first five years beyond menopause. In the five-year period following menopause, calcium supplementation by itself doesn't seem to slow bone loss. In elderly people, both calcium and vitamin D supplements appear to retard bone loss and reduce the incidence of hip fractures.

PALPITATIONS
WHEN THE HEARTBEAT can be easily felt by a hand placed over the heart, and when the beat feels abnormal (very fast, for instance) and can be heard by the sufferer, the term palpitations is usually used. Sudden panic, fear, or nerves are very usual causes of palpitations—the adrenaline released at this time causes a sudden rise in blood pressure, with the palpitations as an immediate result. See Anxiety, and Stress.

SOLUTIONS
Find the cause of the nervousness and ensure adequate supplies of the vitamin B group within your diet. People of a nervous disposition, likely to experience palpitations, should cut down on caffeine in coffee, colas, chocolate, and tea, as this will exacerbate the problem.

Another likely cause of palpitations is low blood sugar or hypoglycemia. Eat little and often and never go for long periods without food. Eat a basic healthy diet and don't eat very large meals, which can in themselves cause palpitations, because the blood supply is diverted to the stomach and digestive system to cope with the amount of food.

Anemia can cause palpitations. If you also feel tired and are pale, weak, and generally lethargic, check with your physician to see if you are anemic.

PEPTIC ULCER

■ A PEPTIC ULCER—either gastric (when in the stomach) or duodenal (when in the duodenum or upper intestine)—is an open sore on the wall of the stomach or intestinal muscle, where the protective lining has worn away, made worse by the acid secretions in the stomach that aid breakdown of food. Peptic ulcers occur in about 2–3% of the population, are more common in men, and also have a hereditary factor.

It is now known that ulcers may often be caused by the bacterium Helicobacter pylori (especially duodenal ulcer), which is passed on through contact (e.g., between family members). Presence of this bacterium needs diagnosing by a medical specialist and treating with suitable antibiotics. Rarely, an ulcer may become so deep that it perforates the stomach or intestinal wall, which is a serious condition requiring immediate medical treatment.

Symptoms of a peptic ulcer are upper abdominal pain and, perhaps, nausea that comes and goes, is triggered by particular foods, and is often worst at night.

SOLUTIONS

Medicines that neutralize the stomach acids will take away the pain. Triggers are frequently spicy foods, high-fat foods, and very rich foods, very hot or very cold foods, alcohol, tea, and coffee (including decaffeinated), and too much candy and chocolate. Smoking and some drugs, such as aspirin, can also cause peptic ulcers. Stress increases acid secretion, so sufferers should practice stress-reduction techniques and learn to relax when eating.

A suitable diet for helping to prevent peptic ulcers is one high in fiber, whole grains, and fresh fruit and vegetables, and with adequate essential fatty acids. Small frequent meals and avoidance of late-night eating, as well as chewing slowly and thoroughly, are also helpful. There may be slight continual blood loss from an ulcer, which may result in anemia, so a diet high in iron-rich foods may be important once an ulcer is formed.

Eradicating the Helicobacter bacterium significantly reduces peptic ulcer recurrence; essential fatty acids are thought to play a role in this by inhibiting the bacteria. EFAs also help by keeping the correct balance of mucus and acids in the stomach.

Post-Viral Fatigue Syndrome, see ME

PMS (premenstrual syndrome), see Menstrual Problems

Respiratory Problems, see Bronchitis and Coughs, and Asthma

Rheumatism, see Muscular Pain and Rheumatism

Rheumatoid Arthritis, see Arthritis

Shingles, see Herpes Simplex 1

Sinusitis, see Colds and Flu

SKIN, DRY

DRY, FLAKY SKIN with no other symptoms (such as rash, redness, swelling, or itching) is a common complaint, and even people who have oily or normal skin in youth and young adulthood may suffer from dry skin as they get older, which may wrinkle more easily.

SOLUTIONS

To help maintain the skin's natural moisture balance, eat the Basic Healthy Diet (page 53), with adequate essential fatty acids from vegetable oils, fish oils, linseed and evening primrose oils, and so on. Don't try to follow a diet too low in fat, e.g., a fat-free diet, as we all need some fat in our diets. Any diet providing less than 20% of its total calories as fat may result in dry skin. Don't try to maintain too low a body weight, either.

Get adequate vitamin E in your diet (for best sources list, see page 24), or supplement your diet with natural-source vitamin E (alpha or a-tocopherol, as opposed to synthetic vitamin E, alpha-dl tocopherol) capsules. In addition, use 2–3 of these every night on your skin as a "night cream"—split the capsules carefully and smooth the oil into the dry areas. To keep facial skin soft and supple, and minimize wrinkles, use the vitamin E "night cream" (again natural-source) every night from your late twenties onward. Once a week or so, make a face mask of ground oats and vitamin E, or EPO or linseed oil, and spread it on your dry patches (or face). Leave for 15 minutes, then rinse off gently with soft water.

Get plenty of all the antioxidants in your diet—vitamins A and C, as well as E, and the minerals selenium and zinc. These help to fight the free radicals that form in our bodies as a result of stress, pollution, illness, and various other reasons, and contribute to the aging process. For best sources of all these, see pages 22–33. For more information on the many different kinds of natural antioxidants, see Section One, page 24.

Drink 4 pints (1.75 liters) of water every day for your skin, and spray your face regularly with a water spray. Both cigarette smoking and too much alcohol can dry the skin and cause premature wrinkling, as can living in a smoky or centrally-heated atmosphere. Exposure to harsh elements, such as wind, sun, and frost, can dry the skin, and a sun-protection cream should be worn before spending time in such conditions.

STOMACHACHE

ABDOMINAL PAIN is a symptom of many different conditions and illnesses. Upper abdominal pain (around and just below the breastbone and to either side of the lower ribcage) may be caused by heartburn and indigestion, hiatus hernia, peptic ulcer, gallstones, or infection. Central abdominal pain (around the front and sides of the waistline) may be caused by food poisoning (see Diarrhea), constipation, irritable bowel syndrome, diverticulitis, appendicitis (see doctor immediately), ulcerative colitis, or Crohn's disease (see Colitis). Lower abdominal pain may be caused by flatulence, constipation, cystitis, or menstrual problems. General stomachaches may also be a symptom of allergies, anxiety, celiac disease, and stress, or, rarely, cancer of the stomach, colon, or bowel, or elsewhere within the body.

Stomachache that cannot be explained and which persists longer than a few days, should be investigated by your physician.

SOLUTIONS

Mild bouts of stomachache caused by problems such as indigestion, flatulence, or over-indulgence can be eased by herbal infusions of basil, dill, fennel, or peppermint.

STRESS

WHEN THE BODY IS UNDER STRESS, particularly long term stress, such as found in people with demanding jobs or perhaps long-term domestic problems or illness, it needs careful handling nutritionally in order both to minimize the stress and ensure that nutrient requirements are met. Stress tends to deplete the body of certain vital vitamins and minerals, and anyone under long-term stress should either be extra careful to incorporate plenty of these into the diet with the right foods, or should take supplements. The vitamin B group is largely responsible for the smooth running of the nervous system, and, as the B group is water-soluble and cannot be stored in the body for long, chronic stress will soon severely deplete it. The same applies to vitamin C, which most experts believe a stressed person will needed in much greater quantities than the RDI of 60 mg a day—200 mg is probably more appropriate.

The minerals zinc (which helps strengthen the immune system) and magnesium (which is excreted in greater amounts from the body when under stress) may need to be supplemented, or zinc- and magnesium-rich foods scrupulously incorporated into the diet (for best sources lists of all vitamins and minerals mentioned, see pages 22–33). Bodies depleted of vitamins B and C and zinc are also at increased risk of getting endless minor infections, colds, coughs, cold sores, and so on, because these are the

SYMPTOMS OF STRESS

Stress can have many other physical symptoms, such as eating disorders, fatigue, migraine, heartburn, impotence, insomnia, irritable bowel syndrome, memory problems, and muscular pain—see individual entries for these. Turn to page 138 for the diet tips for stress reduction. See also Anxiety, Depression.

nutrients that help to protect the immune system. This is why so often stressed-out people complain that they are "run down." The Immune-Strengthening Diet (page 143) will help in this case.

Stressed-out people may turn to alcohol or smoking for relief—both of which will make the nutritional problems worse, as both, like stress, also deplete the body of B and C vitamins and can hinder absorption of many others. The better (food) way to tackle stress relief is to eat plenty of complex carbohydrates, such as pasta and whole grains, which will assist the brain to calm down by helping to release the chemical serotonin. Long-term stress, and the higher levels of adrenaline it produces, raises the level of fats and cholesterol in the blood. This can be a contributing factor in increased risk of circulatory and heart diseases. Blood cholesterol and fats can be reduced by regular aerobic exercise, such as walking or cycling, which, happily, will also reduce stress, release tension, and make you fitter. For a Healthy Heart Diet, see page 142.

Stroke, see Heart Disease and Stroke

SUNBURN

THE BEST WAY TO TREAT SUNBURN is to avoid it—by building up to periods in the sun very gradually, by wearing sun-protection cream, and by wearing suitable clothing. There are also dietary means by which you can lower the risk of sunburn even when exposed to the sun. It is well documented that carotenoids—the orange pigment found in carrots, sweet potatoes, and dark leafy greens—offer protection against the harmful ultraviolet rays of the sun.

In early summer, or before going to a sunny climate, you can give yourself added protection by eating a large portion of carrots every day and including a selection of beta-carotene-rich vegetables and fruits in your diet for two weeks before exposing yourself to strong sun. There are also carotenoid supplement capsules. Extra carotenoids may make your skin look slightly orange, which is evidence that they are working to protect your skin. HOWEVER, it is important not to exceed stated doses for supplements or to eat more than normal quantities of carrots, as carotene toxicity can occur.

Recent research also indicates that essential fatty acids may also offer protection against sunburn. Volunteers took fish oil capsules for three months, by which time their sun-protection factor increased by a factor of three. It isn't clear yet whether it is only the essential fatty acids (omega-3s) in oily fish that achieve this result or whether the same benefit would be gained from eating other EFAs, such as are found in evening primrose oil, and sunflower and olive oils. It is possible that the high vitamin D content of oily fish may play a part, as vitamin D is also produced by the action of sunlight on the skin. But as the EFAs are essential to health in so many ways, with few drawbacks, and many of us don't get enough, it will do no harm to increase intake before exposure to sun.

A diet rich in all the antioxidants is also thought to be important in helping to protect the skin. If you do have sunburn, again eat a diet rich in the antioxidants, which help to fight the free radicals released when the skin is damaged.

Also take plenty of zinc-rich foods, as zinc is important to the healing process. Drink plenty of fluids, as sunburn causes dehydration. In addition, a vitamin E-rich oil applied to the skin will help. Alternatives are aloe vera gel, lavender oil diluted in a base, or, for slightly worse burns, tea tree cream.

Sunburn accompanied by fever, nausea, or delirium should be treated by a physician.

Tension, see Stress

Thrombosis, see Heart Disease and Stroke

Tiredness, see Fatigue

TONGUE, SORE

■ A SORE TONGUE that is smooth and bright or fiery red, may be caused by a type of anemia due to deficiency of vitamin B12 and sometimes iron and folate, or a vitamin B2 or B6 deficiency. Other symptoms such as tiredness may also be present, and your physician should make a diagnosis and then supplement your diet as necessary.

SOLUTIONS
A well-balanced nutrient-rich diet, such as the Basic Healthy Diet (page 53), should prevent this type of problem from occurring. A sore tongue accompanied by furring and, possibly, bad breath is probably caused by oral thrush, which may be linked with vaginal yeast infections (see Candida) and may also be present after you have taken antibiotics. Regular spoonfuls of live yogurt containing the bacteria acidophilus may help.

Ulcers on the tongue may be a symptom of celiac disease, but can also be due to allergies or food intolerances, or possibly sensitization to substances used in dental treatment. See also Mouth Ulcers. Occasionally, sore tongue may be caused by a severe protein malnutrition, but this should be diagnosed professionally.

TONSILLITIS

■ TONSILLITIS is an infection of the tonsils at the back of the throat. Tonsils become infected as a "first line of defense" against infection going down to the chest. Infections are more likely to take hold in someone who has lowered resistance or immunity, perhaps through overwork or stress of another kind, or

TOOTH DECAY IN CHILDREN
Children's teeth are particularly prone to decay, but the mineral fluoride is an important preventer. Tap water usually has fluoride added, as does toothpaste. Fluoride tablets can be bought if water isn't fluoridated. It is also important that children should get enough calcium (from which teeth are mainly formed) and magnesium, which works with calcium, as well as vitamin A. For best sources of all these, see pages 22–33.

perhaps through a diet deficient in the necessary vitamins, minerals, and so on, which we need to maintain a healthy immune system.

At times of stress, our bodies need more of these nutrients, so poor diet and stress together can be a "double blow" to the immune system, and can easily be followed by an infection such as tonsillitis. See Infections.

SOLUTIONS
Sore throat can be eased with drinks of honey and lemon juice diluted in warm water. Lemon contains vitamin C, which is an antioxidant, and honey is a known antiseptic soother. Gargles of infused sage leaves are said to help cure tonsillitis, and a drink of infused meadowsweet tea will lessen the pain.

When tonsillitis is bad, it is hard to eat a normal diet because swallowing hurts—soft foods, such as soups, purées, eggs, ice cream, and custards are, therefore, ideal. To avoid repeated bouts of tonsillitis and other similar throat infections, try the Immune-Strengthening Diet on page 143.

TOOTH DECAY

■ DENTAL CARIES are caused when the teeth become coated with plaque (a combination of food particles and bacteria). If the plaque isn't removed, the bacteria break it down and acid is formed, which may eventually dissolve the tooth enamel and eventually cause tooth decay. Tooth decay can nowadays largely be avoided.

SOLUTIONS
Regular brushing of teeth and flossing thoroughly, preferably soon after every meal and snack, removes the plaque before bacterial action can begin. Diet is also important. Some foods, and the way they are eaten, contribute more to the build-up of plaque than others. Sugary foods are quickly attacked by the bacteria, and acid is soon formed. Refined carbohydrates are also major offenders, as their residues appear to cling to the teeth readily. Any sweet or sticky food that remains in the mouth for a long time—for example, caramels—is particularly bad in this respect.

Poor dietary habits, such as frequently sucking sugary or fruit drinks through straws, will contribute to decay. Some "healthy" foods, such as dried fruits, produce plaque just as much as confectionery and sodas do, and even fruit juices also contain a lot of natural sugars that can contribute to the problem significantly.

If you can't brush your teeth right after eating or drinking something, eat a small piece of hard cheese and chew it thoroughly, as this helps to stop the formation of acid. Chewing on sugarfree gum also helps, as it increases saliva production and this, in turn, helps to disperse the acids.

Thrush, see Candida

Travel Sickness, see Nausea and Travel Sickness

Ulcer, see Peptic Ulcer

Ulcerative Colitis, see Colitis

URTICARIA

URTICARIA (HIVES OR NETTLE RASH) IS A SKIN RASH with, often, large, red, raised, very itchy patches and, perhaps, areas of white, resembling that of a nettle sting. The rash may last for several hours or days, and there may be other symptoms, such as nausea or fever. There are several different causes, of which food allergy is one. Shellfish and strawberries are frequently linked with the condition, but there are several non-food causes that trigger the rash, for example, heat, insect bites, drugs, or hot sun.

SOLUTIONS

Dietary treatment is to avoid the food(s) known to cause problems. In acute cases it is often possible to pinpoint the cause—otherwise, an elimination diet may be the answer (see Allergies). Other reported methods of control are using an "anti-candida diet" (see page 141) or a diet low in food additives and salicylates, including avoiding aspirin.

VARICOSE VEINS

VARICOSE VEINS are veins (most often to be found in the legs) that have become dilated with blood because the system of valves that ensures that the blood is pumped back to the heart through the veins has become weakened. The problem is about four times more common in women than it is in men and it does frequently seem to be hereditary. It quite often starts in pregnancy, and is also much more usually to be found in people who are significantly overweight or, more particularly, obese.

SOLUTIONS

A basic healthy diet, avoidance of too much weight gain at any time, but especially during pregnancy (see Section Three), and a regular program of exercise, which will help to maintain a healthy circulation, will all help to prevent varicose veins.

There is also some evidence that the bioflavonoids found in vitamin C-rich fruits and vegetables act to strengthen the veins, so make sure that your diet includes plenty of citrus fruits, berry fruits, etc. (for best sources of vitamin C, see page 25).

Vomiting, see Nausea and Travel Sickness

WOUNDS, CUTS, AND GRAZES

MINOR WOUNDS, BURNS, AND GRAZES are best thoroughly cleaned and left to heal naturally. Small cuts can be pulled together with a micropore tape, which will also stop the bleeding. Excessive bleeding may possibly be a sign of a deficiency in vitamin K—the vitamin that helps the blood to clot. Vitamin K is found in leafy green vegetables. Wounds are helped to heal with a diet rich in zinc and vitamin C. Honey is a gentle and effective antiseptic when applied to inflamed grazes, cuts, or burns. Vitamin E is said to help wound healing and minimize scarring. Vitamin E capsules can be broken and the oil massaged into healing wounds. It may also be a good idea to get extra vitamin E in the diet, in the form of vegetable oils, nuts, and seeds (see best sources list on page 24).

Yeast infections, see Candida

DIETS FOR PARTICULAR CONDITIONS

The diets that follow are examples of the type of eating that can be used to help prevent or alleviate the specified conditions. They should be used in conjunction with the advice in the preceding Ailments and Solutions section and, where appropriate, should be discussed with your physician or dietitian.   They are not intended to replace any diet that you may be following on medical advice and are for general guidance only.

To begin with, below we set out some quick hints on using diet to help you cope with times of high stress in your lives.

Quick dietary hints for stress reduction

■ Shopping guide
Star foods: legumes, nuts, seeds, leafy green vegetables, fish, liver, milk, brown rice, fresh fruit.

Foods to choose:
In general—complex carbs, especially whole grains and whole-wheat pasta.
■ Rich in vitamin B group—whole grains, nuts, seeds, meat, low-fat dairy products, tuna and other fish, lentils and other legumes, liver, leafy green vegetables.

■ Rich in vitamin C—citrus fruits, kiwi fruit, strawberries, black currants, red bell peppers, leafy greens, snow peas, peas, melon.
■ Low-fat protein sources (preferably non-meat sources)—low-fat dairy products, legumes, white fish, shellfish, tofu.
■ Rich in zinc—oysters and shellfish, liver, wheat germ, seeds, nuts, lamb, beef.
■ Rich in calcium—low-fat dairy products, legumes, nuts, seeds, leafy greens, canned fish, fortified soy milk, and yogurt.

■ Rich in magnesium—nuts, seeds, lentils and other legumes, bulgur wheat, brown rice, whole-grain barley.

Notes
✳ Daily supplements of vitamin B group and C may be taken.
✳ To drink—water, low-fat 2% milk, fresh fruit and vegetable juices, chamomile tea, lemon balm tea.
✳ Snacks—peanut butter on whole-wheat bread, nuts, seeds, low-fat cottage cheese and yogurt, tuna pâté on rye crispbreads, fresh fruit dressed with yogurt.

Anti-arthritis diet

May help to prevent or ease the symptoms of all types of arthritis.

■ Shopping guidelines

Star foods:

mango, sweet potatoes, kale, cantaloupe melon, spinach, broccoli, sunflower seeds and oil, walnuts, tuna, salmon, sardines.

Foods to choose:

■ High in fish oils—mackerel, herring, salmon, trout, tuna.

■ High in vitamin C—black currants, kiwi fruit, strawberries, raspberries, mango, nectarine, peaches, papaya, cantaloupe melon, collard greens, kale, Brussels sprouts, cabbage, broccoli, snow peas, spinach, sweet potatoes.

■ High in vitamin A (beta-carotene)— carrots, orange-fleshed winter squash, sweet potatoes, chard, pumpkin, spinach, kale, greens, broccoli, mango, cantaloupe melon.

■ High in vitamin E—sunflower oil, sunflower/corn oil margarine, sunflower seeds, corn oil, pine nuts, sweet potatoes, avocado, muesli, tuna, salmon, chickpeas, Brazil nuts, hazelnuts, almonds, spinach.

■ High in selenium—walnuts, lentils, tuna, squid, liver, sardines, sole, cod, swordfish, salmon, shrimp, mussels, pork, whole-wheat bread.

■ Anti-inflammatory—ginger, apples, garlic.

Foods to avoid:

Those high in saturated fat, e.g., full-fat dairy, fatty cuts of red meat (limit red meat anyway).

■ Members of nightshade family (only if found to aggravate symptoms)— potatoes, tomatoes, eggplant, and bell peppers.

■ Coffee.

■ Alcohol.

Notes

✳ A minority of arthritis sufferers report a negative reaction to dairy products, wheat, corn, citrus fruits, and nuts, but many other arthritis sufferers can eat these foods with no problem; they all provide valuable nutrients.

✳ You may like to take a daily supplement of omega-3 fish oils, cod liver oil, and/or evening primrose oil.

✳ People on steroids should include plenty of calcium- and iron-rich foods in their diet, and they may need to watch their sodium intake.

✳ Use sunflower oil in cooking.

✳ To drink—water, tea, herb tea, fruit juices, milk, or calcium-enriched soy milk.

✳ Have daily 1 tbsp of sunflower seeds.

✳ Snack ideas—raw carrot, handful of Brazil nuts, almonds, hazelnuts or mixed nuts, slice of whole-wheat bread with corn oil margarine and honey.

ANTI-ARTHRITIS DIET

DAY ONE
Breakfast
muesli with skim milk, peach juice
whole-wheat bread, sunflower spread, honey
Lunch
Lentil and Cilantro Soup, white bread roll
mango and low-fat yogurt
Evening
Salmon and Broccoli Risotto
large green salad, slice of cantaloupe melon

DAY TWO
Breakfast
oatmeal with skim milk and honey
mango juice
slice of whole-wheat bread with sunflower spread and low-sugar jam or honey
Lunch
Hummus, pita bread, salad of avocado and leafy greens with pine nuts
Evening
pork chop with kale, carrot, and sweet potato, Stir-Fried Fruit Salad

DAY THREE
Breakfast
As Day 1
Lunch
Spinach, Parsley, and Garlic Soup
French bread with sunflower spread
slice of cantaloupe melon with ginger
Evening
Sardines with Red-Currant Sauce
green salad
Peach and Banana Fool

DAY FOUR
Breakfast
sheep's-milk yogurt
strawberries or kiwi fruit
handful of mixed chopped nuts
Lunch
tuna and avocado sandwich on whole-wheat bread, small mango
Evening
Spiced Chicken and Greens
brown rice, broccoli, apple

DAY FIVE
Breakfast
As Day 1
Lunch
soup of butternut squash simmered with onion and stock
rye bread with small portion of low-fat cheese, apple
Evening
Herring Fillet with Ginger and Cilantro
spinach, couscous

DAY SIX
Breakfast
As Day 2
Lunch
Seafood and Tropical Fruit Salad
2 rye crispbreads with sunflower spread
fruit yogurt
Evening
Almond, Chickpea, and Raisin Pilaff
snow peas, Raspberry Gratin

Anti-cancer diet

May offer protection against some cancers and may help to control cancer growth. See also page 96.

■ Shopping guide
Star foods:
tomatoes, broccoli, Brussels sprouts, watercress, carrots, sweet potatoes, grapes, cherries, strawberries, citrus fruits, olive oil, oily fish, garlic, Brazil nuts, tuna, whole grains, soy and other legumes.

Foods to choose:
■ All starchy high-fiber foods, including whole grains, root vegetables, various legumes, bread, breakfast cereals, pasta.
■ All fruits, especially cantaloupe melon, mangoes, apricots, oranges, papayas, peaches, nectarines, citrus fruits, berry fruits, cherries, grapes.
■ All vegetables, especially broccoli, Brussels sprouts, kale, collard greens, watercress, carrots, sweet potatoes.
■ Nuts, seeds, oily fish, garlic, Asian mushrooms (fresh).
■ Low-saturated-fat, non-meat sources of protein—such as various legumes, tofu, skim milk, low-fat yogurt, cottage cheese, soy milk, soy yogurt, fish and seafood, various nuts and seeds.

Foods to avoid or cut down on:
■ Saturated fats and meats, especially char-grilled and well-done meats.
■ Salt-cured, pickled, and smoked foods of all kinds.
■ Alcohol.

Notes
* Keep weight at a reasonable level.
* To drink—a glass of red wine or red grape juice daily, green tea, water, fresh fruit and vegetable juices, skim milk.
* Snack ideas—fresh fruit, nuts, seeds, dried fruits, bread, raw carrots with hummus, soy yogurt, sesame seed bar.

ANTI-CANCER DIET

DAY ONE
Breakfast
Branflakes with soy milk, grapes
whole-wheat bread with corn oil margarine and honey
Lunch
Carrot and Orange Soup
whole-wheat bread, Brazil nuts
Evening
Salmon and Broccoli Risotto
mixed salad with tomatoes included
cantaloupe melon

DAY TWO
Breakfast
plain yogurt or soy yogurt
strawberries and lemon
muesli with added chopped nuts
fresh orange juice
Lunch
salad of drained tuna in oil, avocado, tomato, minced garlic and tofu mayonnaise
whole-wheat bread, peach
Evening
Winter Squash with Lentils and Ginger
baked potato, Brussels sprouts
Mango Phyllo Tart

DAY THREE
Breakfast
pink grapefruit
whole-wheat bread with corn oil margarine and honey, yogurt
Lunch
Marinated Shiitake Mushrooms
whole-wheat bread and corn oil margarine
banana and low-fat ricotta cheese with brown sugar
Evening
Pasta with Olives and Sardines
tomato and watercress salad
plateful of grapes or cherries and fresh nuts

DAY FOUR
Breakfast
muesli with extra chopped nuts and dried apricots
skim milk or soy milk
grapes or cherries, fresh orange juice
Lunch
Spinach, Parsley, and Garlic Soup
rye bread with tofu pâté
Evening
Chickpea, Almond, and Raisin Pilaff
broccoli, kale
compote of summer fruits

DAY FIVE
Breakfast
Shredded Wheat
1 tablespoon sunflower seeds
skim milk or soy milk
strawberries or orange
Lunch
salad of grated carrot, hazelnuts, and low-fat Cheddar cheese on a bed of watercress with olive oil vinaigrette, whole-wheat bread
Evening
Potato and Mediterranean Vegetable Bake
peas and lettuce, cantaloupe melon

Anti-candida diet

May help to prevent or minimize symptoms of gut dysbiosis (candida, thrush). See also page 99.

■ Shopping guide

Star foods:
live yogurt, garlic, oysters, green vegetables, peppers, snow peas.

Foods to choose:
■ Zinc-rich foods—wheat germ, calf's liver, oysters, cocoa powder, pumpkin, beef, crab.

■ C-rich foods—broccoli, corn, most salad leaves, spinach, tomatoes, chili and sweet peppers, leafy greens, sprouts, snow peas, black currants, kiwi fruit, strawberries, citrus fruits, papaya.

■ Garlic.

■ Live yogurt.

Foods to avoid:
■ All yeast-containing (leavened) bakery goods, e.g., breads, yeast cakes, and biscuits.

■ All fermented drinks—beers, wines, sherries, spirits.

■ All alcohol-containing products, e.g., some medicines (check label).

■ All vinegars, including apple and wine vinegars, and foods containing these—e.g., pickles, sauces, relishes.

■ All cheeses.

■ All malted drinks, malted cereals, and candies.

■ Mushrooms and fungi of all kinds.

■ Nuts and seeds may also be yeasty or carry molds, so you may also like to avoid these (see note below).

■ Soy sauce.

■ Vitamin B supplements and brewers' yeast tablets, unless they are labeled "yeast-free."

■ Canned, packaged, or frozen fruit juices (home-squeezed are fine).

■ Dried fruits.

■ Sugars, syrups, and high-sugar products.

■ Vegetarians and vegans should not avoid nuts and seeds, but preferably use cashews and pine nuts (which tend to be tolerated better) in preference to other types of nuts.

Notes

✻ You may like to take a daily supplement of the pre-biotic fructo-oligosaccharides (from chilled cabinets of some healthfood stores and by mail order) and pro-biotics containing lacto-bacillus and bifidobacteria. You can eat several portions a day of live yogurt containing the pro-biotic bacteria, too, which will help boost levels.

✻ To drink—water, herbal teas, skim milk or low-fat 2% milk (drink at least ³/₄ cup/200 ml a day), fresh fruit and vegetable juices, cocoa made with skim milk and artificial sweetener.

✻ Snack ideas—live yogurt, rye crispbread with hard-boiled egg, pita with hummus.

✻ Breakfast every day—live yogurt, orange or kiwi fruit, homemade muesli with no dried fruits.

ANTI-CANDIDA DIET

DAY ONE
Lunch
Country Pea Soup, Tzatziki, soda bread
Evening
Rice and Beans, with hard-boiled egg chopped on top, broccoli

DAY TWO
Lunch
Canellini Bean and Basil Spread
rice cakes, banana, green salad
Evening
Pork, Onion, and Pepper Kebabs
brown rice, tomato salad

DAY THREE
Lunch
Spinach, Parsley, and Garlic Soup (omit Parmesan and swirl in some yogurt instead)
chapati
Evening
Potato and Mediterranean Vegetable Bake
Mango and Peach Booster

DAY FOUR
Lunch
Skordalia, soda bread
mixed salad with olive oil and lemon dressing
Evening
Avocado and Turkey Tortillas
apple, pecans

DAY FIVE
Lunch
Hummus, pita bread
Roast Tomato, Garlic, and Pepper Soup
Evening
Baba Ganoush, with crudités
Spanish-style Baked Trout with Chard
snow peas

Healthy heart diet

May help to reduce the risk of heart disease and maintain a healthy circulatory system.

Shopping guide

Star foods:

all fruits and vegetables, especially citrus, apples, black currants, mango, cantaloupe melon, carrots, squash, sweet potatoes, broccoli, leafy greens; oily fish, garlic, oats, legumes, whole grains, nuts and seeds.

Foods to choose:

■ Rich in vitamin C and flavonoids—citrus fruits, black currants, melon, berries, red bell peppers.

■ Rich in carotenoids—squash, carrots, tomatoes, sweet potatoes, chard, spinach, kale, cabbage, broccoli, peas.

■ Rich in vitamin E—wheat germ oil, sunflower oil and margarine, sunflower seeds, corn oil and margarine, sweet potato, avocado, pine nuts, muesli, chickpeas, tuna, salmon, squash, spinach, kale, Brazil nuts, hazelnuts, almonds.

■ Rich in folate—yeast extract, liver, legumes, cereals, muesli, leafy vegetables.

■ Rich in vitamin B6—wheat germ, fish, legumes, nuts, chicken, potatoes.

■ Rich in selenium—walnuts, lentils, sunflower seeds, whole-wheat bread, tuna, sardines, salmon, swordfish, cod, sole.

■ Rich in monounsaturated fatty acids—olive oil, canola oil, peanut oil.

■ Rich in soluble fiber—oats, legumes, many fruits and vegetables.

■ Rich in omega-3 oils—salmon, mackerel, herring, sardines, trout, fresh tuna.

■ Phytochemicals—watermelon, pink grapefruit, onions, broccoli, Brussels sprouts and many more fruits and vegetables, garlic, soy, wine and beer, tea.

Foods to avoid or limit:

■ Too much alcohol (limit).

■ Trans fats and saturated fats.

■ High-cholesterol foods (limit).

■ High-calorie snacks (to avoid obesity).

■ Salt and salt-rich foods.

Notes

* Avoid smoking.
* Supplements of vitamin E, selenium, garlic oil, may be taken.
* To drink—water, fruit and vegetable juices, soy milk, skim milk, tea, green tea.
* One or two alcoholic drinks a day, especially red wine, are allowed.

HEALTHY HEART DIET

DAY ONE
Breakfast
muesli
calcium-enriched soy milk, pink grapefruit
Lunch
Roast Tomato, Garlic, and Pepper Soup
Oat Bread, Rouille
Evening
Pasta with Broccoli and Anchovies
large mixed salad
Peach and Banana Fool

DAY TWO
Breakfast
oatmeal made with skim milk
glass of fresh orange juice
slice of whole-wheat bread with corn oil margarine and marmalade
Lunch
Smoked Mackerel Pâté Salad
Oat Bread, apple
cantaloupe or watermelon
Evening
Potato and Mediterranean Vegetable Bake
peas
strawberries and low-fat cottage cheese

DAY THREE
Breakfast
As Day 1, but with melon
Lunch
Lentil and Cilantro Soup
Oat Bread, banana
Vegetable Cup
Evening
Spanish-Style Baked Trout with Chard
broccoli, Blackberry Ice Sundae

DAY FOUR
Breakfast
As Day 2
Lunch
Thai Salmon Salad, Oat Bread
Evening
Winter Squash with Lentils and Ginger
kale or Brussels sprouts, apple

DAY FIVE
Breakfast
As Day 3
Lunch
Spinach, Parsley, and Garlic Soup
Oat Bread, Hummus
Evening
Sardines with Red-Currant Sauce
potatoes mashed with olive oil
Stir-Fried Fruit Salad

Immune-strengthening diet

Helps to strengthen the immune system generally and fight against disease and infection.

■ Shopping guide

Star foods:

leafy greens, sweet potatoes, Brazil nuts, walnuts, sunflower seeds, tuna, broccoli.

Foods to choose:

■ Rich in vitamin C—citrus fruits, black currants, berries, melon, red bell peppers, leafy green vegetables, broccoli.

■ Rich in zinc—nuts, seeds, wheat germ, All Bran, beef, oysters, crab, lamb, pork, whole-grain barley.

■ Rich in vitamin A (beta-carotene)—carrots, squash, chard, sweet potatoes, spinach, kale, leafy green vegetables, mango, cantaloupe melon, broccoli, tomato.

■ Rich in vitamin B group—whole grains, yeast extract, meat, nuts, seeds, low-fat dairy products, tuna, other fish, lentils and other legumes, leafy green vegetables.

■ Rich in vitamin E—wheat germ oil, sunflower oil and margarine, sunflower seeds, corn oil and margarine, pine nuts, sweet potato, avocado, muesli, chickpeas, Brazil nuts, hazelnuts, almonds, squash, kale, salmon, tuna.

■ Rich in selenium—Brazil nuts, walnuts, lentils, tuna and other oily fish, swordfish, cod, sole, mussels, whole-wheat bread, sunflower seeds.

■ Rich in antioxidants—garlic, thyme, onions, ginger, black and green tea.

Foods to avoid:

■ Low-nutrient foods.

■ Alcohol.

■ Also avoid smoking.

Notes

✳ You may take supplements of zinc and echinachea.

✳ To drink—water, fruit and vegetable juices, yeast extract, cocoa, green tea, black tea, herb tea.

✳ Snack ideas—walnuts, sunflower seeds, whole-wheat bread, hazelnuts, pine nuts, almonds, Brazil nuts, yogurt, pesto on bread.

IMMUNE-STRENGTHENING DIET

DAY ONE
Breakfast
pink grapefruit
muesli with extra nuts and seeds
2 teaspoons wheat germ
Lunch
Tzatziki and whole-wheat pita bread
Spiced Lentils and Mixed Green Vegetables
carrot juice
Evening
Scallops and Mussels in the Pan
Stir-fry of green beans, broccoli, and baby corn, cantaloupe melon

DAY TWO
Breakfast
boiled egg, whole-wheat bread
Brazil nuts, almonds, and sunflower seeds
freshly squeezed orange juice
Lunch
Panzanella with extra garlic
yogurt with banana
Evening
Seafood Risotto with Ginger
salad of romaine, watercress, and arugula
Summer Fruit Compote

DAY THREE
Breakfast
As Day 1, but with melon
Lunch
Warm Broccoli, Red Pepper, and Sesame Salad, rye bread
Evening
Speedy Herbed Swordfish
sweet potato
stir-fried shredded kale
Watermelon Refresher

DAY FOUR
Breakfast
As Day 1
Lunch
Salad of Tuna, Avocado, and Tomato
whole-wheat pita, orange
Evening
Pork, Onion, and Pepper Kebabs
quinoa, mango

DAY FIVE
Breakfast
As Day 2
Lunch
Squash, Potato, and Lima Bean Soup
rye bread, berry fruits
Evening
Tiger Prawns with Rice Noodles
Spinach, Broccoli, and Walnut Stir-Fry
Citrus Granita

Anti-osteoporosis diet

May help to protect bones against osteoporosis. See also page 130.

■ Shopping guide

Star foods:
low-fat dairy products, such as skim milk, low-fat yogurt, low-fat ricotta and cottage cheeses; leafy green vegetables, nuts, legumes, wheat germ, fish, white bread, whole grains.

Foods to choose:
■ Sources of calcium—low-fat dairy products, legumes, tilapia fish, canned sardines, pilchards, shrimp, fortified soy products, e.g., calcium-enriched soy milk, calcium-enriched soy yogurt, calcium-enriched cereals, seeds and nuts.
■ Sources of magnesium—nuts, seeds, legumes, bulgur wheat, brown rice, lentils, whole-grain barley.

■ Sources of vitamin D—sunlight, cod liver oil, oily fish, margarine, fortified breakfast cereals, eggs.
■ Sources of zinc—wheat germ, liver, fish, shellfish, seeds, nuts, lamb, beef.
■ Sources of folate—yeast extract, chicken livers, legumes, fortified breakfast cereals, muesli, nuts, broccoli, Brussels sprouts, kale, leafy green vegetables.
■ Sources of B6—wheat germ, fish, legumes, nuts, chicken, potatoes.
■ Sources of potassium—soybeans and other legumes, dried apricots, dried figs, tomatoes, potatoes, many fruits and vegetables.
■ Sources of essential fatty acids—vegetable, seed, nut, and grain oils, seeds, nuts, and whole grains.

Foods to avoid:
■ Those high in sodium.
■ Those high in alcohol.
■ Excess animal protein.

■ Caffeine—e.g., strong coffee, tea, colas, guarana drink.
■ Foods rich in phytates and oxalates—raw wheat bran, spinach, rhubarb, chocolate, and tea.
■ Sodas, processed foods.

Notes

* To drink—2 glasses of soy milk a day may help to prevent osteoporosis, but use calcium-enriched soy milk. Also drink at least 2 cups (450 ml) in total low-fat dairy or calcium-enriched soy milk a day.
* You may like to use a daily supplement of cod liver oil for vitamin D, or a combined calcium, magnesium, and vitamin D supplement.
* Snack ideas—dried figs and apricots, nuts, seeds, yeast extract on white bread, fresh fruit.

ANTI-OSTEOPOROSIS DIET

DAY ONE
Breakfast
Total cereal with added nuts
glass of skim milk or soy milk
glass of fresh orange juice
Lunch
Smoked Mackerel Pâté Salad
bread roll, mixed salad
Evening
Rice and Greens, with extra Parmesan (use extra broccoli instead of the spinach)
yogurt, Stir-Fried Fruit Salad

DAY TWO
Breakfast
muesli with 2 teaspoons wheat germ and extra nuts, seeds, and dried fruit, skim milk, glass of fresh orange juice, white bread with corn oil margarine and honey
Lunch
Squash, Potato, and Lima Bean Soup
Brie, whole-wheat bread, tomato
Evening
broiled tilapia fish, broccoli
green lentils with herbs, new potatoes

DAY THREE
Breakfast
Shredded Wheat, cantaloupe melon, white bread with corn oil margarine and marmalade
Lunch
sardine and salad sandwich on brown bread
low-fat yogurt or calcium-enriched soy yogurt , Summer Fruit Compote
Evening
Potato Gnocchi with Cheese and Cauliflower
kale

DAY FOUR
Breakfast
As Day 2
Lunch
Feta and Pepper Spread, rice cakes
sunflower seeds
ready-to-eat dried apricots
Evening
broiled lamb, onion, and green pepper kebabs, Tabbouleh
large bowl of mixed salad, ice cream

DAY FIVE
Breakfast
oatmeal made with skim milk, honey
white bread with corn oil margarine and marmalade, orange
Lunch
Thai Salmon Salad, low-fat fruit yogurt
Evening
Pasta with Chicken Livers
1 tablespoon extra Parmesan cheese
salad of romaine and watercress

PMS and diuretic diet

May help reduce symptoms of pre-menstrual syndrome and help to reduce fluid retention at any time.

■ Shopping guide

Star foods:

For minimizing fluid retention, these are some naturally diuretic foods: melon, citrus fruits, salad vegetables, particularly celery, cucumber, watercress, and lettuce, tomatoes, sweet peppers, carrots, tomato juice, carrot juice, mixed vegetable juice.

For helping other symptoms of PMS: all whole foods, fresh fruits and vegetables, legumes, pasta, bananas, nuts, seeds, grains.

Foods to choose:

■ Rich in potassium—bananas, tomatoes, onions, potatoes, whole grains.

■ Rich in vitamin B6—wheat germ, legumes, whole grains, oily fish, bananas, poultry.

■ Rich in vitamin E—most vegetable oils, various nuts and seeds, avocados, tuna, salmon, sardines, brown rice, asparagus.

■ Rich in essential fatty acids—vegetable oils, fish oils, nut and seed oils, grain oils, oily fish, nuts, seeds, and whole grains.

■ Rich in calcium—low-fat dairy products, dark leafy greens, canned fish, seeds, nuts.

■ Rich in magnesium—nuts, seeds, lentils and other legumes, bulgur wheat, brown rice.

Foods to avoid:

■ Salt and all salty foods.

■ Alcohol.

■ Sugary snacks.

■ Caffeine.

■ Refined starches—e.g., cakes, biscuits and rolls, soft white bread.

Notes

* To drink—water, low-fat milk, vegetable juices, fruit juices, herb teas (some herb teas, such as nettle, parsley, and dandelion, may help minimize fluid retention).

* Supplements of evening primrose oil, linseed oil, calcium/magnesium may be taken daily.

* Snack ideas—nuts, seeds, low-fat yogurt, low-fat ricotta and cottage cheeses, fresh fruit.

* Small main meals and plenty of in-between snacks are the key to managing PMS symptoms—i.e., eat little and often.

PMS AND DIURETIC DIET

Breakfast every day
low-fat plain yogurt
handful of no-added-sugar-or-salt muesli, with extra nuts and seeds
2 teaspoons wheat germ sprinkled on top
selection of fresh fruits chopped over, preferably including melon, one citrus fruit, and some banana

DAY ONE
Lunch
small slice of whole-wheat bread
salad of cooked asparagus, avocado, tomato, sliced onion, and tuna in water or oil, well drained, tossed in a little sunflower oil, and lemon juice
Evening
Rice and Beans, slice of melon
Vegetable Cup

DAY TWO
Lunch
large salad, including celery, watercress, lettuce, tomato, cucumber, and onion tossed in dressing as Day 1
small slice of whole-wheat bread with corn oil margarine, Hummus
Evening
Spanish-style Baked Trout with Chard
carrot or orange juice

DAY THREE
Lunch
Warm Broccoli, Red Pepper, and Sesame Salad
Banana and Strawberry Smoothie, apple
Evening
Spiced Chicken and Greens
carrots, Vegetable Cup

DAY FOUR
Lunch
Carrot and Orange Soup
crudités with Feta and Pepper Spread
Evening
Chickpea and Vegetable Crumble
Watermelon Refresher

DAY FIVE
Lunch
small slice of whole-wheat bread
Canellini Bean and Basil Spread
large mixed salad as Day 2
orange
Evening
Salmon and Broccoli Risotto
Vegetable Cup
handful of dried apricots and sunflower seeds

Food supplements — clever aids to health or a waste of money?

Billions of dollars are spent in the US on vitamin, mineral, and food supplements — more than we spend on any other over-the-counter health products except headache remedies — and that is excluding mail-order sources and healthfood stores.

The most popular supplements are fish oils, multivitamins, evening primrose oil, single vitamins, and garlic, but literally hundreds of different products exist in varying combinations, and new products are appearing all the time. Here we look at whether supplements are worth the expense.

Vitamin and mineral supplements

Various types of vitamin and mineral supplement are regularly prescribed by doctors, for good health maintenance, and disease prevention and cure. For example, iron supplements are often prescribed for anemia; folate early in pregnancy; vitamin D for the elderly; vitamin B12 for vegans; and so on. Obviously, then, supplements ARE a necessary and important part of staying healthy — at least, for some of us... occasionally.

Many more vitamin and mineral supplements are, however, sold direct to the consumer who, in buying them, is making his or her own diagnosis about his or her state of health and nutritional needs. Many consumers take supplements regularly, on a permanent basis, as "health insurance"... but is this wise or necessary?

Most doctors and qualified nutritionists will say that, if you eat a basic healthy diet (such as that on page 53) and are in good health, supplements of vitamins and/or minerals are often a waste of money. They will say that if you are not in good health or there is any other reason why you think you should take a supplement, then a visit to your physician will confirm or deny that (and if you need supplements you will be offered a prescription).

They will say that supplementing without professional advice can cause as many problems as it may cure — for example, through overdosing, toxicity, creating nutritional imbalances, or through encouraging the false idea that it doesn't matter how unhealthy your diet is as long as you take vitamin pills. They may say that you can't transfer all the nutritional benefits of food into manufactured pills. They might even quote trials that have shown that sometimes supplements intended to help beat disease may actually have the reverse effect.

Other nutritionists and complementary practitioners will argue that the current RDIs for vitamins and minerals are too low, offering only protection against the deficiency diseases, such as rickets (lack of vitamin D) and scurvy (lack of vitamin C); that for optimum health and protection against disease, much larger amounts of several of the vitamins and minerals are needed; that these amounts are difficult to obtain through an average healthy diet and that supplementation is often the only option.

Here we look at these points of view in more detail.

■ Are the recommended daily amounts too low for people in normal health?

At certain times and in certain situations, you may need more than the RDIs (see pages 22–33), and sometimes it IS hard to get your needs from diet. For example, a woman with iron-deficiency anemia brought on by heavy periods will almost certainly need iron supplementation to bring her back to a suitable level. Someone who smokes and drinks heavily may well be short of vitamins B group and C and may well need supplements, as another example. The chart overleaf lists some typical uses for the main vitamin and mineral supplements.

However, it is extremely hard to find a definitive answer as to whether or not someone in reasonable health, with no illness or deficiency, would benefit from any extra supplements. There is much anecdotal evidence that supplements help people to feel better. For example, someone prone to several colds each winter may begin to take supplements of vitamin C and zinc daily, have no colds, and claim that the supplements did the trick. There is certainly convincing evidence that supplements of vitamin C of at least 1 g daily (much greater than the RDI of 60 mg) can help to minimize severity and duration of colds. There is also good evidence that high doses of vitamin B6 can help with menstrual problems. However, scientific proof of this kind of effect is not extensive.

Another ironic point is that the people

who may well benefit most from vitamin and mineral supplements—the elderly and the poor, both of whom have lower levels of intakes of many nutrients than other social groups in the US—are least likely to be able to afford them.

The consensus is that once your body has its optimum amount of the vitamins and minerals, taking any extra is at best a waste of time and at worst could be toxic.

■ Can high-dose supplements help prevent the major diseases?

For people with more serious problems, such as CHD or cancer, trials to show that supplements can help have had mixed results. For example, supplements of vitamin E have been shown in one major trial to decrease non-fatal heart attacks, and vitamin C supplements have been used successfully in trials too, but other trials have shown negative effects (i.e., increased heart attacks) with both vitamin E and beta-carotene.

Although beta-carotene in the diet, as an antioxidant, is often claimed to help protect against cancers and heart disease, experts now say that beta-carotene supplements should NOT be taken for this purpose. Other experts say that it is nearly impossible to get enough vitamin E in a normal diet to offer health protection and so supplementation is indicated. Selenium is another antioxidant that may be in shortfall in many of our diets, and some experts recommend supplements. The B vitamin folate is also linked with heart disease in some, and supplementation may be the answer in that case.

Anyone thinking of supplementing their diet to help prevent or minimize the severity of disease should get professional advice, as there are so many variables.

■ Can you overdose on supplements and are they toxic?

Yes, you can on some—for toxic levels see Section One. The fat-soluble vitamins A and D are toxic in excess, as they can

be stored in the liver. Too much vitamin A is particularly dangerous for pregnant women. High intakes of iron, zinc, and selenium are toxic, and an excess of vitamin C can cause stomach upsets. While high doses of vitamin B6 are used to treat PMS, mega-doses of the vitamin may cause nerve damage and some countries have withdrawn over the counter sales of pills containing more than 10 mg. Almost all vitamins and minerals will have some side effects if taken in really large doses.

Particular groups of people can be adversely effected by some supplements—for instance, vitamin E supplements shouldn't be taken by those on anti-coagulant drugs, nor calcium supplements if you have kidney stones or cancer.

Sometimes supplements are shown to be toxic for other reasons—for instance, in 1997, some fish oils were found to contain higher-than-recommended levels of synthetic pollutants.

■ Do supplements create nutritional imbalances?

They certainly can do. This is because vitamins, minerals, and other nutrients all work together within the body. Too much of one particular nutrient may have a "knock-on" effect in various ways. Here are some examples:
* If you take calcium supplements, you should also take magnesium supplements as these work together.
* Iron supplements may reduce zinc absorption.
* High zinc intake may mean copper supplements need to be taken, too.
* B vitamin supplements should be taken together, rather than just an isolated B vitamin, as the group works together and an excess of one alters the delicate balance.
* High doses of iron can hinder vitamin E absorption.
The best policy when it comes to supplements, if you're not sure what or

how much to take, or why you're taking them, is to see a professional nutritionist or doctor for advice. High doses of any one vitamin or mineral are best avoided unless you've been advised to take them. A standard multivitamin and mineral preparation is probably the safest way to supplement otherwise. Check the label and make sure that 100% of the RDI of each of the vitamins and minerals needed is offered.

■ Can supplements compensate for a poor diet?

Most nutrition experts now agree that there IS no substitute for a healthy diet of real food, and that nutrients are best taken as part of that diet. In other words, nutrients extracted from foods (or created synthetically, as many vitamins are), probably don't have the same effect on your body as they do when they come naturally packaged as a part of the food itself. A good example of this is beta-carotene, supplements of which seem to increase the risk of cancer in smokers, one trial has shown.

THE MAJOR VITAMIN AND MINERAL SUPPLEMENTS AND THEIR TYPICAL USES

	Typical daily dose	Maximum daily dose**	Typical uses
Vitamin			
A	1–2,000 µg	7,500 µg* women 9,000 µg men	Dry skin, pimples, poor night vision
Beta-carotene	6–15 mg	n/k	As vitamin A. Its use as an anti-cancer, anti-CHD supplement is controversial
B group	100% RDI	n/k	Stress and nervous conditions; smokers, drinkers
B6	10 mg	50 mg	Premenstrual syndrome, fluid retention
B12	100 µg	n/k	Vegans
Folate	400 ug	400 µg	Preconception, pregnancy (helps prevent birth defects)
C	250–1,000 mg	2–3,000 mg	Antioxidant; antibacterial; smokers, drinkers, stress, skin complaints
D	5–10 µg	10 µg	Elderly and those confined indoors
E	400 i.u. (275 mg)	1,200 i.u. (800 mg)	Antioxidant; wound healing; skin complaints
Mineral			
Calcium	800–1,000 mg	1,500 mg	Family history of osteoporosis; insomnia
Iron	14 mg	20 mg fatigue	Anemia, heavy periods, pregnancy
Magnesium	150 mg	n/k	High calcium intakes, insomnia, stress
Zinc	7–15 mg	50 mg	High calcium and iron intakes, immune strengthening; poor appetite, wound healing; acne
Selenium	100–200 µg	500 µg	Antioxidant; HIV, cancer, arthritis
Multivitamin/mineral	50–100% RDI	n/k	Dieters; appetite loss, poor diet

* Avoid in pregnancy   ** Adults in normal health, non-pregnant

When nutrients are obtained through a varied diet, you cannot overdose. Another important factor is that some researchers say that the "active ingredients" in the foods that we eat are many compounds other than vitamins—for instance, the phytochemicals in fruit and vegetables. No doubt in time a range of phytos will be packaged alongside the vitamins, but as yet there are few examples of this, although vitamin C is obtainable "with bioflavonoids."

A third reason why real food is better than pills is that food contains calories, protein, essential fats, fiber, and a whole balance of the things that we need. Take a vitamin C tablet instead of an orange, and you are missing out on many nutrients.

Obviously there are cases when it is better to take vitamin and/or mineral pills than nothing at all—for example, anorexia, or loss of appetite through ill health. However, pill popping alongside a poor diet is not a sensible solution.

■ Are vitamins and minerals in supplements easily absorbed by the body?

Not necessarily. It is well known that many vitamins are hard to absorb. Fat-soluble vitamins (A, D, E) are less well absorbed when taken without food; iron tablets are notorious for being badly absorbed—help absorption by taking with vitamin-C-rich food, drink, or supplement. Don't take mineral supplements with tea or coffee—these hinder absorption.

"Time release" capsules may help vitamin absorption. Mineral supplements are sold with the mineral bound (or "chelated") to other compounds. Minerals that are chelated to organic compounds, such as amino acid chelates, gluconates, picolinates, or citrates, may be more easily absorbed than those bound to inorganic compounds, such as sulfates or phosphates (check label).

■ Is there any difference between natural and synthetic vitamins?

It is usually agreed that natural vitamin E (d-alpha tocopherol) is preferable to synthetic vitamin E (dl-alpha tocopherol), but synthetic vitamin C works as well as the natural extract.

■ What else is in a supplement apart from "active ingredients"?

Capsules may be made from gelatin or a vegetarian substitute. Vegetable oils are usually the base for fat-soluble vitamins in capsule form. Tablets may contain binders, fillers, and other ingredients, including sugar, artificial sweeteners, yeast, colorings, fat. Check the label.

Food supplements

A large—and rapidly expanding—supplement market is that of food supplements other than the traditional vitamins and minerals. Often sold in healthfood stores or by mail order, but increasingly appearing on the shelves of supermarkets and pharmacies, these supplements range from thoroughly tested items, such as garlic and evening primrose oil, through to more exotic remedies like kombucha tea and kava kava. You can even buy fruit and vegetable capsules—for people too busy to eat their "five a day"!

Like vitamin and mineral supplements, their claims vary, but include such things as increased well-being, better health, disease protection, protection against or cure of various ailments, anti-aging, and so on. Most do not have a medical licence and should, therefore, not make medical claims. However, there are FDA-approved "health claims" that manufacturers can put on the label even if most supplements are not regulated.

Below we detail some popular supplements and evaluate, where possible, their worth. Many have not been tested in properly conducted clinical trials, so results can't be evaluated scientifically. Benefits are often anecdotal, and some products (perhaps in their original herbal form) have been used for centuries or more in their countries of origin. (Fresh herbs and herbal remedies are discussed later.)

Acidophilus, see Pro-biotics

Aloe Vera
Aloe vera has been used medicinally since ancient times. The main active ingredient in the plant is said to be mucopolysaccharide, which may help a range of conditions, including infections, allergies, and inflammation. Many skin complaints, including dry itchy skin, rashes, wounds, acne, and psoriasis, are said to improve with oral or applied aloe vera preparations. The plant has also been used for irritable bowel syndrome, candida, ME, arthritis, infections, "detoxifying," and a variety of other complaints. Another active compound in aloe vera, alloin, is said to help constipation. Fresh aloe vera juice can be taken as a drink (often bitter) or in capsule form. Powdered aloe vera in tablet form is said to be less effective. Aloe vera supplements should not be taken during pregnancy.

Amino Acids
Amino acids are the components of complete protein and each has other roles to play within the body. Cysteine is said to be antioxidant and is sometimes used to treat severe viral infections such as HIV. Lysine is said to help treat the cold sore virus, herpes simplex 1 and to help iron absorption. Glutamine is said to help the immune system and relieve digestive disorders. L-carnitine is often sold for fat-burning and arginine for muscle growth. Other individual amino acids are also sold as supplements for a variety of uses. If we have sufficient protein in the diet, however, it is unlikely that individual supplements would be needed, and scientific evidence of the efficacy of these products is scant.

Amino acid supplementation is not advised for pregnant women, children, diabetics, and people with high blood pressure.

Bee Pollen, see Propolis

Bifidus, see Pro-biotics

Blue-Green Algae
Algae from freshwater lakes in mild climates (or, nowadays, "farmed" in tanks) are dried and usually offered in tablet form as a food supplement.

Spirulina and chlorella are two well-known forms of algae. These supplements contain a wide variety of nutrients, including iron, beta-carotene, selenium, and vitamin B12, and also contain EFAs and protein. However, the amount of most of these nutrients in a day's supply of tablets or powder (about 1 gram of dried algae) is small, simply because the dose is so tiny, making them an expensive supplement in terms of nutrient returns.

For example, in one brand, a typical day's supply contains just 350 µg (micrograms) iron, which is a very small proportion of a day's average need of 18 mg. Claims are sometimes made that algae can build the immune system, help speed recovery time after exercise, de-toxify the body, and enhance performance, all of which appear to be anecdotal. Adverse side effects are thought to be rare.

Cat's Claw
(Unicaria Tormentosa, Unade Gato)
Derived from a Peruvian vine, cat's claw in capsules or as a tea is used as a healing

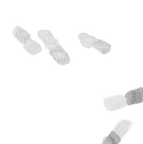

doses should not be exceeded, as vitamins A and D can be toxic in excess. Recently in the UK it was found that levels of toxic chemicals in some bottled fish liver oil preparations could be unacceptably high for toddlers. Cod liver oil supplements should not be taken in pregnancy.

Co-Enzyme Q10

Co-Q10 is said to help the body convert food into energy, strengthen the heart, act as an antioxidant, and even help minimize hot flashes. Our bodies can happily make their own Q10, and it occurs naturally in foods, but it is said by fans that, as we get older or when we're ill, natural levels drop and a supplement may be useful. Many nutritionists think the need for extra is unproved.

Detox Remedies

Several "detox" remedies are available—sometimes as a single liquid supplements, or as a package containing two or more different remedies, usually to be taken for from three days up to three weeks. These are said to help "cleanse" the digestive system, purify the blood and help elimination of "toxic wastes," by improving the action of the liver and sometimes the bladder. (For more on detoxification, see page 156.) They usually contain a range of plant and herbal preparations with these properties and may come with instructions to follow a semi-fast or a particular diet. In unbiased tests these products have mixed results, but may be worth trying.

Echinacea

The benefits of echinacea as an immune-system supporter are well documented, and a short course of tincture or capsules containing the main active ingredient, echinocosides, two or three times every winter may help to prevent colds, flu, and bacterial infections, as well as helping to prevent cold sores. Echinacea also contains mucopolysaccharides (see Aloe Vera).

Evening Primrose Oil

Evening primrose oil is one of the richest sources of the omega-6 (N6) fatty acid gamma linolenic acid, which the body needs for production of prostaglandins that control many vital processes, including fluid balance and the reproductive system. GLA has been shown to help prevent or minimize pre-menstrual syndrome, breast pain, and fluid retention, and is also thought to be anti-inflammatory, thus may help sufferers of arthritis and eczema. Some MS sufferers also take GLA-rich supplements, but the benefit is not proved. The body can convert its own GLA from the essential fatty acid linoleic acid, but sometimes this conversion process may not be efficient, and evening primrose oil is a convenient way to ensure GLA levels. Therapeutic dose may be up to 3,000 mg a day; maintenance dose 500–1,000 mg (1,000 mg of EPO will yield about 100 mg GLA). There are presently no known adverse side effects at the recommended doses.

Flax Seed Oil

This is the richest source of the Omega-3 (N3) essential fatty acid, alpha linolenic acid, and can convert in the body to the fatty acids EPA and DHA, which are those present in fish oils. Flax seed oil is useful for vegetarians wanting to increase their omega-3 intake. Capsules are the best form of flax seed oil to take—one 1,000-mg capsule will provide all your day's requirement of alpha linolenic acid (about 500 mg) and will also provide some of the other EFA, linoleic acid.

Garlic

The possible benefits of the garlic plant are well documented in other parts of this book (see particularly Heart Disease, page 118). However, there is some debate about the protective properties of the manufactured forms of garlic—tablets, capsules, and so on. Some

herb, and is claimed to be antiviral, antibacterial, immune-boosting, anti-inflammatory, antioxidant, and a cure-all for digestive disorders. Said to have been used by Peruvian tribes for centuries, it is relatively untested in Western trials.

Cod Liver Oil

Rich in vitamins A and D and EFAs, cod liver oil has been used as a natural source of these for many years. It is also said to relieve joint pain and arthritis, and help the immune system. Recommended

experts say that the active ingredients in garlic are very volatile and are even deactivated in fresh garlic by cooking. They say that garlic supplements may be far less potent, therefore, and may even be of little use at all.

These theories are being tested, but—until definite answers are found—if you wish to take garlic supplements, avoid those that have been "deodorized," because it is fairly certain that the active allicin in these products will no longer be potent; avoid those that have been heat-treated, which also destroys the volatile compounds; and go for the purest, least "treated" capsules that you can find.

Nobody really knows what the optimum daily dose of garlic is, but some experts say that the equivalent of 2 garlic cloves a day is a minimum—for many brands of manufactured garlic capsules this is 2 capsules. Check labels.

Ginkgo Biloba

The leaves of the ginkgo biloba tree are said to be important in helping to maintain brain functions, such as memory, alertness, and concentration, by maintaining the supply of blood to the brain and therefore oxygenating it. Ginkgo is also said to increase blood supply to the hands and feet. For these reasons it is often promoted as the ideal supplement for older people, and work is being done to see if ginkgo has any effect on Alzheimer's disease.

The quality of ginkgo biloba supplements varies—some are just ground-up dried leaf, and to be effective you would need at least 1,000 mg of this. Other supplements offer standardized extracts of the leaf, where the active ingredients—flavone glycosides, and other compounds—are extracted. A good-quality ginkgo extract tablet will contain about 40 mg extract (of which 24% will be flavone glycosides), and 1–3 tablets a day are normally sufficient.

Manufacturers say that improvement may not be noticed for at least one month after beginning a course of supplements.

Ginseng

The most famous of food supplements from the East, the root of ginseng has been used as a general tonic for at least 7,000 years. There are two main types of "ginseng" available as supplements—*panax* ginseng, sometimes called Korean ginseng, and Siberian ginseng. Both are members of the Aralia family of plants, but *panax* ginseng is a perennial plant while Siberian ginseng (*Eleutherococcus senticosus*) is a shrub. Both are described as "adaptogens," meaning that they can help the body fight, or adapt to, whatever problems it has. For instance, if you are stressed it will help to relax you; if you are tired it will help to stimulate you ... so it is said.

There are slight differences in the claimed actions of these two ginsengs, summarized as follows. *Panax* ginseng is the "classic" ginseng containing ginsenoside compounds that are said to be similar to the body's own stress hormones. As an adaptogen, it is said to help us cope with any kind of physical or emotional stress, as well as being a general tonic, and even a sedative. It may also stimulate the immune system and help liver function. Recent trials show that it has marked antibiotic properties, helping to fight the bacteria that cause lung damage in cystic fibrosis and reducing the severity of lung infection.

Panax ginseng is particularly favored in the East by athletes, by the elderly, and by males. A standard dose is 500–600 mg a day in capsule form, but should be taken for periods of a few weeks at a time only. As a stimulant, *panax* ginseng should be taken in the morning and should be avoided during pregnancy or if you have high blood pressure.

Siberian ginseng is a stimulant and anti-stress tonic with particular physical

benefits—some trials have shown improvement in athletic performance of up to 9%. It also stimulates the immune system and is useful for long-term fatigue. There is also some evidence that it is anti-toxic. A standard dose, which should be taken for a few weeks at a time only, is 1,000 mg in capsule form.

Another less well-known type of "ginseng" is American ginseng, which appears to have a similar, but milder, effect, compared to *panax* ginseng. It may be of use to those people who find the *panax* or Siberian ginsengs a bit too stimulating.

Green-Lipped Mussel

Green-lipped mussel supplements have been taken for some years by arthritis sufferers and seem to have shown benefits. Research appears to have pinpointed the compound that may provide this effect—lyprinol, which seems to be anti-inflammatory, reducing pain and swelling in joints. Lyprinol is one of the mucopolysaccharides, compounds that are also found in aloe vera and glucosamine.

Green-lipped mussel can be taken in capsule form, and results may show after 4–8 weeks.

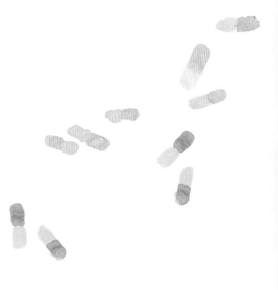

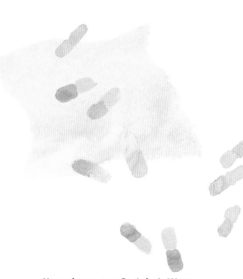

Hypericum, see St. John's Wort

Kava Kava

The root of this Pacific island shrub is a well-known relaxant, which can relieve anxiety, aid sleep, and promote a sense of well-being. The main active ingredient, kawain, is a sedative. Other uses of kava kava are as an antiseptic and analgesic. Capsules are available, and recommended dosage shouldn't be exceeded, as, in excess, they are intoxicant.

Kelp

Kelp (*Fucus vesiculosus*) is a seaweed also known as bladderwrack, rich in iodine and possibly with immune-system-boosting and thyroid-stimulating properties. Some people believe that kelp will aid weight loss, so it is sometimes sold as a dieting aid, but there appears to be little scientific proof of its effectiveness. Kelp is sold in tablet form and a daily dose of about 150 µg is usually recommended. Excess kelp (and iodine) should be avoided, particularly if you have an over-active thyroid.

Kombucha

From Russia and China, kombucha—a fungal brew—has been used for many years there as a tonic, and is said to provide a variety of benefits. Apparently it is anticancer, antibacterial, immune boosting, and a detoxifier, can help arthritis, cataracts, asthma, dandruff, itchy skin, lack of libido... Unfortunately the evidence is, again, anecdotal and not scientific. Kombucha can be brewed at home, or it can be bought as ready-made tea. Various unwanted side effects are being reported in long-term users, including jaundice, nausea, and allergic reactions.

Lactobaccillus, see Pro-biotics

Linseed Oil, see Flax Seed Oil

Milk Thistle

Milk thistle (*Silybum marianum*) contains the compound silymarin, and has been used in Europe for hundreds of years as a treatment for liver disorders. Research seems to back up this claim, and modern herbalists use milk thistle to help in cases of jaundice and hepatitis, and to protect the liver in cases of alcohol abuse or other times when it may be under stress. Milk thistle is available as tincture, in capsule form as extract of silybum, or as powdered milk thistle, which is less potent.

Mucopolysaccharides, see Aloe Vera, Green-Lipped Mussel

Omega-3 Fish Oils

The benefits of fish oils are well described in other parts of this book (see page 16 and Heart Disease, page 118). Fish oil capsules are a convenient way to take the "active ingredients" in oily fish—the omega-3 fatty acids, eicosapentenoic acid (EPA) and docosahexenoic acid (DHA).

They are particularly useful for people who have been asked by their physicians to increase their EPA and DHA intake, but who don't like to eat oily fish. It has been estimated that for full benefit in, say, cases of high cholesterol, two to three portions of oily fish are required a week. Two to three capsules offering about 400 mg of EPA/DHA per capsule daily should be roughly equivalent to two portions of oily fish a week. Exceeding this amount may be even better and will certainly not harm you. Latest research suggests that the effects of fish oils can be boosted by taking them with garlic. Those with raised cholesterol levels should only take omega-3 oil supplements under medical supervision.

Passion Flower

Passion flower (*Passiflora*) is an excellent remedy for insomnia and a mild sedative. In tablet form it is a relatively low-cost, non-addictive "sleeping pill," and, as a supplement, is often combined with other sedative plants, such as hops, chamomile, and valerian.

Pre-biotics

When we take antibiotics to kill bacterial infections, they not only kill the "bad" bacteria, but also the "friendly" bacteria that balance the flora in the body and help to prevent conditions such as thrush, candida, and cystitis. If the numbers of "friendly" bacteria are reduced, they need to be encouraged to re-establish. Pre-biotics are food components called oligosaccharides, a source of soluble fiber that stimulates the growth of the healthy bifido-bacteria by providing a source of food for these bacteria. Particularly beneficial seem to be the fructo-oligosaccharides found in Jerusalem artichokes, onions, and Belgian endive, and also in tablet form. Around 5–10 g is a normal dose per day for 1 or 2 weeks after antibiotics have been taken.

Pro-biotics

The work of the pre-biotics can be enhanced by food supplements containing pro-biotics—the "friendly" gut bacteria, including lactobacillus acidophilus and lactobacillus bifidus. These bacteria can be found in some live yogurts, but taking them in tablet form is a more guaranteed way to get enough of the bacteria to make a difference, as many so-called live yogurts have been shown to have low levels. Pre- and probiotics should be bought from a retailer who stores them in refrigerated conditions, as the bacteria can easily be destroyed by light and heat.

Propolis

Propolis—also known as bee propolis or bee pollen—is made by bees to sterilize their hives, and it is said that, taken in supplement form, it provides antibiotic and antiviral protection for humans, too. It may also be anti-inflammatory, and may help cure gum disease and speed healing. Propolis supplements can be taken by most people, but not anyone who suffers from hay fever or asthma. Propolis lozenges may soothe sore throats.

Royal Jelly

One of the most famous supplements of all in recent years, royal jelly is the sole food fed to the Queen bee by worker bees (who don't eat it themselves). Because the Queen bee lives much longer than the workers (3–5 years as opposed to 6–8 weeks), it is assumed by fans of royal jelly that this is the reason. However, there is little real evidence to substantiate the claims made for royal jelly in human consumption—increased stamina, fertility, and longevity. The only unusual nutrient to have been found in royal jelly is a fatty acid called trans l hydroxydelta 2 decenoic acid, which is found in no other food—proponents say that this is the "magic ingredient," but nothing has yet been proved. Some manufacturers of royal jelly capsules say that you need 150 mg royal jelly for 2–3 months before you will notice an effect, and fresh jelly—rather than other forms—is recommended. This could work out to be quite expensive.

Silymarin, see Milk Thistle

Spirulina, see Blue-Green Algae

Starflower Oil

Starflower (borage) oil is an even richer source of GLA than evening primrose oil, containing approximately twice as much—i.e., 20%, or 1,000 mg starflower oil will yield 200 mg GLA. Though supplements are more expensive than evening primrose oil, obviously fewer capsules need to be taken to achieve the same GLA intake, which may be of benefit to some people. See Evening Primrose Oil.

St. John's Wort

Hypericum perforatum is commonly known as St. John's Wort and is a native wild perennial plant of Europe, including many parts of the UK. The yellow flowers, taken in dried, tincture. or supplement form, are an established treatment in Europe for cases of mild depression and stress, and the plant is gaining in reputation and becoming more used elsewhere.

Conducted trials have shown the efficacy of *Hypericum perforatum* in treating depression; the plant is also thought to be antiviral, and may be of use in AIDS and all viral infections. St. John's Wort is used widely to help cure menopausal symptoms and may also be used for a variety of other symptoms, though results are mainly anecdotal. Doses to treat depression are usually 1,000 µg (micrograms) daily or 10 drops of tincture in water.

Valerian

Another popular supplement for insomnia, this is often combined with passion flower or hops as such.

Wheat Grass

This latest health drink consists of wheat grains sprouted until they become young grass and then puréed. It is said to be antioxidant, immune-boosting, a tonic, and detoxifier, containing many nutrients and chlorophyll, said to cleanse the system. Some American studies suggest that wheat grass may be anticarcinogenic, too, but the evidence is not yet firm.

Herbs for health

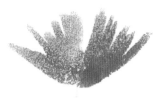

In the West we tend to think of herbs simply as tasty flavorings similar to salt and pepper. We buy them in small jars, ready-dried and -chopped, to be used once or twice, and then they lurk on the shelf for months until we throw them away. However, fresh herbs are not only a wonderful addition to your daily diet but also some of the most potent medicines around.

If you have a windowsill, a pot or two on the patio, or even an area you can turn into an herb garden, it is worth growing at least a few of your own herbs, to cook with or to use in other ways to help your health. Others you can pick from the hedgerow, in the meadow—or even from unweeded areas of your garden... for free!

The main "active" ingredients in herbs are their volatile oils and various phytochemicals, which offer a huge range of therapeutic benefits. Some are sedatives, others digestives, some antibiotics, others stimulant, for example.

Herbs can be used fresh in salads or as a garnish, in cooking, or made into a tea; or they can be dried or frozen and used in cooking; or they can be converted into tinctures that will last a long time. Of course, manufacturers also dry them or extract the oils and convert them into supplement form (see previous pages for more details).

Almost any plant (including its leaves, flowers, buds, seeds, roots, and bark) with a medicinal or therapeutic use can be described as an herb, but for our purposes here an herb is an annual, biennial, perennial plant, or small shrub, the leaves of which you use, and that you can grow in a small area and/or that would look fine as part of an herb garden—with the exception of the two "weed" herbs we have included, nettle and dandelion, which may not be so welcome amongst the rosemary and thyme! Both of these are best picked from a "wild" patch, inside your garden or out.

■ Picking and storing fresh herbs

It is best to pick herbs in the early morning, when they should be at their freshest and most potent. Once picked, they should be taken indoors very quickly, especially if the weather is hot, as they will soon wilt. Leaves can be picked at any time of year if they look green and healthy (some herbs, such as thyme and rosemary, are evergreen and can be picked all year round), especially for cooking purposes. To retain maximum medicinal properties, however, leaves are best gathered before the plant flowers.

If possible, pick enough for immediate use, or, if you pick extra to use fresh at another time, pick whole stems (not just the leaves), immerse these in water as you would a bunch of flowers, and keep them in a cool spot indoors until required, changing the water daily. Herbs that have been de-stemmed will also keep well in a plastic bag in the salad drawer of the refrigerator. Don't chop fresh herbs until the last possible moment before use.

■ Drying fresh herbs

Pick the herbs as above. If you have a dry, warm, and airy room, you can simply hang stemmed herbs up in bunches to dry. You can, if you like, tie large paper bags around the bunches so that if leaves fall off they fall into the bags.

You can also dry small sprigs of herbs on a baking sheet in a very cool oven or in an airing cupboard. Turn once or twice and remove them as soon as they seem completely dry—stems should break

easily if they are dry enough. Once dry, either hang the sprigs up in bunches or de-leaf them, storing the dried leaves in airtight containers in a cool, dark place.

■ Freezing fresh herbs

Some herbs you can simply de-stem, pop into small freezer bags, and freeze as they are. Parsley works well this way—when frozen, you can crumble it and save the bother of chopping it when it is thawed. The softer-leaved herbs, like mint and cilantro, can be frozen in ice-cube trays with a little water, and used in cooking simply by putting a cube into your cooking pot. Basil doesn't freeze very well; it is better dried.

■ Infusions

For medicinal purposes you can make an infusion of fresh or dried herb leaves, just as you would a pot of ordinary tea. See the recipe on page 255. Infusions will not keep—drink them the same day.
NOTE: Herbal remedies should not be taken for more than a few weeks at a time.

■ Infused oils

Herbs can also be chopped, covered with a good-quality olive oil, and left in an airtight jar in a warm place for two to three weeks. Then the oil is strained off to be used medicinally, or even in cooking or on salads, depending upon which herb has been infused.

For example, infused oils of thyme, rosemary, and tarragon make excellent cooking oils.

Some popular herbs for health

Angelica *Angelica archangelica:*
Hardy biennial, up to 8 ft (2.5 m).
Damp soil, needs plenty of space.
Culinary Uses: Stems can be crystallized; leaves chopped and added to salads.
Medicinal Uses: Root and seeds, as well as the stem and leaves, used as a powerful digestive, tonic, expectorant, and circulatory stimulant.

Basil, Sweet *Ocimum basilicum:*
Half-hardy annual, up to 20 inches (50 cm).
Dry, sheltered, sunny, good in pots and tubs, window-boxes.
Culinary Uses: Leaves used in salads, good with tomatoes, major constituent of traditional Italian pesto and French pistou, good in most pasta dishes.
Medicinal Uses: Infusion of leaves can aid digestion, flatulence, nausea, stomach-ache, mildly sedative. Oil infusion can be used as insect repellent and sting relief.

Chives *Allium schoenoprasum:*
Hardy perennial, 1 ft (30 cm). Sunny, well-drained bed or pot, window-sills and -boxes.
Culinary Uses: Chopped into salads, dips, soups, sauces, omelets, a constituent of bouquet garni or *fines herbes*, use as onions. Add at end of cooking.
Medicinal Uses: From the same family as garlic and onions, with similar (though less potent) allium compounds. Rich in vitamin C and iron, acts as digestive, can help lower blood cholesterol if eaten in quantity.

Dandelion *Taraxacum officinale:*
Hardy perennial, to 1 ft (30 cm). Will grow almost anywhere.
Culinary Uses: Leaves are excellent in salads; root ground as "coffee."
Medicinal Uses: Strong diuretic, potassium-rich, blood detoxifier, root is aid to liver action and has also been used to treat arthritis, eczema, and constipation.

Lemon Balm *Melissa officinalis:*
Hardy perennial, to 2 ft (60 cm).
Culinary Uses: Excellent tea, leaves can be used in salads.
Medicinal Uses: Calming; antiviral (infusion good for treating cold sores); may also help over-active thyroid.

Lovage *Levisticum officinale:*
Hardy perennial, to 6 ft (2 m).
Needs plenty of space, sunny, well-drained.
Culinary Uses: Tasty addition to salads, good in soups and casseroles.
Medicinal Uses: Warming tonic that stimulates circulation; digestive; diuretic; can help cystitis, period pains.

Mint *Mentha spicata, spearmint:*
Hardy perennial, to 3 ft (90 cm). Pot or bed (invasive).
Culinary Uses: Spearmint is the traditional English mint, peppermint (*M. piperita*) and apple mint (*M. rotundifolia*) are similar in use—in sauces, relishes, as vegetable and fruit garnish, as tea and in cold drinks.
Medicinal Uses: Mint contains menthol, used widely for an indigestion remedy, and for clearing congestion in colds and chest infections. It also helps purify the breath, an infusion applied to the skin can help relieve pain, and oil infusion can be used as a massage balm.

Nettle *Urtica dioica:*
Hardy perennial, to 3 ft (90 cm).
Culinary Uses: Young leaves—said to be rich in iron, potassium, vitamin C, and carotenoids—can be used as a green vegetable similar to spinach, lightly cooked or made into a soup. Nettle tea is also good.
Medicinal Uses: Diuretic, cleansing and detoxifying herb; to help relieve the pain of arthritis, bites and stings, nettle and nappy rash; helps excretion of uric acid in gout; calms hay fever and rhinitis. Nettle root is being used to treat enlarged prostate.

Parsley *Petroselinum crispum:*
Hardy biennial, to 1 ft (30 cm). Most situations, except shade, including window-sills and -boxes.
Culinary Uses: Parsley is rich in iron, carotenoids, and vitamin C, and uses are many, including sauces, soups, salads, in herb blends, and with pasta.
Medicinal Uses: Diuretic and stimulating to the liver; breath freshener; can help arthritis and gout.

Rosemary *Rosmarinus officinalis:*
Semi-hardy shrub, to 4 ft (1.25 m). Sheltered, dry, sunny border or pot.
Culinary Uses: Pungent herb ideal for cooking with meats, chicken, fish; also good in herb bread.
Medicinal Uses: Tonic and circulation stimulant; said to enhance memory and help mild depression, headaches, and migraine.

Sage *Salvia officinalis:*
Shrub, to 2 ft (60 cm) Dry, sunny borders, pots.
Culinary Uses: Ideal with duck, goose, pork. Savory stuffing ingredient and blends well with other herbs, in omelets, onion, and mixed vegetable dishes.
Medicinal Uses: Antiseptic, digestive, and stimulant, but is also a calming herb. Said to be tonic for the liver, memory, and nerves. Infusion makes a good mouthwash and gargle for sore throats and gum problems.

Thyme *Thymus vulgaris:*
Sub-shrub, to 1 ft (30 cm). Dry, sunny banks, pots, window-boxes.
Culinary Uses: Herb widely used in meat cooking, in stuffings, herb blends, omelets and egg cookery.
Medicinal Uses: A powerful antiseptic, infusion helps bronchitis and respiratory infections, asthma, thrush; anti-flatulence; oil infusion helps bites and stings and fungal skin complaints. Thyme is an antioxidant and tonic.

Demystifying detoxification

Everybody's doing it—detoxing. A "detox" diet seems to be the millennium's answer to taking the waters or food combining. For anyone who feels run down, tired, or in any other way under par, detoxing appears to be the answer. So what exactly IS a "detox" diet—and does it really work?

Toxicants can enter your body in or on what you eat (e.g., pesticides, herbicides, hormones, preservatives, etc.) and even a "healthy" diet may include more of these "hidden extras" than you would think. Even "healthy" foods, in the wrong quantities, may become toxins. For example, you can overdose on carrots or cod liver oil. You may also be mildly intolerant to a food without realizing.

Viral and bacterial organisms can enter in or on food, too, or via the skin and lungs, and these are "toxic" in that the body fights them off. Frequent or recurring minor—and less minor—ailments may be indicative of the immune system's inability to cope. Swollen lymph glands (in the neck or up the arms, for instance) when you aren't exactly ill but feel "under par" are indicative of too much "detox" work to do.

Tobacco smoke contains toxins that we breathe in (even if we don't smoke). Alcohol is toxic in large quantities or in moderately large quantities on too regular a basis. Medicines and drugs can be toxic—even over-the-counter painkillers can have a strong effect on the stomach, liver, and so on.

Stress—both physical and emotional stress—can compound the problems. So, if you feel "under the weather" and have been subject to more than one or two of these factors, you may possibly feel a lot better for "detoxing."

■ How can a detox diet work?

It is the job of the lymphatic system—a network of glands and tubes—to drain excess fluids from all body tissues. At the lymph nodes (glands), foreign material and any unwelcome microorganisms, such as infections, are filtered out before the lymph fluid joins the blood. A healthy lymph system is, therefore, important in detoxing the body. Outward signs of a sluggish lymph are swollen or puffy eyes, swollen ankles, and dull skin and eyes.

Perhaps the most important of the "detoxing" jobs are carried out by the liver, probably the most hard-working and versatile organ in the body. One of its jobs is to convert the body's own waste materials—such as ammonia (a poison produced when the body proteins are broken down) and outside toxins such as drugs, alcohol, inhaled toxins, and food-borne toxins—into harmless, or less harmful, components, for excretion.

To help this process, a healthy gallbladder and urinary system are also important, and an eating and exercise program that helps speed up removal of wastes from the body in the urine could also then be regarded as a legitimate part of a "detox" routine. Unwanted body material is also disposed of through the bowels and, therefore, regular bowel movement is important. Waste material is, lastly, excreted in sweat and breath, two processes that can also be enhanced through diet and exercise.

A useful "detox" diet will, therefore, aim to help by providing dietary items that will encourage the processing and elimination of toxins—and by, as far as possible, avoiding all dietary items likely to be toxic. Lastly, a diet high in antioxidant phytochemicals will help to de-oxidize the body and neutralize harmful free radicals that will be produced during a detox regime. Regular exercise will also help by increasing lymph activity (lymph flow increases up to 15 times during exercise), by creating urine, by encouraging the bowels to work, and by increasing blood circulation, liver activity, sweating, and exhalation.

FOODS AND HERBS FOR DETOXING:

To help liver and/or gallbladder function: dandelion root, marigold (flowers and leaves), parsley, burdock (leaves or root), milk thistle (can be taken as a supplement), peppermint, dock root, globe artichoke, apples, olive oil, cucumber, onion.

To help stimulate lymphatic system and circulation: angelica, lovage, marigold, oregano, rosemary, dock root, echinacea, ginger, cayenne.

To help fluid elimination: dandelion, lovage, nettles, parsley, tarragon, apples, cucumber, onion, dock root.

To help purify the blood: garlic, chives, onion, leek, dandelion, nettles, echinacea.

Laxative effect: olive oil, burdock, dock root, aloe vera juice.

To increase body heat/perspiration: marigold, thyme, garlic, onion, chives, mustard, green tea.

NOTE: Herbal regimes shouldn't be followed for more than 6 weeks without a break of 6 weeks, unless advised by a qualified practitioner.

SAMPLE OF HOW A DAY'S EATING ON A GOOD SHORT-TERM DETOX DIET MAY LOOK:

Glass of pure water 6 times a day

On rising
Water and fresh apple juice; two milk thistle tablets

Breakfast
Fresh fruit salad with live yogurt and sesame seeds
Dandelion and burdock decoction

Mid-morning
Aloe vera juice

Lunch
Large fresh mixed salad, including marigold petals, cucumber, onion, nettle leaves, with olive oil and lemon juice dressing
Fresh walnuts and almonds
Dandelion and burdock decoction

Mid-afternoon
Green tea

Evening
Globe artichoke dressed with olive oil and lime juice
Selection of crudités with live yogurt, cayenne, and chive dip
Apple and sunflower seeds
Dandelion and burdock decoction

Bedtime
Chamomile tea
Small slice of organic wholegrain bread (optional)

NOTE: For detoxes of more than a few days, add starchy vegetables and/or whole grains to at least two meals a day.

EXERCISE: Take two 20-minute walks and/or swims a day, concentrating on your breathing.

■ So what kind of diet to follow?

Some detox diets are little more than fasts with water. These may help in avoiding toxin intake, but may also be dangerous if followed for more than a day or two.

A good program needs to be one you can stay on for more than a day or two—so for most of us, who want to carry on leading a normal active life, it needs to contain a wider range of foods and more calories. Such a diet is more helpful if it contains plenty of the foods, herbs, etc., thought to help the body detoxify itself.

A list appears opposite—choose one or two from each category to eat or drink regularly while on your "detox" diet.

Several are herbs or roots—see page 255 for how to make infusions and decoctions.

Foods to eat happily are all organically grown fresh fruits, fruit juices, salads, and unstarchy vegetables, raw, steamed, or, occasionally, very lightly cooked; fresh herbs, olive oils, and other uncooked pure vegetable and seed oils, organic live yogurt, and raw nuts and seeds.

Such a diet can be followed for a few days if you are doing light work and light exercise, and will provide plenty of antioxidants. For longer-term detox, add whole grains and starchy vegetables—e.g., brown rice, quinoa, and a little organic wholegrain bread, potatoes, etc.

Foods to cut right down on—or out completely—include: animal products, all dairy products except yogurt as above, caffeine, alcohol, all processed foods. Also avoid drugs, other than necessary prescription medicines, and smoking.

Drink plenty of pure spring water—3 pints (1.75 liters) a day—and freshly squeezed fruit and vegetable juices. You can also drink homemade or organically produced herb and green tea.

Go to bed early and sleep with a window open, or use an ionizer to purify the air. You should spend at least part of each day outdoors in the clearest air you can find, and learn to breathe deeply.

■ How long before I feel better?

If you are intolerant to one or more foods and you carry out a detox that eliminates it, you may experience a withdrawal "headache," or flu-like feeling. Caffeine addicts may experience moderate to severe headache for up to 4 or 5 days on withdrawal. If there are considerable levels of toxins (e.g., pesticides) stored in body fat, a water-only fast may release large amounts at once, causing other symptoms.

This is one good reason not to go headlong into a strict fast without a few days' preparation, by gradually easing yourself into the regime—say, giving up alcohol or smoking. A low-cal, low-carb regime in itself can cause headache. After perhaps feeling worse and tired for a few days, maybe with a bad taste in the mouth, however, most people report an enhanced sense of well-being, feeling much more vital and alert after a week.

■ When should it end?

Rather than just abruptly stopping a detox, it is best to reintroduce a few other foods every day until eating a wide range of healthy foods again. If the detox has benefited you, it is wise to keep to its main principles, using fresh natural organic foods and drink, and avoiding sources of toxins as far as possible.

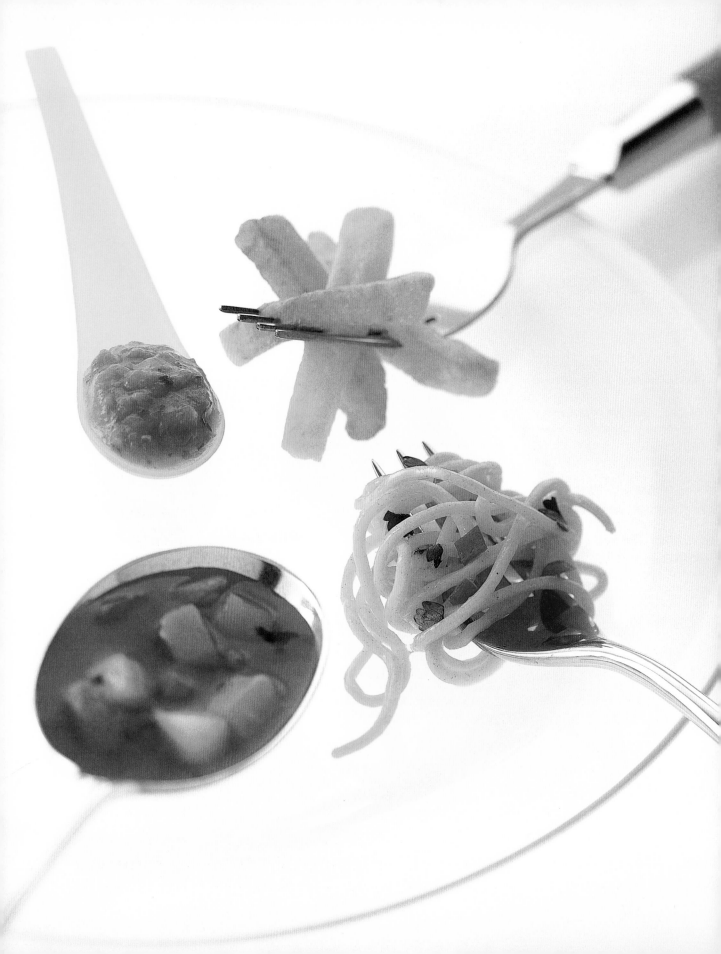

Food for the time of your life

Everyone knows that a baby needs different food from an adult—and that there are special dietary requirements for pregnant women. However, eating right for the time of your life is important at ANY age. Hardly any two decades, from birth to old age, will present the same set of nutritional problems. What you need now may well not be what is right for your health in several years' time. So here we look at all those different needs. For example, we examine the many problems that parents face in getting their children to eat well. Then there are the typical teenage food problems—like faddy eating and silly diets.

In the twenties and thirties, many people don't consider nutrition at all, but take their health for granted. Yet, with a little thought, one's "prime" can be even better—and adults can be better prepared for the years ahead. These may include pregnancy and getting food right before, during, and after the birth is the kindest thing a woman can do for her body—and her baby.

We move on to the middle years and, for women, the menopause. Many of the less wanted symptoms of these years can be reduced or prevented with a suitable diet. For men—well, there is menopause, too. A large number of doctors now believe that there IS such a thing as the male menopause, and so we look at what men should be doing to help smooth their passage through mid-life.

We also examine the importance of diet in the middle years to help prevent the problems that beset older people. For every 65-plus person who has ever thought, "It's too late now—it won't make any difference what I eat or drink," we prove them wrong! It is never too late to begin getting it right.

CHILDHOOD AND TEENAGE YEARS

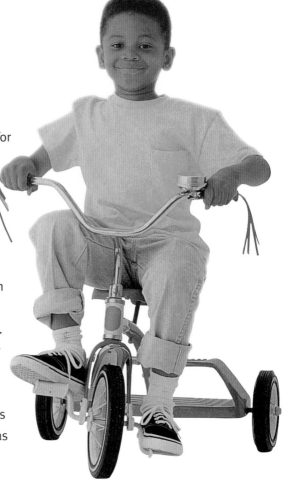

How much does your child's diet affect his or her health, growth, and future well-being? And what IS a healthy diet for most children? The importance of a suitable diet in childhood is recognized by every health professional, and yet the people who should care most—the parents—sometimes seem less concerned. In this country, only 22% of mothers breast-feed their babies until four months of age. By the age of $4^{1}/_{2}$, less than 40% of children eat any green vegetables except peas, and even fewer eat any salad. Yet cookies, sodas, potato chips and candies are eaten by more than 70% of preschool children. Studies show that children consume an excessive quantity of high-calorie fruit drinks and sodas. The average teen drinks about 65 gallons of soda a year! Thus, it is not surprising that a large proportion of children and teenagers are deficient in major minerals, while eating almost twice as much salt as is recommended.

Birth to four months

At this point, most babies need nothing other than breast milk, apart from vitamin K, which is routinely given at birth by injection. Few will need vitamin supplements or any other food (there are always exceptions, particularly if nutrition during pregnancy was inadequate). Breast feeding is beneficial to the baby's health in many ways:
* Breast milk contains some useful compounds, including lactoferrin and lysozome, which reduce risk of gastroenteritis, and ear and respiratory infections.

* It provides protection against asthma, eczema, and jaundice.
* Breast feeding may offer protection against other health problems, such as cows'-milk-protein allergy or intolerance, and against other food allergies in the longer term by building up immunity in the baby. (In atopic families, breast feeding is recommended for six months or longer.) It may also offer protection against diabetes and it is speculated that it may delay the onset of celiac disease.
* Breast milk is high in the long-chain omega-3 polyunsaturated acids, e.g., DHA (contained in fish oils), and this may

have an effect on "cognitive" (brain) development. For this reason—or perhaps other, as yet undiscovered, reasons—breast-fed children appear to have a higher IQ than bottle-fed children.
* Breast milk is natural, free, convenient, and easily digested, with a perfect balance of nutrients in a highly available form. For instance, the iron in breast milk is 70% absorbed, while that in formula milk is only 10% absorbed.

Bottle feeding, however, is necessary for some and adequate without further nutrition, again, normally, until the baby is around 4 months old, although one report has suggested that babies fed exclusively on formula milk may be at risk of selenium deficiency. An approved infant formula should be used (NOT ordinary cows'-, sheep's- or goats'-milk). About 2% of babies develop an allergy to the protein in cows' milk, which can cause vomiting, diarrhea, skin, and respiratory problems. Some also are intolerant of the lactose in cows' milk, which will also result in intestinal upsets (see Allergies, page 88).

Alternatives in these cases are infant formulas based on goats' milk (to which some are also intolerant or allergic) or soy milk, to which up to 10% of cows'-milk-intolerant infants are also intolerant. Soy milk is also higher in natural estrogens than formula milk and thus should only be given to babies on medical advice. Cows'-milk intolerance may be only temporary in infants, and medical advice should be taken.

Weaning

Weaning between the ages of 4 and 6 months is recommended by health experts. Earlier weaning has been linked with the development of celiac disease, with infection, and possibly with obesity in infants, and there is no advantage for most babies in introducing solids at an earlier age. However, between 4 and 6 months—by the time a baby has doubled his or her birth-weight—breast milk supplies of iron, zinc, copper, and vitamin D and A, protein, and energy supplied may not be adequate for the growing infant. By 6 months all babies will need some solid foods.

Research indicates a link between poor growth rate in infancy and disease in adult life. Low-weight infants at 1 year old have an increased risk of coronary heart disease in later life, for example. Breast feeding may continue to advantage until 1 year old or even longer,

COMMERCIAL BABY FOODS

It is possible for a weaned infant to get all his nutritional requirements from a diet based on commercial, ready-made (or dried) baby foods and formula milk. Artificial flavorings and other additives are normally not allowed, and sugar content should be stated on the label. Organic baby foods are available.

However, health experts recognize the importance of home-prepared food for the infant and suggests that it is ideal if home cooking is introduced to the diet early. There is evidence that infants fed only, or mostly, on commercial baby foods may be reluctant to change to home cooking as they grow older. It is also likely that the range of phytochemicals present in fresh foods, which we now know are so important to health, are just as important whatever one's age.

but if breast feeding is discontinued at weaning, the baby should receive infant formula to the age of one. Cows' milk should not be given as a main drink until 1 year old, although it can be introduced (though not recommended) in small quantities as part of the baby's food.

First weaning foods are usually bland, puréed gluten-free cereals, such as rice, potatoes, and some vegetables. These can be home-cooked or commercial, and a wider variety of items can be introduced from day to day—yogurt, custard, fruit, legumes and other vegetables, cereals, and meat can be offered, all still puréed. Water or milk should be the main drink; fruit juices (although most contain good amounts of vitamin C) also contain extrinsic sugars and should be limited, diluted, and offered only with a meal, (when the vitamin C will help iron absorption in the food), unless no fresh fruit is eaten. Fruit drinks, cordials, and sodas, tea, or coffee should not be offered, and neither should "diet" drinks containing artificial sweeteners. Sweet drinks should not be given in a bottle—infants can drink out of a cup after 6 months to avoid tooth decay. Bottles containing sweet drinks should never be given at bed- or nap-time.

Second-stage weaning foods (from the age of 6 to 9 months) can include

finger foods and foods with more texture, to encourage chewing, and wheat-containing foods and bread can also be introduced.

Third-stage (9 to 12 months plus) infants can begin to eat a diet similar to that of the rest of the family, with three meals a day plus snacks, and infants should be encouraged to feed themselves as much as possible. However, an infant diet shouldn't mimic the diet of a healthy adult exactly—a high-fiber, low-fat diet should be postponed. Salt should not be added to weaning foods at all.

Preschool children

From weaning to the age of five, children need more of some nutrients than adults and less of others. They need:

* More fat. Breast milk is over 50% fat; follow-on milks about 42% fat. Children should only gradually reduce the amount of fat in their diets, down to the recommended adult level of 30–35%. From 1 to 2 years old, whole milk should be given, and from 2 to 5, low-fat 2% milk can be given, but skim milk should not be used until after 5.

Whole-milk yogurts and cheeses are also preferable. The higher fat levels are important because of the high energy needs of young children (fat is the most calorie-dense food), and fats provide the fat-soluble vitamins A, D, E, and K. Children up to 2 can also cope only with moderate amounts of starchy foods.

* Less fiber. Young digestive systems are not equipped to deal with large amounts of high-fiber foods. High-fiber diets may hinder absorption of vital minerals, such as iron and calcium, and because high-fiber foods tend to need more chewing and appear to satisfy appetite more quickly than low-fiber foods, may also mean that a child may have trouble consuming enough food at each meal to take in adequate calories.

* Children should not be given whole nuts until age 5. They can choke on them—and nut allergy, particularly to peanuts, is a growing problem in children.

Most of all, small children need to enjoy their food and be encouraged to eat as wide a variety of new foods as possible. Young children are sometimes more willing to do this than school-age children. Almost any child dislikes some foods, but using Section One you can easily find replacement foods for all the nutrients. Often, a few weeks or months later, the refused food will become acceptable. It is important not to make an issue of food refused or the occasional meal when a child doesn't seem hungry. Negative associations with food can begin through a child being made to feel "naughty" or guilty.

How do you tell if a young child is getting all the nutrients he or she needs? If the child is growing well, has a good appetite, seems strong and active, and is neither fat nor thin, then all is well. A child who doesn't appear to be thriving, eats only a few foods, has an under- or overweight problem, is ill a lot, or suffers problems that may be linked to food intolerance, should see a physician and perhaps be referred to a dietitian. Poor growth-rate in young children has been linked with heart disease, stroke, and diabetes in later life. A survey of US preschool children revealed that 8% have lower-than-recommended levels of vitamin A intake, and 9% have low iron intake, with one in about 10 of all under-five-year-olds anemic, and 40% have intakes less than 70% of zinc RDI.

Ages 5 to 11

When a child reaches school age, good groundwork in previous years pays off. By this time, he or she should be enjoying a wide variety of meals, including plenty of fruits and vegetables. Normal healthy children of this age usually have very healthy appetites and, if plenty of activity is undertaken, may eat as much as an adult in order to gain enough weight and growth. The chart below lists nutrient requirements of children aged 1 to 11.

■ Packed lunches vs school meals

School meals should provide adequate nutrition, however, the nutritional content and value of school meals varies tremendously—not only according to the policy of the area and school but also the choices made by the child. The government tries to enforce strict nutritional standards for school meals but it is not easy. To be sure of what your child is getting at lunch, a packed lunch is a sensible answer.

A packed lunch should be similar in style to those recommended for adults on page 47, containing at least one high-carbohydrate item (e.g., sandwich, pasta), some protein (e.g., cheese, tuna), some fruit, something sweet but nutritious (e.g., a slice of fruit cake), and a drink of milk or pure juice. To that you can add what your child will need to satisfy his or her appetite (e.g., dried fruit, a hard-boiled egg). In winter, a small flask of soup is good. It is also important to vary contents as much as possible from day to day—otherwise the child gets bored and may not get a complete range of nutrients.

Remember that young children don't need a very low-fat diet, so don't feel guilty about contributing to the calorie content with fat—for instance, spreading bread with real butter, adding mayonnaise to a sandwich, giving whole milk, even a chocolate bar if the school allows it. What you need to do is pack a lunch containing plenty of fresh items and not too many highly refined, colored, additive-heavy items. Just make sure things are colorful and tasty.

SELECTED NUTRITIONAL NEEDS OF CHILDREN (RDI 1980)

Age	Calories	Protein g	Folate µg	C mg	A µg	D µg	Calcium mg	Iron mg	Zinc mg
1–3	1,300	23	100	45	400	10	500	15	10
4–6	1,700	30	200	45	500	10	800	10	10
7–10	2,400	34	300	45	700	10	800	10	10
11	2,200–2,700	45/46	400	50	800	10	1,200	18	15

■ Weight control

Parents often worry about their children getting overweight but, in fact, statistics show that there are also many malnourished, underweight children in the US. Despite the fact that our children are on average 1 inch (2.5 cm) taller at age 5 than they were in the sixties and average weight has increased, a large proportion of all child admissions to hospital are related to malnutrition. (Malnutrition is not just simply underweight, however, but also deficiency in nutrients.)

If your child looks fat (compare with the other children in the class to get a sensible comparison), however, the best course of action is to reduce portion sizes slightly, cut back a little on the very-high-fat and sugary items, like puddings, cakes, cookies, chocolate, and candies, and offer slightly more lower-calorie items like yogurts, fresh fruit, and so on. Don't mention the word "diet" to your child; there's no need. Over the months, most children will grow taller, while staying the same weight or losing a little—and so look much slimmer.

Without appearing over-anxious about childhood overweight, it is more sensible to do something about it early on, in as relaxed a way as possible, rather than leaving it and hoping the child will "grow out of it."

Children's high energy needs in comparison with their age should not become an excuse to feed them exclusively on a high-saturated-fat, high-sugar, low-fresh-food diet.

More importantly, exercise and good nutrition will help to prevent heart disease and other health problems in adulthood. Although low birth-weight and low infancy-weight can increase risk of CHD, research shows that a child who is overweight at 6 to 9 has a ten times greater chance of being obese in adulthood, and a child overweight at 10 to 14 has a 28 times greater chance.

The height/weight charts for children given here are only a guide—there is much individual variation. Weight for height is a better guide than weight for age. Use common sense in interpreting this chart: if your child is in the center of the lower and upper figures there is no problem; if right at the maximum average, there may be a weight problem in the making. If he or she is right at the minimum weight, care should be taken that weight does not fall farther.

AVERAGE WEIGHTS AND HEIGHTS OF CHILDREN

Age	Weight			Height		
	Bottom	Average	Top of range	Bottom	Average	Top of range
Girls						
5	29 lb (13.05 kg)	40 lb (18.00 kg)	60 lb (27.00 kg)	3 ft 1¾ in (0.94 m)	3 ft 6½ in (1.06 m)	3 ft 11¼ in (1.18 m)
6	32 lb (14.40 kg)	44 lb (19.80 kg)	69 lb (31.05 kg)	3 ft 4¼ in (1.01 m)	3 ft 9¼ i (1.13 mn)	4 ft 2¼ in (1.26 m)
7	35 lb (15.75 kg)	51 lb (22.95 kg)	82 lb (36.90 kg)	3 ft 6 in (1.05 m)	3 ft 11½ in (1.19 m)	4 ft 5 in (1.33 m)
8	39 lb (17.55 kg)	56 lb (25.20 kg)	97 lb (43.65 kg)	3 ft 8 in (1.10 m)	4 ft 2 in (1.25 m)	4 ft 7½ in (1.39 m)
9	42 lb (18.9 kg)	63 lb (28.35 kg)	112 lb (50.40 kg)	3 ft 10 in (1.15 m)	4 ft 4 in (1.30 m)	4 ft 10¼ in (1.46 m)
10	46 lb (20.7 kg)	71 lb (31.95 kg)	128 lb (57.60 kg)	3 ft 11½ in (1.19 m)	4 ft 6¼ in (1.36 m)	5 ft 1 in (1.53 m)
11	51 lb (22.95 kg)	79 lb (35.55 kg)	143 lb (64.35 kg)	4 ft 1 in (1.23 m)	4 ft 8¾ in (1.42 m)	5 ft 3¾ in (1.60 m)
Boys						
5	31 lb (13.95 kg)	40 lb (18.45 kg)	60 lb (26.10 kg)	3 ft 2 in (0.95 m)	3 ft 7 in (1.08 m)	3 ft 11¾ in (1.19 m)
6	33 lb (14.85 kg)	46 lb (20.70 kg)	69 lb (30.60 kg)	3 ft 4 in (1.00 m)	3 ft 7 in (1.08 m)	4 ft 2¾ in (1.27 m)
7	38 lb (17.10 kg)	51 lb (22.95 kg)	82 lb (35.55 kg)	3 ft 6½ in (1.06 m)	4 ft (1.20 m)	4 ft 5 in (1.33 m)
8	41 lb (18.45 kg)	56 lb (25.20 kg)	97 lb (41.40 kg)	3 ft 8½ in (1.11 m)	4 ft 2¼ in (1.26 m)	4 ft 8 in (1.40 m)
9	44 lb (19.80 kg)	62 lb (27.90 kg)	112 lb (48.60 kg)	3 ft 10¼ in (1.16 m)	4 ft 4¼ in (1.31 m)	4 ft 10½ in (1.46 m)
10	49 lb (22.05 kg)	68 lb (30.60 kg)	126 lb (56.70 kg)	4 ft (1.20 m)	4 ft 6¼ in (1.36 m)	5 ft 1 in (1.53 m)
11	53 lb (23.85 kg)	77 lb (34.65 kg)	143 lb (63.45 kg)	4 ft 1¼ in (1.23 m)	4 ft 8¼ in (1.41 m)	5 ft 3¼ in (1.58 m)

Data from Child Growth Foundation, 1995

Childhood eating problems

The nutritional needs of children, as outlined on the previous page, are fairly straightforward. For many parents, however, putting those needs into practice—in the form of an everyday diet that their children will actually eat—is far from straightforward.

From toddler to twelve-year-old, how do you persuade your child to eat what you want him or her to eat, rather than the "junk" he or she seems to want? And what can you do with a child who will eat only one or two types of food for weeks at a time, or the child who will hardly eat at all?

■ The junk food dilemma

You want your child to eat fresh fish, green vegetables, citrus fruits, and whole-wheat pasta, but he or she hates all that and only wants commercial hamburgers, pizza, French fries, baked beans, ice cream, chocolate, and candy. In truth, your ideas on good food and his or hers

are so far apart that you can't see how you're ever going to reach a compromise... but you will. You simply need to understand why children like "junk" food and then apply the same criteria to the kinds of food they should eat for good health—if that proves to be necessary. For the fact is that much of what we dismiss as "junk" is a perfectly acceptable part of your child's diet (see the panel on the opposite page).

First, let's look at the reasons why most children like "junk" food and how you can deal with that:

✱ They are familiar with it. Children like to experiment with new foods to a certain degree, while wanting to find something familiar on their plate at each meal. Children who have been raised on hamburgers and French fries can't be expected to forsake them overnight and turn to lentils and brown rice.

Solution: "Starting as you mean to go on" is a sensible idea when it comes to feeding your family. Children who are weaned onto a healthy varied diet, with plenty of fresh fruit, vegetables, and

salads, will tend to carry on being happy to eat this way even if in later years they crave the occasional "junk" item.

If, in your child's case, it is too late for that, you need to introduce the healthier foods into the diet very slowly and in small amounts, disguised, as necessary (see the next point).

✱ It is easy to eat with minimal chewing. Many children hate anything at all difficult to chew or swallow—lumps of meat, fibrous vegetables or fruits, even bread crusts. This is understandable because, of course, children are one stage on from babies whose diet is mainly liquid.

Solution: All "healthy" foods can be served in child-palatable form without much trouble. If you want your child to eat meat, offer it in ground form as homemade burgers, meat pies, lasagnes, soups, pasta sauce, and so on. Most vegetables and fruits can be puréed or mashed, or the tougher bits of stalk, etc., removed—children don't need to eat them to get their fiber. You can get most children to eat fresh fruit by converting it

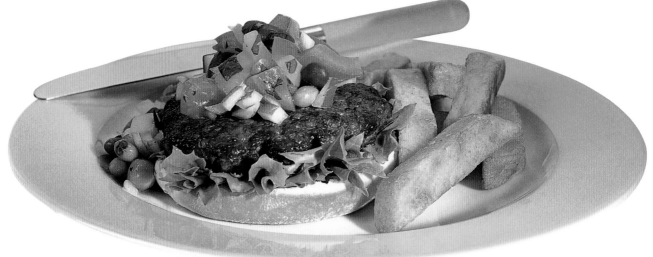

BURGERS USING LEAN MEAT AND BROILED OR DRY-FRIED ARE AN EXCELLENT SOURCE OF IRON, B VITAMINS, AND PROTEIN FOR CHILDREN. HOMEMADE IS A BETTER BET THAN COMMERCIAL BURGERS.

into homemade fruit juices, fruity milk shakes, popsicles, ice creams, and fruit jello. You can also cut crusts off bread and feed the birds or grind them into crumbs and freeze them for savory toppings, gratins, etc.

✱ Children like attractive colorful food— junk food isn't always, but it often is, with golden fries, crimson tomato ketchup, golden crumbed fish fingers or golden pastry, and brightly colored drinks and desserts.

Solution: Try to present all food attractively and use plenty of the more colorful fruits and vegetables, cut into small pieces. Don't serve over-boiled, soggy vegetables—besides looking and tasting totally unattractive, they have hardly any of their inherent nutrients left in them anyway.

✱ Children like tasty food. They like things that really hit the palate and quickly learn to mistake the high salt content of most savory junk foods, and the high sugar content of most sweet junk foods, for "taste."

Solution: Make your own healthy offering as tasty as you can by using natural flavors and healthier items. Make full use of the sweeter fruits, dried fruits, raw cane sugar, Greek-style or plain yogurt and honey for homemade desserts. When cutting down on salty and sweet items, do so slowly a little at a time. The average child's palate can be re-educated to accept less salt and sugar in a few weeks.

■ Junk food—the truth

The fact is that a lot of the foods that you may consider to be complete junk actually contain a lot of valuable nutrients for growing children. Children need plenty of energy (calories), protein, and calcium, as discussed earlier. In fact, when "health food" eating became widely popular in the 1980s, the children of many "health food" converts became nutritionally and calorifically deficient

because the parents' so-called healthy diet was depriving them of all three vital elements.

There have also been many documented cases of children who have existed for months on only one, two, or three different types of food—for example, jelly sandwiches and milk, or bananas and orange juice—and on later examination have proved to be in perfectly good health and making normal good growth.

So, instead of fighting with a child over yet another request for hamburger and fries for their evening meal, perhaps the sensible answer is to look for ways to make that hamburger and fries more acceptable to you both, by, say, making the burger at home out of extra-lean pork or lamb, by using large fries that are brushed with oil and baked (or by offering baked potato skins instead), by adding a small colorful salad or, if that is refused, a glass of fresh citrus juice, or a dessert of fresh strawberries.

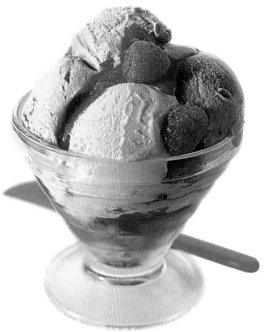

ICE CREAM IS A GOOD SOURCE OF CALCIUM AND PROTEIN. TOP WITH A HOMEMADE FRUIT PURÉE FOR A HEALTHY TREAT.

JUNK FOOD—OR IS IT?

French fries: Can be a good source of vitamin C, calories, and some fiber and, if cooked well in fresh oil (or brushed in oil and oven-baked), have no negatives unless your child tends to be overweight, in which case deep-fried fries should be limited as they are high in calories.

Burgers: Made with lean meat and broiled or dry-fried are an excellent source of iron, B vitamins and protein for children. Homemade is a better bet than commercial burgers, which are usually higher in fat. If choosing beef, you may prefer to use organic.

Baked Beans: High in protein and fiber and low in fat.

White Bread: Good source of calcium and ideal for children who generally don't need as much dietary fiber as adults. Try to buy good-quality bread made from hard wheats.

Chocolate: Contains iron and calcium and, if a child isn't overweight, is a better occasional snack than candies.

Pizza: Good food for children, containing calcium, vitamin C, and fiber. Go for vegetable-topped pizza rather than the high-fat meat and salami versions.

Ice cream: Good source of calcium and protein. Top with a homemade fruit purée for a healthy dessert for children.

White pasta: Fine for children, who don't necessarily need the extra fiber that whole-wheat pasta provides.

The truth is that there are few genuine completely "junk" foods. The exceptions are the sweet and sugary products that offer little if any nutritional benefit, but too many additives for comfort—the colored sodas and fruit drinks, brightly colored candies, commercial popsicles, and packaged dessert mixes that line our supermarket shelves. Don't buy them, and don't give your child the impression that these are "treats" for special occasions—take time to explain in the simplest terms that they are poor food lacking in real substance.

It's also wise to limit the amount of commercial pies, pastries, cookies, cakes, and bakery items that you let your child eat, especially the cheaper ones. They are often extremely high in saturated fat and/or hardened margarines (trans fats), and (in the case of sweet items) sugar, but little else in the way of good nutrients, and are also often high in salt (both the savory and the sweet ones).

Active children may be able to eat these foods and stay slim and apparently healthy, but a diet high in saturated fat is linked with heart disease and obesity in adult years. Tests have also shown that children as young as 10 who eat such a diet already show signs of atherosclerosis (the "furring" of the arteries that is an early sign of possible heart disease). It is, therefore, best to keep an eye on saturated fats in your child's diet right from the early years.

Those items apart, most other foods can be eaten and enjoyed by your child as part of a varied diet without you having to feel guilty in any way, as long as you always remember to add some fresh fruit, and fresh or frozen vegetables to every meal of the day.

Think of your child's diet as something you are constantly trying to improve. It may not be perfect now—but children's tastes evolve and can be manipulated with patience and a "softly softly" approach.

SPECIAL POINTERS TO CHILD HEALTH THROUGH FOOD

Sweet tooth: Children have a naturally sweet tooth, probably because breast milk and formula milk is sweet. Try to satisfy this throughout childhood with fruits first, offering refined sweet products as little as possible. It is best to get away from the idea that candies and chocolate and desserts are "reward" foods. Sweet foods are one of the major causes of tooth decay.

Asthma: Childhood asthma, coughing, and wheezing has been shown to be reduced in children who eat enough fresh fruits and vegetables. There is also evidence that a diet low in vitamins E and A may increase risk of asthma-type illnesses. For foods high in these vitamins, see the lists on pages 24 and 22.

Breakfast: This is an important meal for children, tests show. Energy, concentration, and brain power are all better in children who get a good breakfast. They are also more creative and have more physical endurance. If a child is having a packed lunch, a hot breakfast such as oatmeal or a boiled egg and toast is a good idea. A small bowl of highly refined sugary cereal does not really provide enough calories.

Nutrients: Most likely to be in shortfall in schoolchildren up to age 11 are folate and zinc. At age 11, calcium and iron deficiencies are fairly common.

Soy milk: Soy milk and soy products are regarded as safe as part of a general and varied diet for children, despite the recent findings in animal tests of a link between soy-based infant formula and problems with reproductive development.

The teenage years

Teenagers (especially those aged between 14 and 18) have greater nutritional needs than any other age-group in terms of calorie, protein, vitamin, and mineral requirements. This is the crucial time for making height and muscle, for building bone mass, and for sexual development. Health problems later in life, including osteoporosis and heart disease, may be influenced by what people eat in their teens. Yet, sadly, many teenagers get a poorer diet than most other social groups. Here we discuss the main areas of concern in the teenage diet and offer solutions.

■ Girls and iron intake
The iron RDI for female teenagers is higher than that for boys of the same age (see the chart on the right) because iron is lost each month in the blood during menstruation, and young teenage girls tend to have heavier periods than women in their 20s and 30s. However, research suggests that optimum iron intake is actually being met by few girls. Since many girls are worried about weight gain and/or are becoming semi-vegetarians, iron intake can be well below the RDI.

All the general notes on the importance of iron in the diet (see page 30) also apply to teenagers, but the shortfall is of particular importance because it has been shown in more than one scientifically controlled trial that iron deficiency in the teens can affect academic performance.

One 1989 trial showed that in schoolchildren with moderate iron-deficiency anemia, a three-month course of supplements measurably improved both physical and academic performance. Another 1997 trial showed that iron-deficient teenage girls have IQ scores almost ten points lower than others, and that a ten-week course of supplements

DAILY ENERGY REQUIREMENTS AND RDIS FOR SELECTED NUTRIENTS FOR TEENAGERS

Age	Calories** g	Protein mg	Calcium mg	Iron mg	Zinc µg	A µg	Folate mg	C
Boys								
12–14	2,500	45	1,200	12	15	800	200	50
15–18	3,000	59	1,200	12	15	800	200	60
(19 plus as adult)								
Girls								
12–14	2,200	46	1,200	15*	15	800	180	50
15–18	2,200	44	1,200	15*	15	800	180	60
(19 plus as adult)								

* 10% of girls may need more than this.

** Calories are just estimates and vary according to body size and lifestyle.

this time of life to help build bone mass during the period of enormous growth spurt (12–16 for girls and 13–18 for boys). Folic acid intake is also low in both sexes in the teens, just as in younger children, and this important nutrient is also found in many similar foods to those high in iron (e.g., variety meats and dark leafy greens). Deficiency in folate and its best sources are discussed on page 28.

leveled out the difference.

Why do so many teenage girls not get enough iron from their diets? There seem to be four reasons: one, many follow faddy low-calorie diets so they don't eat enough food to provide the iron; two, many are vegetarian or semi-vegetarian, and some of the richest and most easily absorbed sources of iron are meats and meat products; three, many others eat a "junk" diet low on variety and particularly low on green vegetables (another good source of iron).

Such a "junk" diet also affects iron absorption—tea, coffee, caffeine drinks, and lack of vitamin C in the diet all lower the amount of iron that can be absorbed. Finally, school meals chosen by many teenagers tend to be below the recommended iron content and, for many teenagers, a school meal may be the main meal of the day.

Iron-rich foods (see the box below and the chart on page 30) should be introduced at each meal to help prevent teenage anemia, and, if you suspect that your daughter is already anemic, a doctor can do a blood test and prescribe iron tablets as necessary, which should be taken with food including items rich in vitamin C, such as fruit or fruit juice.

Of course, however, the four problems listed left may mean the task is difficult.

IRON-RICH FOODS:

Liver, red meat, liver pâté, dark green leafy vegetables, whole-wheat bread, seeds, fortified breakfast cereals, seaweed, cocoa powder, textured soy protein, vegetable burger mix, quinoa, lentils, pulses, cashew nuts, whole-grain barley, dried apricots and peaches, whole grains, eggs, baked beans in tomato sauce, curry powder.

■ Other teenage nutritional deficiencies

Teenagers with poor or insufficient eating habits are likely to be deficient in a range of important nutrients, but, importantly, research shows that many teenagers (both boys and girls) are significantly deficient in calcium, which is vital at

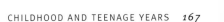

AVERAGE WEIGHTS OF TEENAGERS

Boys

Age	Average Weight
12½	92 lb (42 kg)
13½	106 lb (48 kg)
14½	118 lb (53.5 kg)
15½	130 lb (59 kg)
16	142 lb (64.5 kg)

Girls

Age	Average Weight
12½	97 lb (44 kg)
13½	106 lb (48 kg)
14½	105 lb (52 kg)
15½	122 lb (55.5 kg)
16–19	125 lb (57 kg)

(Based on information from the Department of Health growth charts)

■ Weight problems

Calorie intake is also too low in many teenage diets. In one survey, 25% of older teenagers and young women had a BMI (Body Mass Index, see page 188) lower than 20, meaning that they were clinically underweight, whereas throughout all adult age groups of women only 12% were lower than 20.

However, about 25% of people between the ages of 6 and 17 are overweight, this is probably due to lack of exercise, (particularly in girls), and is more common in teenagers who follow a high-fat, "junk"-type diet. Overweight teenagers will be unlikely to develop into slim and fit adults unless encouraged to take more exercise and eat a healthy diet. For more information, see Section Four.

■ Vegetarianism

An increasing number of teenagers are vegetarian and those between 16 and 24 have a higher concentration of vegetarians than any other age group. The guidelines on a safe and enjoyable vegetarian diet which appear on pages 60–63 also apply to teenagers. Special points to watch if your child decides to give up meat are:

✱ Make sure that the protein content of the diet remains reasonable by replacing meat with dairy products (sometimes the lower-fat versions, especially if the teenager inclines toward overweight), legumes, and other acceptable sources (see lists of protein sources on page 21).

✱ If your teenager is female, pay special attention to ensuring that she eats plenty of iron-rich foods and folate-rich foods.

✱ Find out what provision is made at school/college for vegetarian meals. If these meals are not adequate, the teenager should take a packed lunch.

✱ Make sure that your child is aware of what constitutes a healthy diet for vegetarians and knows how to prepare simple nutritious meat-free meals.

■ Anorexia and eating problems

The incidence of anorexia, bulimia, and over-strict dieting is high among teenagers, particularly teenage girls. There is a large article on these problems in Section Two (see page 107). If you feel that your teenager may have an eating problem, it is always best to attempt to sort it out at the earliest opportunity first by discussing what you perceive to be the problem with the child, and secondly by taking medical advice or other appropriate action (e.g. counseling or nutritional advice) and by contacting an eating disorders association, who can give plenty of help.

The following range of obvious danger signals will help you decide if your child does have, or may soon have, an eating problem:

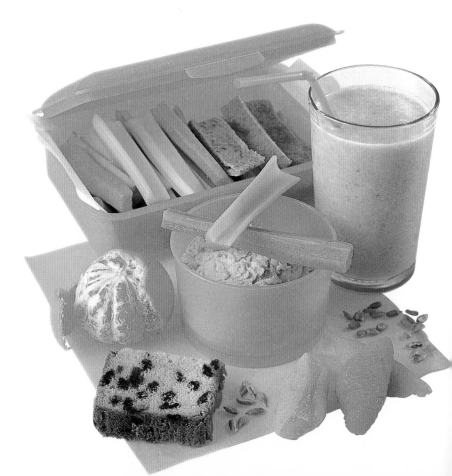

AN IDEAL VEGETARIAN LUNCH-BOX FOR TEENAGERS — SLICED WHOLE-WHEAT PITA, HUMMUS, CRUDITÉS, FRUIT CAKE, SMALL PACK OF SUNFLOWER SEEDS, DRIED APRICOTS, BANANA MILK SHAKE, TANGERINE.

✶ Wanting to diet although not over-weight.

✶ Preoccupation with calories and food.

✶ Eating too little and making excuses for not eating.

✶ Fluctuating body weight.

✶ Over-activity.

✶ Disappearing after meals (may have bulimia).

✶ Secretiveness, moodiness.

✶ Wants to hide their body from you.

■ **Refusal to eat a varied healthy diet**

For every teenager who is faddy about her or his diet in one way—wanting, for instance, no red meat and lots of healthy salads—there is another who tends to want nothing but foods like potato chips, fries, fried foods, pies, pastries, sweet things, and sodas, and will balk at having to eat anything like fresh vegetables, salad, and fruit.

Much of what has been said on page 164 about the "junk food dilemma" also applies to teenagers. They are, however, less likely to be compliant to your solutions than younger children! Teenagers also spend more time outside the home and outside the control of parents, and have more money to spend on the kind of food and snacks they wish to buy.

Appeals to vanity may work ("Your teeth will decay if you carry on eating so much sweet food!") or the official approach may do the trick—getting leaflets from school or your doctor on the importance of getting a healthy diet in the teenage years, for instance, or finding a dietitian to outline to him or her the possible dangers of a poor diet.

The key is, perhaps, to build on any areas—even if only one or two—of common ground. If possible, cook the things the teenager enjoys most yourself—e.g., he loves pies and French fries, well your homemade pies and fries are likely to be much better for him than those bought outside at the supermarket.

THIS MACARONI CHEESE, MADE WITH LOW-FAT 2% MILK AND INCLUDING PARBOILED BROCCOLI, PEAS, AND SLICED TOMATO, FORMS THE HEART OF AN EVENING MEAL WHICH ALMOST ANY VEGETARIAN TEENAGER WILL ENJOY—SERVED WITH A CRISP SIDE SALAD, AND FOLLOWED BY ICECREAM, AND FRESH FRUIT SALAD.

Research shows that children who receive a high proportion of home-cooked food tend to choose a better diet for themselves in later life.

Lastly, if all else fails make sure the teenager gets a daily multivitamin and mineral tablet.

■ **Acne**

Teenage acne is very common indeed; few boys are likely to escape completely. The subject is covered in Section Two on page 86.

■ **Anti-social behavior**

There is new evidence emerging from a long term UK-Government-sponsored study into violence and anti-social behavior in young people, that diet has a part to play, particularly deficiencies in vitamins, minerals, and essential fatty acids.

Other previous studies from other parts of the world have also indicated this—a variety of nutrients are lacking in the blood of criminals, for instance, and incidence of criminal acts falls sharply when extra nutrients are given. Exact advice on how to feed a potential teenage monster is not yet in hand, but it seems that a good general varied healthy diet may indeed help your children and young adults to behave better.

■ **Academic performance**

As we've already seen, lack of iron in teenage girls can cause lowered mental ability and performance. Other trials have shown that there may be a link between lack of a wider range of vitamins and minerals, and poor academic performance, but the evidence on this varies considerably.

The most likely conclusion is that if children and teenagers are falling short on nutrients then their performance may be impaired, but that if they already have a healthy diet and get their RDI of all the nutrients, then giving them more won't make any difference. Moreover, as with any age group, it is better to get nutrients within a healthy diet rather than as supplements.

ADULTHOOD

That period between the teens and the start of "middle age" in the mid-forties is a time when many people ignore, or even abuse, their health—eating poorly, drinking too much alcohol, coping with stress, lack of sleep, an over-busy lifestyle, and so on. Yet how you treat your body in this period has a very important bearing upon health later in life. This is the ideal time to look after yourself and your diet, so that middle and old age can be enjoyed in robust, optimum health, with as few illnesses and physical problems as possible.

Ages 20–35

These are the years when people tend to take fitness and good health for granted, and yet it is wise to use this time sensibly to build up a healthy body, fit for anything you care to do, including, for women, the stresses of pregnancy and child-care.

The Basic Healthy Diet and healthy eating guidelines described in Section One will ensure that such needs are met, but it is worth emphasizing here some of the most important nutritional points for young adults:

Bone building: At this age you are still building bone until peak bone-mass is reached around the age of 35. Optimum peak bone-mass means that the effects of osteoporosis in later life will be minimized. It is therefore vital to get enough calcium in the diet and to absorb enough calcium from that diet so that adequate bone is made. You won't get another chance to do this! Regular weight-bearing exercise, such as walking, will also help build bone. Follow all the guidelines on pages 28–9, eating plenty of lower-fat dairy products, tofu, legumes, leafy greens, nuts, and seeds.

Weight control: Many previously slim people tend to begin putting on weight, especially around the midriff, as they reach the mid- to late-twenties. This is usually because activity levels have slowed (e.g., many men give up playing regular sport at this time) and with, perhaps, marriage and more home cooking, and more money to be able to afford to eat out often, calorie intake increases.

A very gradual and small weight gain from the 20s to middle-age is acceptable (up to 14 lb/6.5 kg), but it is sensible to watch diet and exercise if weight seems to be escalating more quickly than this as maintaining a reasonable weight is one simple way to help prevent many ills, including CHD, arthritis, mid-life onset diabetes, breast cancer in women, and others. It is also easier to keep weight off for most people than it is to lose pounds that have been in place for years.

Up until the age of 30 or so, your metabolic rate remains constant (all other factors being equal), but after that age it begins to slow down. It has been estimated that you need 50 calories a day less for every five years you are over 30. For example, at 40 you will need 100 calories a day less than you did at 30, and by 50 you will need 200 less. See Section Four for more information on weight control and dieting.

Family planning: In the 20s or 30s many people plan a family. For women, this means following a healthy diet and maintaining a reasonable body weight, as a low BMI may increase the risk of periods ceasing and therefore will reduce fertility. Before actively trying to conceive, women should consider pre-conceptual care for optimum health for mother and baby during pregnancy and afterward—a subject discussed overleaf. For men, a healthy diet high in zinc, selenium, and vitamins E and C has been shown to help fertility. Incidentally, one Spanish study in 1997 showed that women who drank more than 5 cups of strong coffee a day took significantly longer to get pregnant than women who didn't, and that heavy coffee drinkers are 45% more likely to take 9 months or more to conceive.

Women's needs: Menstrual losses mean that throughout the reproductive years, women will always need more iron intake than men (for a list of good sources, see page 30) to prevent iron deficiency diseases, including anemia. They may also have to cope with problems such as PMS, menstrual problems, and fluid

retention. All these topics are discussed in detail in Section Two. Here are a few more pointers for women in adulthood:
* Diet should be adequate in calories and all nutrients. It is not wise to follow a diet too low in fats as the role of the essential fatty acids, found in a variety of plant foods, is important not only for health but also to keep skin soft and supple, and hair in good condition.
* Women on the contraceptive pill may find they gain up to 7 lb (3 kg) in weight. This is partly due to fluid retention; the PMS and Diuretic Diet on page 145 will help minimize this, as will exercise.
* Drinking more than one alcoholic drink a day may increase the risk of breast cancer in young women.

Ages 35–45

As the metabolic rate begins to slow, it is important to keep a watch on the intake of high-density, low-nutrient foods, such as many desserts, pastries, candies, and animal fats, and to take adequate exercise. A weight gain of 7–14 lb (3–6.5 kg) over your weight at 20–25 is acceptable.

The basic healthy diet should still be followed, paying particular attention to the "superfoods" highlighted in the Food Charts at the back of the book. These are the foods that seem to offer most protection against the major diseases of middle and old age, and against the aging process. Plenty of fresh fruits and vegetables is vital, not only for the well-known antioxidants, vitamins C, E, beta-carotene, and selenium that they contain, but also for the other phytochemicals, which are protective too (see page 34).

A healthy diet at this time can also give a perhaps much-needed boost to brain power. Research has shown that various dietary factors can influence how well our

brains work. A diet low in saturated fat encourages circulation of blood through the brain, and eating a diet slightly lower than average in calorie content has been shown to help prevent the brain from deteriorating as we get older, as well as helping to improve mood, memory, and other factors.

Brain power can also be adversely affected by eating a big meal OR by crash dieting, so that blood sugar levels fall too low. As Section One explains in detail, mental powers can also be improved by eating a breakfast high in protein and not too much carbohydrate at lunch. Lastly, "eat little and often" is the best way to benefit your brain and keep one step ahead.

A good night's sleep also becomes very important in the 30s and 40s, both to help the body rest and repair itself, and to keep the brain alert. If having trouble sleeping, see Insomnia on page 123.

See also: Eating Out (page 64), Fast Food (page 55), and Alcohol Abuse (page 86).

Pregnancy and pre-conceptual care

We now know that your health and nutritional status both before and during pregnancy may have a bearing not only on your baby's health in infancy but on his or her health right through to adulthood, and even on the length of his or her life.

■ Pre-conceptual care

If a pregnancy is planned, it is now accepted that it is sensible for the prospective mother to prepare herself for the pregnancy with suitable diet, folate supplements, exercise, and weight control. She should also give up, if necessary, smoking and cut back on alcohol. The reason for the importance of pre-conceptual care is that this will reduce the risk of birth defects and of giving birth to a low-weight infant, which is a proven risk factor in various lifelong health problems. Here we look at the various pre-conceptual factors that can influence ease of conception, a healthy pregnancy, and baby.

Weight: If you have a BMI (Body Mass Index, see page 188) within the accepted normal range of 20–25 you have a greater chance of becoming pregnant. With BMIs under 20 and over 30, the rate of conception is lower. Most research also shows that mothers with a low pre-pregnancy weight (BMI under 19) are at increased risk of having a low-birth-weight child (for the disadvantages of this, see right) even if they gain satisfactory weight during pregnancy. Although one major research project published in the US in 1998 appeared to show the opposite to be true for first-time mothers and debate about these latest results is still continuing, the consensus of opinion is that a pre-pregnancy BMI of 20–26 is still the ideal. For information on weight control see Section Four.

Diet: The mother's diet both before conception and during the first few weeks after conception (when many women still don't realize that they are pregnant) is important for the growth and proper development of the embryo, since from conception for the first few weeks it grows more rapidly than at any other time. Any abnormal cell development also seems to happen at this early stage.

To help prevent neural tube defects, such as spina bifida, adequate amounts of the B vitamin, folate should be taken. The normal RDI for non-pregnant adult women is 400 µg a day, but pre-conceptually and for the first three months of pregnancy it is sometimes recommended that a supplement of 400 µg is taken and that an extra 100 µg is taken in the diet. (More than this will be prescribed for women who have already given birth to a baby with a neural tube defect.)

This means eating a basic healthy diet containing plenty of naturally folate-rich foods, such as green vegetables, legumes, nuts, fruits, and potatoes, and fortified breakfast cereals. For a more detailed list of rich sources of folate, see page 28. Even with a healthy diet the supplement is important, though. There is some evidence also emerging that supplements of the compound inositol can also help to reduce possible neural tube defects.

It may also be a good idea to take in extra calcium and iron during the pre-conception period, as women with low iron stores at the start of pregnancy may become anemic, and there is evidence that the fetus will deplete maternal bone if calcium runs short.

Fitness: The mother-to-be should aim to get fit for pregnancy, taking regular walks or similar, and cutting out smoking (one of the major causes of low-birth-weight babies).

Alcohol: An overview of 5,000 pregnancies in the US published in late 1997 concluded that moderate drinking before pregnancy didn't increase the risk of miscarriage, but found that even moderate drinking during the first ten weeks of pregnancy did increase the risk of miscarriage fourfold. The UK's Royal College of Obstetricians and Gynaecologists also advised in 1997 that moderate drinking of one unit of alcohol a day for pre-conceptual and pregnant women will not harm the unborn baby and that there is no proof that up to 15 units a week will have a detrimental effect. The cautious woman would probably opt to avoid alcohol altogether, at least during the time of conception and up to the first three months of the pregnancy.

■ **Pregnancy**

Once a pregnancy is confirmed, it is important to continue to live healthily, eating a balanced, healthy, and adequate diet. This is not only for the sake of the growing fetus but also in the interests of the mother's own health, and in order to avoid such potential problems as excessive tiredness, constipation, nausea, and so on.

ADDITIONAL DAILY NUTRIENT REQUIREMENTS FOR PREGNANCY

(For nutrients not listed here, requirement is the same as for RDIs.)

Calories	+400
Protein	+60 g
Vitamin B$_6$	+2.2 mg
Folate	+400 mg
Calcium	+1,200 mg
Phosphorus	+1,200 mg
Iron	+30 mg *
Iodine	+175 µg

* The increased need for iron cannot be met by a typical American diet; therefore, supplements should be taken.

ADDITIONAL DAILY NUTRIENT REQUIREMENTS FOR LACTATION

(For nutrients not listed here, requirement is the same as for RDIs.)

Calories *	
up to 1 month	+450
1–2 months	+530
2 to 3 months	+570
4–6 months	+480–570
over 6 months	+240**
Protein	+65 g***
Vitamin B1	+1.6 mg
Vitamin B2	+1.8 mg
Vitamin B3	+2 mg
Vitamin B6	+2.1 mg
Vitamin B12	+2.1 µg
Folate	+280 µg
Vitamin C	+95 mg
Vitamin A	+1300 µg
Vitamin D	+10 µg
Calcium	+1200 mg
Phosphorus	+1200 mg
Magnesium	+355 mg
Zinc	+19 mg****
Copper	+0.3 mg
Selenium	+75 µg

* Estimated calorie needs are +400 calories per day above normal intake
** Assuming non-breast milk foods form majority of baby's diet
*** 6 months plus, reduces to +62 g (due to weaning)
**** 6 months plus, reduces to +16 mg

Surprisingly, the need for many nutrients doesn't need to be over the RDI during pregnancy, but there is a need for more of some of them. The chart above lists the recommended nutrient intake for all major nutrients in pregnancy and when lactating.

The lists on pages 22–33 show rich sources of all the extra nutrients needed in the charts above. Authorities in some European countries think that there is no extra need for calcium or iron in pregnancy. This is because absorption of both iron and calcium rises during pregnancy. In addition, loss of iron through the process of menstruation ceases, but if iron stores are low at the start of pregnancy, supplements may indeed be prescribed.

Less calcium is also excreted in the urine during the period of pregnancy, thus conserving supplies, and if more calcium is needed the mother's bone mass will supply this. However, extra calcium intake is, in fact, recommended in the case of teenage pregnancies.

"Eating for two" during most of the course of pregnancy is also not necessary. A mere 400 calories extra a day for the last three months will be enough for most women's needs—representing a baked potato with cheese or ¼ cups (300 ml) of skim milk and a sandwich.

It is thought that part of the reason why pregnant women don't need to eat a lot extra is that the metabolic rate slows down during pregnancy, and also that they naturally become less active. However, women who are significantly underweight at the start of their pregnancy may need to consider eating more than this.

OILY FISH, SUCH AS SARDINES, ARE A GOOD SOURCE OF VITAMIN D, AND ESSENTIAL FATTY ACIDS—AS WELL AS MANY OTHER NUTRIENTS—FOR THE PREGNANT WOMAN.

Although vitamin A need is increased during pregnancy (especially in the last 3 months), most women can get plenty in their diets; and, in excess (above 3,300 µg a day), vitamin A (in the form of retinol, not pro-vitamin A beta-carotene) is toxic in pregnancy and can cause birth defects. For this reason, pregnant women are warned not to eat liver, as liver contains potentially toxic amounts of vitamin A. They should also not take supplements containing retinol (e.g., cod liver oil) unless prescribed by their physician.

Extra vitamin C is needed in pregnancy, especially in the last three months. Vitamin D intake should be increased, and often it is supplied by fortified milk as it is hard to get this amount from the diet unless quite a high-fat diet is followed (vitamin D is found in butter, eggs, oily fish, full-fat dairy products, and fortified foods, such as cereals and margarines).

There are no additional requirements for total fat or carbohydrate during pregnancy (except as a means of increasing calorie intake), but the essential fatty acids and their derivatives such as GLA, EPA, and DHA, found in plant and fish oils, may be very important to a healthy pregnancy and baby. Research has linked a diet rich in EFAs

with longer pregnancies (and therefore higher birth-weight, see below), a reduced risk of high blood pressure in the mother, and optimum brain and eye development in the baby—and therefore intelligence. EFA intake in the last three months of pregnancy, when the brain of the fetus increases in weight by four or five times, is believed to be the most crucial.

There is no official recommendation for fiber increase in the diet for pregnancy, but many pregnant women experience constipation; increasing fiber intake (see list of rich sources on page 14) as well as water will help prevent this, as will regular gentle exercise.

■ Healthy pregnancy and the importance of the baby's birth-weight

Almost all research to date shows that a baby's weight at birth has great relevance to its future health, both in the immediate- and long-term. Low-birth-weight babies are more at risk of CHD, high blood pressure, stroke, and diabetes in later life. They also appear to suffer poorer cognitive (brain) function in childhood. Low-birth-weight babies are also more likely to die at—or soon after—birth or suffer poor health in infancy. Some of these connections may be related to restricted fetal growth. Low birth-weight is 5½ lb (2.5 kg) or less. Nutritional factors that may produce a low-birth-weight baby include:

* Excess alcohol intake during pregnancy. One to two drinks a day is the maximum recommended.

* Smoking—this should be stopped.

* Inadequate calorie intake. Most researchers agree that thin mothers and mothers who fail to put on adequate weight and/or fail to eat adequate calories during the pregnancy may run greater risk of having a low-birth-weight baby. The ideal weight that should be gained varies depending upon the weight of the mother at the start of the pregnancy (see chart below). In general, the heavier she is at the start, the less weight she needs to gain.

* Poor diet. A shortfall of all the nutrients required as outlined above can result

WEIGHT GAIN GUIDELINES FOR PREGNANCY

BMI at Start of Pregnancy	Total Optimum Amount of Weight to Gain
under 20	27–38 lb (12.5–18 kg)
20–26	25–34 lb (11.5–16 kg)
26–30	15–25 lb (7–11.5 kg)
over 30	minimum of 13 lb (6 kg)
	maximum to be decided in individual consultation

Gaining too much weight is not a good idea—gains over those listed are associated with several complications in pregnancy, such as high blood pressure and prolonged labor, as well as overweight after the pregnancy.

DIET TIPS FOR A TROUBLE-FREE PREGNANCY

The three most common complaints mentioned by pregnant women and how to deal with them:

Morning sickness: This can occur at any time of day but is usually worse in the morning. Probably caused by low blood-sugar levels and so eating several small high-carbohydrate snacks throughout the day will probably effect a cure, or at least minimize the nausea. Sickness on waking may be helped by eating such a snack as soon as you wake (have it ready by your bed). Ideal snacks: a banana; a slice of whole-wheat bread and jelly; graham cracker; oatcake. See also the ideas on curing nausea on page 129.

Tiredness: This is especially common in the first three months of pregnancy and is often the first sign that a woman is pregnant. Good pre-conceptual care will help, including a healthy energy-giving diet and an exercise program to increase heart/lung capacity. Follow this on with a healthy diet for pregnancy (Basic Healthy Diet, page 53, plus supplements as necessary) and make sure to get enough calories. Dieting is out. Alcohol and caffeine will increase fatigue. Adequate rest is essential. Check with a doctor that you aren't iron-deficient. For more information see Fatigue, page 111.

Food cravings: Many women do find themselves craving foods that they possibly wouldn't even usually consider. These cravings can be for almost any food, from pickles to oranges, and some women want strange combinations of foods. There is little scientific basis for the idea that the cause of such a craving is the need for a food high in a particular nutrient that the mother is lacking; e.g., if she craves oranges she must be lacking vitamin C.

If such cravings are for reasonably nutritious food then there is no great problem, unless the craved food is eaten regularly and to such an extent other types of foods are avoided, which will create nutritional shortages, or to such an extent that too much weight is gained, in the case of the higher-calorie foods.

If cravings are for the less nutrient-dense foods and/or "junk" foods, the pre-natal dietitian should be told and she or he can then work out a suitable strategy, which may include supplements.

There is no guaranteed way to cure cravings but a basic healthy diet, taking on board all the points raised in these pages, and snacking "little and often" may help to decrease the problem to some extent.

---

in low birth-weight. Shortages of B vitamins, magnesium, iron, phosphorous, and zinc in the first three months of pregnancy have been associated with low birth-weight.

■ Avoiding Food Poisoning

When pregnant, it is even more important than usual to avoid getting food poisoning; such bacteria as salmonella and listeria can seriously affect the unborn baby.

* Avoid soft mold-ripened cheeses, like Brie and Camembert, and unpasteurized cheeses, such as most Parmesan, and blue-veined cheeses like Stilton and Danish Blue, which may harbor the listeria bug. Cheddar cheese and cottage cheese are fine.

* Avoid pre-packed salads, deli salads in dressings, and other items sold loose from chill cabinets in stores and restaurants.

* Avoid raw or lightly cooked eggs and anything containing them, e.g., real mayonnaise, tiramisu, in case of salmonella.

* Avoid pâté, unless pasteurized, in case of listeria. (Liver pâté should be avoided in any case, because of high levels of vitamin A.)

* Avoid raw or partly cooked meat, unpasteurized milk, soil-dirty fruits and vegetables, to avoid toxoplasmosis.

See page 68 for more information on food safety.

BANANAS AND WHOLE-WHEAT BREAD MAKE IDEAL FIRST-THING-IN-THE-MORNING SNACKS TO HELP ALLEVIATE MORNING SICKNESS.

THE MIDDLE YEARS

For most people between the ages of 45 and 65 the good health of youth is eroded, and problems like arthritis, atherosclerosis, obesity, diabetes, and general physical deterioration take its place. With dietary and lifestyle intervention, however, it really is never too late to make significant improvements to long- and short-term health and to keep many of the typical signs of aging at bay. Experts are also unlocking the secrets of increasing life span through diet!

In the middle years, some changes—such as the menopause in women—are natural and inevitable, while others that many people regard as natural may, in fact, be undesirable and possibly preventable. Our health in so-called "middle age" is, in part, dependent upon what has gone before, and obviously good diet, enough exercise, and a healthy lifestyle throughout youth are important factors. However, many people don't, in fact, "look after themselves" until their youth is gone. It isn't until they hit 40 or 50 that they begin to realize that perhaps their own body deserves a regular service as much as their automobile does! Even if you do leave it this late to begin paying attention to what you put in your body for fuel and other lifestyle factors, however, you can still see great benefits.

One recent twenty-year international study published in the British Medical Journal, which examined the link between the diet of men aged 50 to 70 and their death rates, found that a healthy diet (as laid down by the WHO) is associated with a reduction of 13% in all causes of death in men of those ages.

Other important US and UK studies on mice, rats, fruit flies, and monkeys have found that life span can be increased by up to 50% on a calorie-restricted but highly nutritious diet and that such a diet also reduces the risk of CHD, cancer, stroke, and diabetes, and increases the functioning of the immune system (see Anti-Aging, opposite).

On a more mundane level, we now know that all kinds of health problems and signs of "getting older"—from Alzheimer's and osteoporosis to hair-loss and lack of libido—can be minimized, or even prevented, by particular diets or foods. Middle age really is the time to pay attention to your diet.

■ Your Starting Point

If you don't know where to begin, the best place is the Basic Healthy Diet on page 53. A complete health check-up by a physician is a good idea—this should reveal any health problems you may have; or perhaps you already know what they are. In that case you should follow the particular type of diet that suits your ailment. You will find all the information and special diets for major ailments in Section Two.

Many more people will be in reasonable health now, but perhaps have higher than average risk factors for a particular disease or ailment. Here are the major risk factors for the most prevalent ailments of middle and old age:

Arthritis: Family history; obesity; lack of exercise.

CHD and stroke: Smoking; heavy drinking; obesity; family history of coronary heart disease; diet high in saturated fat and low in fresh fruits and vegetables; stress; lack of exercise.

Cancer: Smoking; heavy drinking; diet low in fresh fruits and vegetables; family history of some cancers; possibly high-meat or -animal-fat diet; possibly obesity (link between breast cancer and obesity in post-menopausal women established).

Diabetes: Obesity.

Alzheimer's: Smoking; heavy drinking; poor diet.

Osteoporosis: Low BMI throughout life; family history; insufficient calcium/magnesium/vitamin D in diet; lack of exercise; female.

A: If you have one or more risk factors, apart from obesity, for any particular ailment, the corresponding diet in Section Two may be right for you, though you should see your doctor and discuss those risk factors.

B: If you are obese, with no other risk factors, then you should lose weight by following a sensible diet plan. Obesity, even moderate overweight, is a risk

ANTI-AGING AND CALORIE RESTRICTION

If you want to live to be 120—or more—there is fascinating evidence emerging that the way to do it is to restrict your calorie intake on a permanent basis. Three different research trials—two in the US and one in the UK—have discovered that if calorie intake is restricted to between 30 and 70% of normal calories, life-span in mice, rats, fruit flies, and monkeys can be extended by from 20% up to 50%.

It also seems that a calorie-restricted diet can have many beneficial effects on health, including much reduced risk of certain cancers, heart disease, and stroke, as well as increased energy levels and improved efficiency of the immune system. The scientists who conducted these experiments see no reason why the same effects won't apply to humans—and the US government is so impressed with the research that it is funding an official trial for 120 volunteers who will aim to restrict their calories to about 1,800 a day on average (for men) and reduce their body weight by 10–20%.

The concept of calorie restriction is not without its risks, however, and shouldn't be undertaken by people of normal weight until the results of the trials come through and are evaluated, a task that will take some years. The risks include malnutrition (although the humans in the experiment will be fed carefully to ensure this doesn't happen), increased risk of osteoporosis, and lack of menstruation and fertility in younger women.

Perhaps some time in the future, calorie-restriction will prove to be a safe method of extending healthy life for all—meanwhile, the message for most people in mid-life is to think thin, but not too thin!

factor for so many illnesses and problems in later life that it really is worth getting a grip on your size as soon as possible. All the information you need about weight and health, your optimum weight and weight-loss information is in Section Four. (See also Anti-Aging above.)

C: If you are obese, with other risk factors, you should lose weight as in B. After you have lost weight, you should revert to plan A.

D: If you have no risk factors, follow the Basic Healthy Diet, taking into consideration any further information in this article that applies to you; or, if in the menopause, try the diet overleaf.

■ The male menopause and other problems

Up to 40% of doctors believe that, yes, there really IS a male menopause. Many more middle-aged males know that there is. It may not carry clinical symptoms, as the female menopause does, but there

are indeed symptoms. Here are those most frequently mentioned:

* Diminished sex drive (libido).
* Depression and/or negative mood or mood swings.
* Lethargy/fatigue.
* Weight gain.
* Loss of hair and skin-tone.
* Problems getting or maintaining an erection even when aroused.
* Loss of muscle-tone/strength.

Many of these problems can be helped by the Basic Healthy Diet (see page 53). Extra help can be found in the relevant entries in the Ailments and Solutions section (e.g., fatigue is discussed on page 111, depression on page 103, skin problems on page 134, and libido on page 122). Surplus weight can be lost by using the advice in Section Four, and muscle- and skin-tone can be improved and/or maintained by regular weight-bearing exercise. Skin tone can be improved further with good diet, including plenty of fresh fruits, vegetables, essential fatty acids, and water. With improvement in general well-being, appearance and mood, the sex drive generally tends to improve too. Stress levels can be helped with the right diet—if this is a major part of your life, try the anti-stress diet hints on page 138.

A high proportion of middle-aged men begin to have prostate troubles—an enlarged prostate gland can be uncomfortable and tests show that a diet high in zinc and vitamin E can help (for rich sources, see pages 31 and 24). To help prevent prostate cancer, avoid heavy drinking and a diet that is high in saturated animal fats.

One area of health often forgotten in mid-life is the care of teeth and gums. Regular dental checks, thorough cleaning twice daily and a diet low in sugar and refined produce and high in natural, crunchy, fruits and vegetables will help to avoid problems later. Almost nothing ages you more than a set of teeth that aren't your own.

■ The menopause

For every woman the menopausal years—when hormonal changes in the body bring about the gradual decline in her fertility and an end to her ability to bear children naturally—are an inevitability. For many, the menopause brings a variety of symptoms, ranging from the mildly upsetting to those severe enough to disrupt their lives.

The majority of these symptoms—such as hot flushes, tiredness, mood swings and depression, libido problems, and insomnia—can be alleviated by correct diet or, on the other hand, made worse by a poor diet. We look at the dietary options here and consider also the long-term effects on your health in old age of what you eat at this time. We also provide solutions to the "male menopause" dilemma.

As 50% of the human population will one day face the menopause, it is difficult to understand why so little information is available on the prevention of the symptoms and consequences of the female menopause by natural methods. Medical intervention through hormone replacement therapy—and often through prescription of anti-depressants and tranquillisers—may provide relief for quite a lot of women, but the side effects of HRT are, for many, almost as unpleasant as the symptoms of the menopause themselves, and the long term effects are still uncertain, though it is now generally agreed that HRT does increase the likelihood of breast cancer.

One of the major benefits of HRT is that it helps to prevent the loss of bone density which accelerates greatly in menopausal and postmenopausal women, causing osteoporosis. HRT works mainly by replacing the female hormone estrogen, which allows calcium to be absorbed more effectively. There are, however, various dietary means by which bone loss can be slowed in susceptible women. A diet high in soy and soy products has been shown in studies to mimic the effects of estrogen in maintaining bone density. Other foods that may have an estrogen-like effect include nuts, yams, linseeds, legumes and grains, and most fresh fruits and vegetables.

Adequate calcium intakes during menopause and beyond are essential—1,500 mg per day may be beneficial. Good sources of calcium are dairy products (which should be low-fat versions, rather than full-fat, because there is evidence that saturated fat "binds up" calcium and inhibits its absorption), calcium-enriched soy milk and yogurt, tofu, seaweed and other dark green leafy vegetables, nuts, sunflower seeds, white flour, soy flour, legumes, sardines, whitebait, and shellfish.

Even if calcium intake is adequate, absorption is affected by various factors. It is hindered by eating raw bran at the same meal; by oxalic acid in spinach and rhubarb; by high alcohol intake; by caffeine found in tea, coffee, cola, cocoa, chocolate, and some herbal supplements; by smoking; by saturated fat, and possibly by a diet high in highly processed junk foods.

It also appears that calcium is leached from the bones by a high intake of protein—particularly animal protein—so it makes sense to choose more plant proteins in your diet and not to eat more protein than your body needs for good health and maintenance (see page 20 for more detail).

Calcium absorption is helped by adequate vitamin D. Zinc—found in shellfish, nuts, wheat germ, seeds, soy, whole grains, legumes, and cheese—and magnesium—found in nuts, whole grains, soy and other legumes, seeds, wheat germ, and fruits and vegetables—are also important for bone status. Absorption of all the minerals, including calcium and zinc, is helped considerably by eating vitamin C-rich foods at the same time.

Calcium is also important in the diet for menopausal women as it helps to maintain a healthy nervous system and a healthy heart and blood pressure.

Osteoporosis, and its prevention and management from childhood through to old age, is dealt with in more detail on pages 130–32.

MENOPAUSE MANAGERS

Moderate alcohol consumption can delay the menopause by up to 18 months, and in postmenopausal women a little alcohol can protect against coronary heart disease. Smoking induces an earlier menopause.

■ Hot flashes and other menopausal symptoms

In the West, approximately half of menopausal women suffer from severe or prolonged "hot flashes," with flushing of the face and neck, a feeling of suffocating heat and sweating, often followed by chilling. Yet in Japan and China, hot flashes and many of the other symptoms of menopause are almost unknown. Research indicated that this is because Japanese and Chinese women regularly eat soy-based foods such as tofu, which contain powerful phyto-estrogens, and other estrogenic foods, like yams, linseeds, beansprouts, and other fresh vegetables. One leading UK expert says two glasses of soy milk a day can reduce hot flashes by up to 50%. Japanese and Chinese women also eat plenty of foods rich in the amino acid tryptophan, known to help the brain produce serotonin, the "mood-calming" chemical. Vitamin E is also said to help minimize hot flashes.

Weight gain is not an inevitable consequence of the menopause, but a change in body shape happens to many women—the waist may thicken and mid-body fat increase, due to altered levels of hormones. It is important not to attempt to maintain a very low body-weight as thinness will have a detrimental effect on bone loss and calorie intake needs to be sufficient to give your body all the nutrients it needs. Yet it is also important not to put on too much body fat during and after menopause, as obesity in postmenopausal women is linked with an increased risk of breast cancer as well as increased risk of heart disease (one of the biggest killers of women aged 50-plus in the US), high blood pressure, diabetes, and arthritis of the weight-bearing joints. Most women who were thin in their teens and 20s should aim for a weight approximately/no more than 14–21 lb (6.5–9.5 kg) heavier in their late 40s and 50s. The best way to maintain a

sensible weight is to eat healthily and cut back on all highly processed and junk foods.

Lack of libido may improve if your overall diet and lifestyle improve and your menopausal symptoms diminish—tiredness and depression are passion-killers at any age. A diet rich in zinc is said to help libido. The "anti-aging" mineral, selenium, may also help, and adequate essential fatty acids and vitamin E may help minimize vaginal dryness.

Mood swings, depression, and insomnia can be helped by adequate intake of B vitamins, zinc, magnesium, and tryptophan. A calcium-rich snack before bed can induce sleep.

Headaches can be minimized by

regular meals and snacks, including complex carbohydrates, such as whole grains, and foods rich in vitamin B group.

Fluid retention can be largely avoided by a diet low in sodium, junk foods, and highly refined foods, and high in natural diuretics like parsley, celery, and asparagus.

Dry skin and poor hair condition is improved by eating plenty of the antioxidants selenium (found in shellfish, dairy products especially butter, avocado, whole grains, legumes, and leafy greens) and vitamin E (found in plant oils, seeds, nuts, wheat germ, cabbage, tuna in oil, and asparagus), as well as omega-3 fats found in fish oils and flax seed (linseed) oil, and GLA oils found in evening primrose and starflower oil.

SUPPLEMENTS FOR THE MENOPAUSE

If one or more of your own menopausal symptoms is severe, it may be worth considering a food supplement, along with the menopause diet overleaf. Actual scientific evidence for their worth is fairly scant, but anecdotal evidence for all is quite strong.

Hot flashes: Vitamin E supplements (look for d-alpha tocopherol on the label, which is the natural vitamin E, rather than the synthetic, which is less effective)—minimum 200mg a day.
Herbs—try black cohosh, marigold, hawthorn, and sage.

Depression, mood swings: Korean ginseng, trytophan (available from healthfood stores), St. John's Wort (*Hypericum perforatum*).

Nerves: Motherwort, calcium, B complex.

Insomnia: Kava kava root (from health-food stores), melatonin, chamomile. See also Ailments and Solutions section, page 86.

Fluid retention: Hawthorn, motherwort, dandelion.

Libido: St. John's Wort (*Hypericum perforatum*).

■ The menopause diet plan

This plan is a sample of the kind of eating that should help reduce menopause symptoms as well as minimizing bone loss. After the menopause is over it is acceptable to continue with a similar diet.

Instructions:

✱ Substitute calcium-enriched soy milk (widely available) for cows' milk at least 50% of the time. When using cows' milk, try to choose skim as much as possible.

✱ Drink only decaffeinated tea and coffee and avoid all cola drinks and cocoa. Keep all types of chocolate for only a very occasional treat.

✱ Drink a maximum of 1 or 2 glasses of wine a day.

✱ Drink plenty of water, freshly squeezed fruit and vegetable juices, and soy milk.

✱ Eat as much fresh fruit and vegetables as you can, getting a wide variety.

✱ Avoid junk food—any processed foods high in saturated fat/sugar/phosphates (read labels).

✱ Keep salt to a minimum—use sea salt when you do.

Unlimiteds:

Drinks as left; fruits and vegetables as above (plainly cooked or with pure vegetable oils); fresh and dried herbs and spices.

Breakfast every day:

Have either fortified soy milk OR yogurt with a portion of wholegrain low-salt cereal—e.g. muesli, oatmeal, Shredded Wheat.

Add one orange, a few chopped nuts, preferably Brazil nuts, a tablespoon of sesame and/or sunflower seeds, and a tablespoon of wheat germ.

For a change, have a pink grapefruit or 1 or 2 tangerines, or other citrus fruits instead of the orange.

If still hungry, have a slice of whole-wheat bread with a small amount of butter and honey.

Snacks every day:

Twice a day between meals have a small snack of any of the following:

Fresh nuts; seeds; fresh fruit; dried fruit; fortified soy milk; low-salt rye rice cake with a little low-salt peanut butter or hummus.

SPINACH, BROCCOLI, AND WALNUT STIR-FRY (SEE PAGE 244).

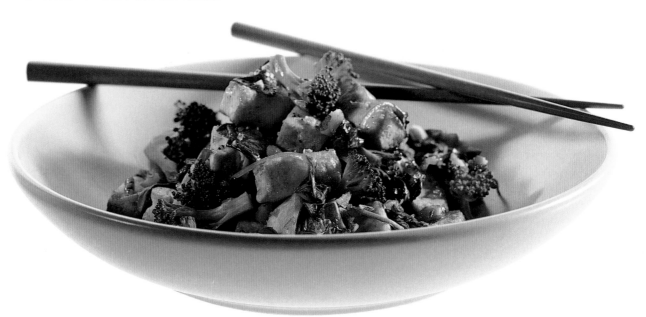

THE MENOPAUSE DIET

DAY ONE
Lunch
salad of mixed green leaves (some dark green, e.g., arugula, romaine, watercress) with celery, cucumber, tomato, one hard-boiled egg and two anchovies, dressed in olive oil and vinegar dressing
whole-wheat, rye, or white bread
1 banana
Evening
Chicken Cacciatore
brown rice
Brussels sprouts or collard greens
fruit and soy yogurt

DAY TWO
Lunch
salad of drained tuna in oil mixed with cooked butter beans, sliced ripe tomatoes, red onion and lightly cooked asparagus tips, garnished with chopped parsley and olive oil and red wine vinegar
French bread
Evening
Stir-Fried Tofu
Spinach, Broccoli, and Walnut Stir Fry
brown rice
berry fruits with yogurt

DAY THREE
Lunch
Lentil and Spring Green Soup
rye bread
dried apricots
Evening
omelet
pepper and onion salad
1 banana

DAY FOUR
Lunch
Smoked Mackerel Pâté Salad
rye bread
coleslaw made with white cabbage, carrot, onion, dried apricots, and mixed nuts, dressed with low-fat yogurt mixed with lemon juice and a little honey, and black pepper
Evening
Pasta with Broccoli and Anchovies
mixed salad with balsamic vinegar dressing
1 orange

DAY FIVE
Lunch
Hummus
pita bread
salad of cucumber, olives, tomatoes, onion, dark green lettuce leaves
Evening
broiled sardines or herring fillets dressed with ginger and cilantro
peas
new potatoes
fresh fruit of choice

DAY SIX
Lunch
salad of slices of ripe avocado, tomato, and low-fat cheese, dressed with olive oil and red wine vinegar, seasoned and flashed under grill for a minute
Italian bread
selection of seeds and dried fruits—e.g., pine nuts, sunflower seeds, dried figs, dried peaches
Evening
salmon fillet with a herb and ginger crust
brown rice
snow peas
Green Lentils with Herbs

DAY SEVEN
Lunch
feta cheese, stir-fried in sunflower oil to brown, and served with black pitted olives, and lemon juice
salad of fresh beansprouts, carrot, celery, watercress, spinach, and mixed chopped nuts in classic vinaigrette dressing
white bread
Evening
small amount of extra-lean organic beef, cut into strips and stir-fried in sesame oil with a selection of fresh mixed vegetables, including bok choy, with ginger, garlic, and soy sauce
egg-thread noodles
fresh fruit salad with yogurt

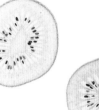

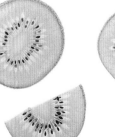

SIXTIES PLUS

The nutritional needs of older people are not all that much different from those of younger adults. However, the practicalities of eating such a balanced diet seem to become increasingly harder as we get older. This means that many older people in the US do suffer deficiencies in some areas. Here we look at healthy eating in the later years and suggest ways in which diet can be improved— and enjoyed more.

The average requirements for nutrients in older people are similar to those in younger adulthood. The main differences are that older people require fewer calories (2,330 for males and 1,900 for females aged 65–74, 2,100 for males and 1,810 for females aged 75+) because their lean-body-mass decreases and lifestyle becomes more sedentary. Older women also need less iron (at 8.7 mg/day compared with 15 mg in younger women) due to cessation of periods. Most people still will require dietary vitamin D, and the 10 µg/day RDI can be met by consuming fortified milk products.

■ Energy and nutrients

Energy requirements decline slightly with age as body metabolism slows down; but, in general, the requirements for the micronutrients don't. This can pose a problem, as absorption of some of the vitamins and minerals seems to decrease in older people, added to which many of the elderly are on prescription drugs, which can also hinder absorption.

This means that, if deficiencies aren't to occur, food needs to be selected carefully on the reduced-calorie diet that the average older person will eat.

Fat, protein, and carbohydrate can be eaten in similar proportion to that of younger adults (see pages 170–71), with up to 30% calories from fat, up to 15% from protein, and the balance made up from carbohydrates.

■ Vitamin D

Vitamin D is vital to maintain bone health in the elderly. In younger adults, this vitamin is obtained via sunlight on the skin, but older people tend to go out in the sunlight less often, and absorption through the skin may also be less efficient. For these reasons, for those aged 65 plus, vitamin D needs to be taken in the diet. 10 µg a day is recommended, an amount that might be hard to get in a normal diet (if fortified milk is not part of your diet), so a daily supplement (e.g., a spoonful of cod liver oil) may be needed. Good dietary sources are margarine, eggs, and fatty fish.

■ Nutritional problems in the elderly

Although requirements may not appear excessive, many older people in the US do suffer nutritional deficiencies, according to research, because their eating habits differ considerably from younger people. According to the USDA's Continuing Survey on Food Intake, people over 60 appeared to eat considerably less vegetables, meat, and cheese than younger adults, but considerably more ready-made foods and beverages.

According to some surveys, main areas of deficiency seem to be the B vitamins, especially vitamins B6, B12, and folate. The USDA l996 report suggests that the over 60s have especially lower intakes (than the RDI) in calcium, magnesium, B6, and zinc; while some older people are likely to be deficient in vitamin C, iron, and beta-carotene.

We look at the reasons why the diets of many elderly people are inadequate and offer solutions (right).

■ *Keeping the diseases of age at bay*
Cancer, CHD, and stroke: 64% of new cancers occur in people aged 65 plus, and a similar proportion of new cases of coronary heart disease and stroke. This means that following the kind of diet which can help to prevent these ills, or minimize their effects, is well worth following, whether one is 40 or 80. This means a diet high in antioxidants, fresh fruits and vegetables, plant oils, fiber, and oily fish, and low in animal fats. Weight should also be watched. For more information see pages 96 and 118.

TYPICAL EATING HABITS AND HEALTHY SOLUTIONS

Eating habits	Reasons	Problems this may exacerbate	Solutions
High sugar	Easy to eat, tasty, low-cost long shelf-life, no cooking	Weight gain and associated symptoms, e.g., high blood pressure, deficiency in nutrients,* dental problems	Nutrition education, supplements, dental advice
Low-fiber processed foods	Easy to chew and swallow; low-cost	Deficiency in vitamins, minerals, fiber Constipation, hemorrhoids, increased risk of bowel cancer	See Easy Eats, overleaf
Narrow range of foods	Habit; fear of change, lack of interest in food, loss of appetite; shopping difficulties	Nutritional deficiencies, possible deficiency in energy intake (under-weight)	See Easy Eats and Pantry Stand-bys, overleaf
High-fat diet	Low-cost, easy to eat, habit, frying cheaper than baking or broiling	Deficiency in nutrients,** obesity, increased risk of CHD/stroke	More bread and potatoes, use reduced-fat items,** exercise if appropriate
Low on fruits and vegetables	Expense, shopping/ storage problems, can be hard to chew/ swallow/digest	Deficiencies in vitamins, e.g., C and beta-carotene, fiber. Constipation; hemorrhoids; increased risk of CHD; some cancers	Long-life fruit juices, dried apricots, baked beans; see also Easy Eats, overleaf

* A diet high in sugars and fats means there is less "room" for other more nutritious foods, unless the person overeats and then obesity will be a problem.

** See Section Four for advice on swapping high-fat foods for lower-fat foods.
Slim or thin elderly people can eat a higher-fat diet, but should include more plant fats in their diets, e.g., vegetable oils for cooking rather than lard.

There is evidence that the immune system becomes weaker in old age, which may also lessen immunity against cancer—a diet high in zinc (see page 31 for rich sources list), will help to boost the immune system.

Osteoporosis: Adequate calcium (perhaps with supplements, especially for women, who are four times more prone to osteoporosis than men) and vitamin D intake will help to prevent or minimize osteoporosis, which can result in hip and other fractures in the elderly. Smoking is a major factor in loss of bone density in postmenopausal women—it increases the risk of hip fracture by an amazing 50%. (Smoking before the menopause, however, has little effect.) Body weight is also a factor—thin people are at greater risk of bone fractures. Lack of exercise also increases the risk—if possible, a regular walk will help keep bone mass intact.

Alzheimer's disease: This is dealt with in full on page 90 but, briefly, research indicates that a diet high in antioxidants and estrogen, with moderate wine consumption, and a diet such as that for CHD, which helps to lower levels of LDL blood cholesterol, may help stall the progress of the disease.

Alcohol: As with younger adults, there is no harm in older people drinking in moderation. All the advice

REFRIGERATOR AND PANTRY STANDBYS

Low-cost items
* Canned sardines, tuna, mackerel, rollmop herrings.
* Canned beans, legumes, carrots, tomatoes.
* Canned fruits.
* Long-life milk, cream, custard, yogurt.
* Part-baked bread.

Concentrated sources of energy and nutrients
* For protein and calcium: milk, cheese, eggs, yogurt, custard.
* For vitamin C: fruit juice.
* For iron, B vitamins: red meat, eggs.
* For calories: whole milk, Cheddar and cream cheeses, eggs, whole-milk yogurt, red meat, oily fish.

EASY EATS

For people needing to increase their intake of fruits and vegetables
* Cooked purées of vegetables, such as rutabaga, parsnip, carrot, with other vegetables mixed in as appropriate, e.g., peas, spinach, shredded cabbage.
* Canned tomatoes.
* Raw purées of fruits, skinned if necessary, and confectioners' sugar added as necessary, sieved—e.g., strawberries, raspberries, peaches.
* Fruit juices, long-life if necessary.
* Canned fruit salad.
* Baked or stewed fruits—e.g., cooking apples, pears, in season.
* Vegetables added to casseroles and stews.

For people needing to increase their intake of fiber
* Baked beans on toast or on mashed potato.
* Canned legumes added to casseroles and stews or puréed with meat.
* Ready-to-eat dried apricots.
* Canned stewed prunes or rhubarb.
* Extra fluids to make the extra fiber "work."

FISH PIE USING OILY FISH LIKE TUNA, WITH A TOMATO SAUCE, ADDED LEGUMES AND VEGETABLES, AND MASHED POTATO TOPPING, MAKES EXCELLENT FARE.

about alcohol (see pages 66 and 86) applies to older people, although as body mass and total body fluid content decrease with age, alcohol tolerance may also decrease. It makes sense, if necessary, to drink alcohol in later years at the minimum end of the safety guidelines rather than the maximum, especially if alcohol is bought at the expense of other, nutritious foods.

See also: Alzheimer's Disease (page 90) and Arthritis (page 93).

SAMPLE 3-DAY DIET FOR AN ELDERLY PERSON

This plan represents an ideal food intake for a female aged 75+, assuming she is of reasonable body weight. All portions are medium unless otherwise stated. Overweight females could choose lower-fat versions of the foods marked with an *. Males in the age range could increase portion sizes and add an extra snack a day.

Every day

Allowance of low-fat 2% or whole milk * of 1 cup (250 ml). Unlimited water, diluted fruit juices. Several cups of tea or coffee allowed a day, with milk from allowance and sugar unless obese. Unlimited salad items, fruits, and vegetables in addition to those listed, although the amounts listed should be adequate for provision for vitamin C, fiber, etc.
* If butter used instead of margarine, have 1 tablespoon cod liver oil daily.

DAY ONE

Breakfast
glass of orange juice
medium bowl of oatmeal made with half milk* and water
milk from allowance to cover
sprinkling of sugar or maple syrup
1 slice of whole-wheat bread ,
with margarine and jam or marmalade

Light meal
(lunchtime or evening, as preferred)
2 medium eggs scrambled with milk and a little margarine on 1 slice whole-wheat toast (chopped tomato stirred in toward end of cooking, if liked)
OR
hard-boiled egg and tomato sandwich
1 medium banana

Main meal
(lunchtime or evening as preferred)
chicken casserole made with chopped tomatoes, tomato purée, chicken stock and onion
frozen peas
baked potato
thick and creamy fruit yogurt*

Snack
toasted bun with margarine
grapes or apple

DAY TWO

Breakfast
glass of orange juice
Medium bowl All Bran with milk from allowance and sugar
1 slice of whole-wheat bread, with margarine and jam or marmalade

Light meal (as before)
medium bowlful of ready-made or home-made lentil soup (preferably green or brown)
1 small roll
OR
baked beans on toast
portion of strawberries with light cream* and sugar or 1 tangerine with a small piece of Cheddar cheese

Main meal (as before)
1 portion of cod in butter sauce (ready-made, frozen)
potato mashed with milk from allowance and margarine
portion of frozen green beans or spinach
banana, honey, and light cream*

Snack
handful of ready-to-eat pitted prunes
slice of bread and peanut butter

DAY THREE

Breakfast
glass of orange juice
1 boiled egg
2 slices of whole-wheat toast, with margarine and jam, or marmalade

Light meal (as before)
sandwich of 2 slices of whole-wheat bread with margarine
filled with canned sardines OR tuna in oil*, drained, plus cress and cucumber if liked
fruit yogurt

Main meal (as before)
ground lamb* stewed with ready-prepared stewpack vegetables, lamb stock, and tomato purée, with 1½ oz (40 g) dried pasta shapes added for last 15 minutes of cooking time
carrots
stewed apples and custard

Snack
small slice of fruit cake
grapes or apple

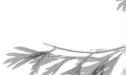

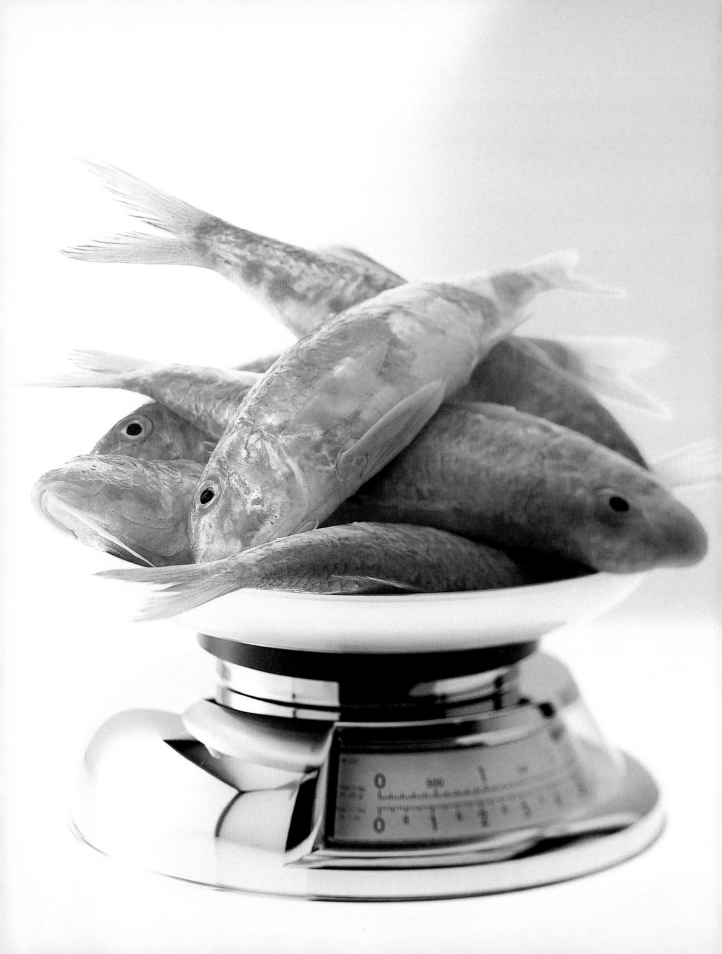

Food for weight control

Average weight in the Western world is on the increase and has been since the 1950s. 97 million American adults are currently thought to be overweight, that is 55% of the population! The prevalence of obesity (those severely overweight) has increased from 13% in the 1960s to 22.5% in the 1990s, and most of this increase has occured in the past decade. These figures are worrying because overweight and obesity are linked with many health problems, such as high blood pressure, Type II diabetes, coronary heart disease, stroke, osteoarthritis, respiratory problems, and prostrate, breast, colon and other cancers. Obesity is the second leading cause of preventable death in the US, and in fact, obesity has now been declared an endemic disease by the WHO and is recognized as one of the most common avoidable causes of death.

With all the health advice on offer, just why are so many of us overweight? It appears that we aren't actually eating any more calories per day. However, we are much less active, taking a third less exercise than we did in the 1950s, largely because of a sharp decline in the amount of everyday physical chores. Our hobbies, too, have become more sedentary—we spend four hours or more a day watching TV rather than walking or playing sport. Decreased activity means that we don't need as many calories—and yet we haven't reduced the amount we eat to compensate. So surplus food is stored as body fat.

The cure, therefore, is not only to eat fewer calories, but also to exercise more, which will redress the balance. It only takes relatively minor regular adjustment to the energy out/energy in balance to achieve steady and healthy weight-loss. In the following pages we will look at how best to achieve this, and will discuss the questions most often asked about diet and weight control.

We will also examine the problems of the minority of people (nevertheless representing millions) who have the opposite dilemma—how to put ON weight.

Your top 20 questions on weight control

To set the scene for this section, here we attempt to answer some of the questions most frequently asked about the whole vexed area of weight control. By doing so, we will, to a large extent, cover most of the background information you need to know to get to grips with the subject.

1 What is the accepted definition of being overweight?

There is a fairly broad band of "acceptable weight" for your height, within which you're not, clinically, over- or underweight. The scale used by most professionals to determine acceptable weight is Body Mass Index (BMI). Your BMI is easy to work out with the formula: $BMI = Weight (kg) \div height (meters)^2$. The result is then interpreted as follows:

below 20 = underweight
20–25 = acceptable weight range
25–30 = clinically overweight
30–40 = clinically obese
over 40 = morbidly obese

The acceptable range of 20–25 allows, for example, a woman of 5 ft 6 in (1.65 m) to weigh anything between 120 lb (54.5 kg) and 150 lb (68 kg). An acceptable maximum weight for health, then, is higher than many people realize and means that many people who feel they are overweight aren't really—a lot of people trying to diet may be having difficulty because they're aiming too low.

Another good indication of genuine overweight is the "waist circumference" test, because surplus weight around the waist ("central fat distribution") is more likely to be linked with health problems (particularly CHD and non-insulin-dependent diabetes) than surplus weight around the hips, bottom, and thighs.

A waist measurement of less than 37½ in (94 cm) for men and 32 in (80 cm) for women is all right; 37½–40½ in (94–101 cm) and 32-34¾ in (80–87 cm) respectively indicates further weight gain should be avoided and perhaps weight should be lost; and over 40½ in (101 cm) and 34¾ in (87 cm) indicates weight should be lost. If you are "borderline" on the BMI system (say, just on or over 25), then the waist circumference theory may help you decide, or vice versa.

2 How can I be overweight when I don't overeat?

There is this common idea that overweight people are greedy, but in most cases that is far from the truth. Most people lead fairly sedentary life-styles, and calorie (energy) needs may not be great. Eating just a small amount more than those needs will result in a slow but steady weight increase.

For example, it is estimated that a moderately active woman needs 2,200 calories a day to maintain a reasonable weight. Eating just 100 calories a day more than her needs (represented, say, by a banana or one large chocolate cookie) will result (all other factors being equal) in an annual weight gain of 10 lb (4.7 kg)!

As we get older, our metabolic rate also slows down a little, very gradually (see Q 5), which can result in slow weight-gain in people aged 30 plus.

3 Couldn't my weight problem be due to some reason other than overeating—perhaps hereditary?

"It's my genes!" is an "excuse" for overweight that doctors have been listening to—with some degree of scepticism—for years. Now more research is being done to indicate that the tendency to put on weight can certainly be inherited.

After extensive research on twins, it is now known that body-fat distribution is at least 60% inherited (meaning that most people are stuck with their basic body shape and "fat profile" for life). It also seems possible that our genes control other factors in the weight balancing act, such as how well our body responds to exercise. One leading UK obesity expert says that 25% of obesity may be caused by "minor gene defects".

However, all this doesn't mean that it is impossible to stay a reasonable size, even if you have more trouble staying slim than most. What it does mean is balancing your own equation—more exercise, less calories—until you reach a weight that is acceptable. This may be heavier than that considered normal.

In the future it may be possible to reprogram "faulty" genes so staying slim is no longer a problem. California scientists have already isolated a gene (UCP2) that helps burn off excess calories rather than allowing them to convert to fat. Work is also currently being done on the hormone leptin, the product of a defective gene in obese mice.

Lastly, it should be pointed out that many people with no inherited tendency to put on weight easily do still get fat, simply by not balancing their energy in/energy out equation correctly (see Q 2).

4 Could I have a slow metabolism?

A lot of overweight people believe that their problem lies in a slow metabolic rate—that they burn up calories slower than slim people. In fact, the opposite is normally true. The most important factor governing energy metabolism is how big you are—the heavier a body is, the more work it has to do, the faster its metabolic rate and the greater its calorie needs. That is why a 225 lb (101 kg) woman needs much more to eat than a 125 lb (57 kg) woman in order to maintain weight. Once the heavier woman begins to lose weight, her metabolic rate will gradually slow down, and, if she dieted down to 125 lb (57 kg), her metabolic rate (other factors being equal) would be similar to the lighter woman.

Research has also proved that it is not a slow metabolic rate that makes most people get fat, but simply eating more than the person who doesn't get fat.

5 Isn't it natural to put on weight as you get older?

Our basal metabolic rate (the rate at which we burn up calories when doing no physical activity at all) does very gradually begin to slow down over the years, once we reach the age of thirty or so. It is estimated that for every five years older than 30 we are, we need to consume about 50 calories a day less in order to maintain the weight we were then. That means by the age of 60, if you haven't reduced your daily calorie intake by about 300 calories a day less than at 30, you will have slowly put on weight. (After sixty, body fat percentage tends to slowly decrease again, naturally.)

Part of the reason for this slow-down is that we lose lean tissue mass (muscle) as we age. Muscle is more metabolically active than fat and other body tissue. Another reason is that we tend to use up less energy in activity as the years go by. There is also some natural slowing down through the aging process itself.

The only way to stop or minimize this slowing down of the metabolism is to increase the amount of exercise that you do, and include toning/strengthening exercise to keep muscle mass. It can be done—but, it seems, few manage it.

For your health's sake, a few pounds on your slim early-adulthood weight won't harm you, as long as you eat healthily and stay as fit (although plenty of new research indicates that calorie restriction is a key to longer life). Trying to maintain the very slim weight of your youth may be an unrealistic target.

6 I am fat—and happy with my size. Why should I change?

The feminist and politically correct movements have done much in recent years to persuade many overweight people that they shouldn't bow to what they see as social pressure to lose weight. Many overweight people take fitness tests, come through well, and see no reason to change. However, the overwhelming majority of evidence demonstrates quite clearly that a high BMI (particularly over 30) is a major cause of ill-health, disease, and early death. When people are young and overweight these risks are less evident, and, of course, there will always be some obese people who lead healthy, happy, and long lives.

7 So what is the best diet to follow in order to lose weight?

The best diet is one that hardly seems like a diet at all—one where you have a varied diet and at least three meals a day, plus snacks. It needs to be healthy, containing all the major nutrients, fiber, and so on. As a rough guide, for men 1,500–1,750 calories a day and for women 1,250–1,500 calories a day are suitable. Very overweight people will be able to eat more than that and still lose weight, particularly if activity levels are stepped up.

8 How do I lose weight quickly?

All recent research has come to the same conclusion—that there is no fast-track to permanent weight loss. There are three main reasons for this. One, in order to stick with a diet, it needs to contain enough calories to ensure you don't feel hungry, bored, or over-restricted in what you can eat. On these calorie levels, you can't lose weight quickly, but it has been shown that those who allow themselves a more generous amount of calories do better at weight-loss long term.

Two, in order to get all the nutrients you need while losing weight, you need a reasonable amount of food, again, meaning you can't lose weight quickly.

Three, there is considerable research to show that people who lose weight quickly are more likely to put the weight back on again, or become serial "yo-yo" dieters, than those who lose it slowly. There is also some research to show that people who crash-diet are more prone to depression and poorer mental function.

9 Should I count calories or just cut fat?

In effect, the two come to the same thing. In order to lose weight, you have to create a calorie "deficit," burning up more energy (calories) than you take in as food. On a good calorie-counting diet you will cut down on the high-calorie foods, things like cakes, pastries, fatty meats, mayonnaise, sugar, alcohol, and so on. There is no point in cutting down on low-calorie foods, like fruits and vegetables, because, firstly, you won't save enough calories to make much difference and, secondly, they are healthy foods your body needs. Neither is there any point cutting out the starchy carbohydrates, such as bread, potatoes, pasta, and rice, as these are also healthy foods, although if counting calories you may cut down on portion-size a little.

On a good fat-cutting diet, you simply avoid the foods you know to be high in fat, like cakes, pastries, and fatty meats.

10 Would I have more success on one of the more specialized diets, such as a high-protein one, or the Hay system (food combining)?

There is an appraisal of some of the most popular methods of dieting on page 202–3. Briefly, both a high-protein diet and food combining only work to help people lose weight by creating a calorie deficit. An analysis of a typical diet on either regime shows them to be very low in calories overall—bordering on dangerously low levels in some cases. A high-protein diet can be dangerous in itself (see page 202), compounded by the low amount of carbohydrate allowed on such regimes, and there is no scientific evidence to back up the theory behind food combining. For most people, these are not diets to be recommended.

11 What can I do to control hunger pangs when I diet?

Habit can be mistaken for hunger—we tend to eat before real hunger manifests itself, if the clock tells us we should eat. If that isn't the case, however, and you follow the guidelines above for sensible dieting (and the Four-Week Retraining Program on page 192), hunger shouldn't be a problem.

Cutting calories by only a little will help to prevent hunger, as will following a diet high in foods that have a low Glycemic Index. More about these appears on page 194–5, but basically they are carbohydrate foods that have a high "satiety value," because they are broken down into blood sugars slower than other carbohydrate foods and will keep you feeling full for longer than foods with a high GI. These include pasta, legumes, oats, citrus fruits, and yogurt. Each meal should also include a little fat and some protein, both of which have a similar effect on slowing down food absorption as low-GI foods. A diet high in natural fiber will also help to control hunger pangs.

Women often feel hungrier in the week before their period. This is a natural occurrence, and such women should eat a little more (healthy foods) at this time, if necessary, reverting to a maintenance diet rather than a weight-loss diet.

12 What can I do to control specific food cravings, e.g., for chocolate?

A small amount of any food can be included in a healthy diet, so there is no need to give up completely foods you enjoy. Sugary foods can be eaten after a meal. A small bar of chocolate or a chocolate mousse dessert, for instance, after a healthy low-fat main course would be fine, even on a diet.

It is important, when dieting, not to miss meals, go long periods without food, or indulge in over-strict calorie control. This could result in low blood-sugar levels producing cravings for sweet and/or high-carbohydrate foods, such as chocolate or cookies, with the effect of very quickly raising the blood sugar. Such a craving shouldn't be indulged with a sugary snack, though, as excess insulin may be released to cope with the sugary influx, and the result may be an even lower dip in blood sugar levels—and another craving for more sweet food!

The way to get off this "yo-yo" of crave-indulge-crave is to eat regular small meals high in healthy and low glycemic index foods (see Q 11). These keep blood sugar levels on a more even keel and cravings at bay. Ensure every meal also includes small amounts of protein.

13 Are there any special foods that will help me burn up fat?

Whole books have been written about so-called "fat-burning" foods, which are said to release enzymes that burn up fat, and whole books have also been written about "miracle" foods that take more calories to digest than they provide in the first place. Sadly, however, neither theory holds up under scientific examination.

14 So is there any short-cut way to lose weight without dieting?

Unless by surgery (as in liposuction, for example, where melted fat is sucked out of your body), the answer at the moment is no—however many mail-shots you receive telling you otherwise.

Prescription drugs that dull the appetite can help you lose weight, but most doctors will only supply these as a last resort, and strict guidelines now apply to their use (and you still need to diet). In the US, a new pill called Orlistat (awaiting FDA approval), causes 30% of the fat in the diet to be excreted without absorption. There are said to be no major safety issues, but side effects can be unpleasant and vitamin absorption can be affected.

15 How can I eat out and still lose weight?

Much of what you eat when you lunch or dine out isn't really essential to the spirit of the occasion, and that is the best attitude to take if work or a busy social life means that you have to eat out a great deal. If you only eat out occasionally, simply cut back a little for the rest of the day and enjoy yourself, while attempting to eat sensibly.

The pages in Section One on healthy eating out (page 64–5) are useful to provide more background information.

16 How can I stick to a diet when I miss my favorite foods too much?

The re-training program on the following pages will help you to adapt to healthy tastes. For instance, high-fat savory foods are often also high in salt—e.g., cheeses, crackers, and potato chips. It takes only two weeks to train your taste buds into disliking high-salt foods. High-sugar foods are often also high in calories and fat—yet, again, it takes only weeks to train yourself to find them far too sweet.

If your favorite foods are things other than those high in sugar and salt, then they can almost certainly form part of your healthy weight-loss diet.

If the re-training approach doesn't suit you, then another method of incorporating favorite foods into a diet is to allow yourself a number of "treat" calories a day and use these up on whatever you like. So that this doesn't lead to a binge, see Q 12.

17 Are the new calorie-free fat products a good idea?

Fat substitutes such as Olestra are used instead of fat in traditionally high-fat foods like ice creams, desserts, cakes, and cookies. Because of the way Olestra is formulated, the body doesn't absorb it and so calories are saved.

Olestra has been permitted for use in several products in the US. Drawbacks are possible depletion of the fat-soluble vitamins A, D, E, and K, and carotenoids, and possible side effects such as loose stools and anal leakage. Olestra is a sucrose polyester, but other types of fat substitute are also available. Simplesse, made from milk protein, is used in a wide range of products for a smooth, creamy taste. It is not calorie-free, but, at just over 1 calorie per gram, is much lower in calories than fat (9 calories a gram) or sugar (3.75 calories a gram). In the past few months a new, natural, oat-based fat substitute—Nu-Trim—has been developed and is currently being investigated by the USDA. Since Nu-Trim is all natural it is thought not to have the side effects of Olestra.

Various other products are available in various countries, and more of these fat substitutes are likely to appear in our foods all the time.

There is, though, some evidence that, overall, such highly processed low-fat products don't help us to eat any less or indeed to stay slim, because of their low content of essential fatty acids—natural oils found in plants and fish. This may apply to processed low-fat products in general, not just those containing fat substitutes.

18 Why does weight loss slow down after a while on a diet?

When you begin a diet, in the first week or two you will lose several pounds of weight which are fluid, not fat. After this, weight loss will be mostly fat.

For long-term dieters, the main reason is that when you lose weight, your metabolic rate gradually slows down simply because you are getting smaller. As explained in Q 4, when you are overweight you will have been eating more than average to maintain that weight. For example, a woman of 168 lb (76 kg) may well have been eating 2,500 calories or so a day rather than the "average" of 2,200. All she needs to do is cut down to, say, 1,450 calories a day for a daily "deficit" of 750 calories, resulting in a weekly weight loss of 1½ lb (675 g). At 140 lb (63 kg), however, she will be a fairly average weight and a daily diet of 1,750 calories is not much under the normal calorie intake (2,200) for a woman of her weight. To continue with good weight loss, a diet of, say, 1,500 calories a day would be more appropriate. That would result in a daily calorie deficit of 700 calories and a loss of just under 1½ lb (675 g) a week.

For weight loss to continue at a steady rate throughout any diet, therefore, you need gradually to cut the calorie content of the diet accordingly. In practical terms, it is probably best to be happy with slower weight loss as you near target-weight and to increase your exercise levels a little to compensate.

Other reasons why weight loss may slow down are that you have reached a reasonable body weight (you may have been aiming too low; check your BMI) or that you have begun eating more calories again—check your diet carefully. Also, weight does fluctuate from day to day and week to week for a variety of reasons, including hormones, fluid levels, etc. Most women in the week before a period won't lose weight at all and may indeed put a little on; this will disappear within days of the start of menstruation.

19 How often should I weigh myself?

As we've seen in Q 18, weight does fluctuate on a daily—and sometimes weekly—basis, so frequent scale-hopping is not advised, as the results may not present a true picture. For men, a weekly weigh-in is plenty. For women of menstruating age, it is probably more sensible to limit the weigh-in to once a month, directly after a period.

20 Why is maintaining a new slim body so hard?

It is true that, often, keeping weight off is harder than losing it in the first place. Research indicates that a high percentage of successful dieters do, eventually, put the weight back on again. However, this seems more to do with social, lifestyle, and psychological factors rather than being, as so many people believe, a consequence of dieting having artificially lowered the metabolism.

Research at a leading UK center for research into obesity clearly demonstrates that people who were once overweight and who slim down, have a similar metabolic rate to other people of the same (slim) weight who have never been fat.

However, a slim person's basal metabolic rate, as explained in Qs 4 and 18, is always going to be lower than that of an overweight person. In other words, once you are slim, you can't eat as much as you did when you were fat. People who do manage to keep weight off long-term seem to be those who followed a sensible healthy diet to lose the weight slowly, including behavior modification and exercise, and who continue to eat healthily and take regular exercise.

Four-week retraining course

For all those people who have battled with their weight for some time, yet another quick-fix diet really isn't ever going to be the answer... but this easy-to-follow four-week eating retraining course could be just what is needed to change things for good.

The four-week course is designed so that by the end of it most people will have little trouble in sticking to a healthy reduced-calorie program until they are down to a reasonable weight. Each week we will examine different aspects of eating for weight control, including strategies for behavior modification and practical dietary advice. At the end of the four weeks, two diet plans are laid out as a sample of how you could be eating to lose weight.

For the course, all you will need is enough time to give to the program, a notebook, and a degree of enthusiasm! Once the course is over, and whenever you have reached a suitable weight, the Basic Healthy Diet and all the information in Section One will help you to maintain that weight—along with the behavior modification you will learn in the four-week course.

Week one—getting started

Goals for the week:
* Read Section One and understand what makes a healthy diet.
* Decide on sensible targets.
* Check out motivation (see box on the right).
* Cut calories and fat in snack foods.

If you have tried, and failed, to lose weight on various "fad" or "crash" diets in the past, don't be deterred. The basis of any good weight-loss diet is varied and healthy eating. Any diet that isn't based on such principles is likely to fail, certainly in the long term.

During Week One, don't think about "dieting" as such at all. All you need to do is read through Section One and spend the week preparing practically and mentally to begin adjusting your eating accordingly. Sort out your pantry, and shop for a healthier range of foods; look through the recipe section and find a few recipes that appeal to your taste-buds. Try one or two.

Meanwhile, also work out your own BMI (see Question 1, page 188); work out what weight will achieve a sensible BMI, then decide on a sensible time-scale for achieving your ideal BMI.

Example: you are 5 ft 6 in (1.65 m) tall and 168 lb (75.5 kg) now, with a BMI of 28. You decide you will be happy with a BMI of 24, which will be achieved when you weigh 144 lb (64.8 kg). You have 24 lb (11 kg) to lose. You can adjust this target later—a good gauge of being a reasonable size is the waist circumference test (Question 1, page 188).

You lead a busy lifestyle and eat out regularly, so it would be sensible to achieve that weight-loss slightly more slowly than average. Allowing 1–2lb (0.5–1 kg) a week loss on average, it will take you 16–24 weeks to achieve.

> **FACT:**
>
> To gain 1 lb (450 g) of weight you need to eat around 3,500 calories more than you need. That is represented by just seven standard chocolate snack bars and an 8 oz (225 g) bag of potato chips.

■ Take a look at your snacking habits.

One major cause of slow-but-sure weight-gain is wayward snacking habits. We live in an era when grabbing food on the run has become normal; busy lives mean that it seems easier to eat a burger or bag of potato chips than bother with healthier food. On other occasions, a quick snack fills a gap between meals and we don't stop to consider what a large contribution such items can make to the total calories in the diet. Just one unwise snack a day could put over 8 oz (225 g) on your waistline every week—and do more damage to a diet than you

> **MOTIVATING YOURSELF**
>
> Use this week to complete a list of all the reasons why you would like to be a reasonable body weight. Divide them into health reasons (check the index for all the ailments linked with overweight), practical reasons (e.g., getting into favorite clothes, being able to play your favorite sport better) and social and other reasons. Most people should be able to come up with a list of at least twenty reasons they would like to lose weight.
>
> If you have tried and failed previously to lose weight and/or keep it off, agree with the following three statements:
> * I didn't fail on past diets, the diets failed me.
> * I will not dwell on my past disappointments.
> * Now I am willing to take responsibility for what I eat.

may think. Take a look at your snacking habits—use your notebook to write a list of all the "non-meal" foods you eat this week. Analyze your reasons for eating that particular food (e.g., nothing else available when hungry, speed, ease of eating) and think of better alternatives for each occasion.

However, don't try to give up snacks altogether; simply swap them for better alternatives. One or two small but nutritious "mini-meals" a day will help to keep hunger at bay (see Week 2) and will provide useful nutrients. Ten low-calorie, yet filling, snacks are listed below. Fresh fruits, dried fruits, and small amounts of shelled raw nuts are always easy to eat —plan ahead and carry some with you.

The box on the right shows three examples of how high in calories snack foods can be. Most are high-calorie because they are high in fat (and sometimes sugar) and yet, because you don't think of them as a "meal" (and neither should you because useful

nutrient content tends to be low), they are eaten as "extras." Instead of each of the snacks—eaten in a few mouthfuls— you could have a complete meal, as the illustration shows. Alternatively, for many

calories less, you could have a more balanced snack that would fit in well with a reduced-calorie diet. (See the Ten Low-Calorie Healthy Snacks box below.)

CALORIES AND FATS IN COMMON SNACKS

High-calorie snack	Low-calorie meal
1 standard Snickers bar (2.16 oz)	1 medium banana; 1 3/4 oz (50 g) no-added-sugar dried peaches; 1 triple rye wafer with 1 tablespoon (15 g) part-skim cottage cheese, herbs
277 calories and 13.6 g fat	248 calories and 2.2 g fat
1 hot dog on bun	1 x 2 oz (50 g) whole-wheat roll; 1 oz (30 g) part-skim ricotta cheese; 80 g homemade coleslaw, (using 1/2 cup (40 g) white cabbage, 1 1/2 tbsp (10 g) each grated carrot and onion; 1 1/2 tsp (6 g) golden raisins, and 1 tbsp (15 g) light Miracle Whip; 2 3/4 oz (75 g) tomato, cucumber, and celery salad; 1 apple
419 calories and 14 g fat	480 calories and 13 g fat
2 oz bag of dry-roasted salted peanuts	Sandwich of 2 slices of bread from a large sliced whole-wheat loaf; 1 medium hard-boiled egg, sliced; 2 teaspoons (10 g) 70% fat-free mayonnaise; plenty of salad greens and sliced tomato
327 calories and 27 g fat	270 calories and 14 g fat

TEN LOW-CALORIE HEALTHY SNACKS

(All around 100–150 calories each and none contains more than 6 g fat.)

* 1 triple rye wafer spread with 1 table- spoon (15 g) hummus; 1 tangerine.
* 1 small slice of wholegrain bread with a little mustard and 1 slice lean ham; small kiwi.
* 1 small tub of plain yogurt; 1 table- spoon chopped walnuts.
* 1 oak cracker; 1 apple.
* 6 shelled almonds; 1 kiwi fruit, 1 plum.
* 1 shredded wheat with skim milk.
* Ready-made fresh fruit salad; 1 small tub of plain yogurt.
* 1 small banana; 1 triple rye wafer with 1 tablespoon low-fat cottage cheese.
* Portion of Baba Ganoush (page 215) with mini pita.
* Mango and Peach Booster (page 253).

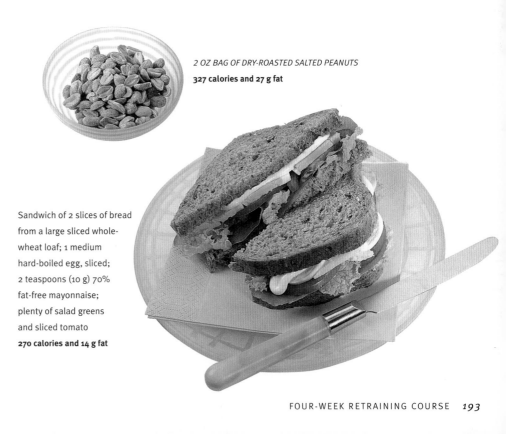

2 OZ BAG OF DRY-ROASTED SALTED PEANUTS
327 calories and 27 g fat

Sandwich of 2 slices of bread from a large sliced whole- wheat loaf; 1 medium hard-boiled egg, sliced; 2 teaspoons (10 g) 70% fat-free mayonnaise; plenty of salad greens and sliced tomato
270 calories and 14 g fat

Week two—taking control

Goals for the Week:
* Learn that you—and only you—have control over what you eat, despite outside influences.
* Learn how to avoid hunger while reducing your overall calorie intake.
* Start retraining your taste buds to less salt.
* Examine your breakfast eating habits.
* Begin to build more activity into your life.

If you want to be slimmer, you need to control your food intake. Nobody else can do that for you. Often it seems that almost everyone is trying to influence what, when, where, and how much you eat. It is for precisely that reason that you need to make the positive decision that you are going to eat what YOU want, what is good for YOU, and when you want it.

This week, take note of every time you are offered food or drink that you hadn't planned on eating. You'll be surprised how often it happens. You'll also be surprised how the typical reaction is to accept the food.

This week, start to say "no" to food you don't want, food you don't need, and food that isn't going to do your body much good. Keep a diary and note your achievements.

Also take note of how many times during the week you eat something you hadn't intended to eat because hunger

FACT:

If you removed from your diet all food that you didn't actually eat through genuine hunger and pre-planned decision, most people would save enough calories in a week to lose weight steadily without doing one other thing.

THE ANTI-HUNGER FOODS

Many people dislike the idea of dieting because they fear hunger. In fact, on a sensible diet, such as that outlined in the answer to Question 11 on page 190, hunger is much less likely to be a problem than on faddy diets or diets too low in calories.

An anti-hunger diet, just like a normal healthy diet, will contain plenty of complex carbohydrates, adequate protein, and some fat. A normal non-weight-loss diet should contain 30% or less fat; a weight-loss diet can reduce this to around 25%, the rest of the diet being made up from up to 15% protein and 60% carbohydrate. An extremely low-fat diet, such as is sometimes recommended, can exacerbate hunger and is also very impractical to follow.

Importantly, a hunger-free diet will contain plenty of the carbohydrate foods that have a low Glycemic Index. The Glycemic Index was invented to help professionals treat diabetics, and it measures the rate at which blood glucose levels rise when a particular carbohydrate food is eaten. Given that glucose itself has a GI rating of 100, then the nearer to 100 a food's rating is, the quicker it will be absorbed; the lower a food's rating is, the slower it will be absorbed. Foods with a low GI rating will help you to feel full for longer than high-GI foods and will help keep your blood sugar levels constant.

Protein and fat aren't measured on the Glycemic Index, but both have the effect of lowering a food's GI rating when eaten at the same time, which is why each meal and snack that you eat should contain a small to moderate amount of protein and a small amount of fat. See the Glycemic Index, opposite.

has taken you by surprise. Most high-fat snack foods are eaten this way. In the quest to control your own eating, it helps to plan ahead as much as you can. Decide where and what you're going to eat in advance. Make sure you are well stocked up with healthy, easy-to-prepare food items so that you aren't tempted by others.

Lastly, take note of all the times that you eat simply because food is there in front of you—reasons of habit and availability (e.g., at the newsstand, or while you are preparing food for others). This all, too, is food you don't really need. When you have time on your hands, food "surplus to requirements" can easily find its way into your mouth. Waiting at a station when the train is late, you get a chocolate bar from the vending machine; sitting at home waiting for guests to arrive, you nibble at a bowl of salted nuts.

BOILED EGG; 1 SLICE OF WHOLEGRAIN BREAD WITH 40% FAT MARGARINE.

■ Salt reduction

Most of us eat much more salt than we need (see page 33) and many of the high-salt foods are also those that contain a lot of fat. In order to give your taste-buds a better chance to enjoy natural foods, you need to retrain them to need less salt. This is very easy to do.
∗ This week, stop adding salt to food at the table, and cut down by half all the salt that you add in cooking. If you see low-salt versions of products you usually buy (e.g., baked beans), buy those instead.

■ Better breakfasts

Mid-morning can be difficult for many dieters. Hunger pangs creep up and that donut can be very tempting. This is usually because many people skip breakfast when trying to lose weight.

As we saw in Section One, breakfast is important for everyone, but particularly so for weight control and avoidance of hunger. A sensible breakfast for dieters will contain 250–300 calories a day and consist of some carbohydrate, some protein, and a little fat. The following healthy low-calorie breakfasts will all keep hunger away until it is time for a "legitimate" snack or lunch. Carbohydrate-only breakfasts, based on white or whole-wheat bread and jam, are high-GI and should be avoided. This week, improve your breakfast habits and their quality.
∗ 1 small box All Bran (35 g) with 2% milk; blueberries.
∗ Half a grapefruit; low-fat plain yogurt; teaspoon of honey; medium slice of wholegrain bread with a little 40% low-fat margarine.
∗ Old-fashioned oatmeal with skim milk and water; teaspoon of honey; orange or nectarine.
∗ Citrus fruit, apple, and grape salad; low-fat yogurt; 2 tablespoons of muesli.
∗ Boiled egg; 1 slice of rye bread with a little 40% fat margarine; apple.

■ Begin some exercise

Start doing a daily walk of at least 20 minutes. Try to build more activity into your normal routine, e.g., stair climbing, washing the car by hand, using the stairs rather than the elevator. A diet cannot be successful long term without regular exercise.

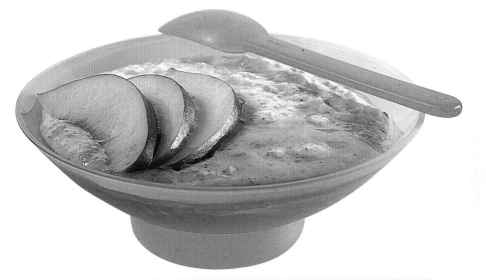

OLD-FASHIONED OATMEAL WITH SKIM MILK AND WATER; TEASPOON OF HONEY; NECTARINE SLICES.

THE GLYCEMIC INDEX

Low-GI foods (long-term energy; try to include plenty of these in your diet):

All legumes including lentils, soybeans, kidney beans, chickpeas, lima beans, cannellini beans.
Barley, buckwheat, bulgur, couscous.
Apples, dried apricots, peaches, grapefruit, plums, cherries.
Avocado, zucchini, spinach, sweet peppers, onions, mushrooms, leafy greens, leeks, peas, green beans, fava beans, Brussels sprouts, snow peas, broccoli, cauliflower.
Plain yogurt, milk, peanuts.

Medium-GI foods (medium-term energy; eat freely):

Sweet potatoes, boiled potatoes, yams, raw carrots, corn, peas.
White pasta, whole-wheat pasta, oats, oatmeal, Grapenuts, All Bran, noodles.
Wholegrain and rye breads, rye crispbreads, pita bread, buckwheat, bulgur, white and brown rice.
Grapes, oranges, kiwi fruit, mangos, beets, fresh dates, figs, apple-and-date bars.

High-GI foods (quick-release, short-term energy; eat as part of a meal containing protein/fat/low-GI foods):

Glucose, sugar, honey, pineapple, bananas, raisins, watermelon.
Baked potatoes, mashed potatoes, parsnips, cooked carrots, squash, rutabaga.
White rice, brown rice, whole-wheat bread, white bread, rice cakes, bread sticks.
Cornflakes, Bran Flakes, instant oat cereal, puffed cereal, popcorn, wheat crackers, English muffins.
Fruit drinks, watermelon, dried dates, bananas, sweetened yogurt.

Week three—eating to lose weight

Goals of the week:
* Learn to listen to body signals about food.
* Build up a more detailed picture of how to cut calories sensibly.
* Retrain taste buds to prefer less sugar.
* Look at your main meals and see how they can be re-balanced to provide fewer calories.
* Continue with exercise and control techniques.

If, for years, you have been eating from habit, overeating just because food is there, eating without paying attention to what you were doing, then this week you need to get back in touch with what your body is telling you about its needs.

Few of us actually feel genuine hunger any more—mealtimes and snack-times come around well before real hunger has time to set in. This week, see if, instead of eating exactly by the clock, you can get that slightly hungry feeling before tucking in. If you find it is lunch-time and you don't have that hunger, but you can't eat later because of, say, your work, just have a little and save some more for mid-afternoon.

Few of us are truly in tune with the moment when we feel full and should stop eating. Instead, we just eat all that is on the plate because it is there, and usually there is more of it than we would genuinely need to satisfy hunger.

This week, pay attention when you eat. Chew thoroughly, take your time, and decide to stop when you feel full enough. If you do this a few times and find you always have food left on your plate, give yourself smaller portions, especially of the high-fat foods.

If you don't override your body signals, soon you will get back in tune with your real needs, and weight loss should become much more natural.

■ Calorie-cutting without pain

By cutting surplus fat from the diet, in the form of high-fat snacks, high-fat meats, high-fat dairy products, and too much fat used in cooking, and by following the behavior techniques you have learned so far, it is likely that you can be saving enough calories to effect a steady weight loss without having to do much else. If that doesn't prove to be the case, though, sugars and alcohol should be cut next, because these provide calories with virtually no nutrients.

You can retrain a sweet tooth in just the same way as a salty tooth—by gradually cutting back: firstly on sugar added to drinks and cereals, then on sweet drinks themselves, then on sugary items such as cakes, cookies, and confectionery. High-calorie desserts are best avoided by dieters except now and then. Nutritious desserts based on fruit and low-fat dairy products are ideal. Artificial sweeteners save calories by replacing sugar, but do little to help a sweet tooth in the long term.

If calories still need to be saved, you need, finally, to look at the amount of protein and starchy foods on your plate. An overall slight reduction in portion size can save enough calories in a day to make a difference.

Remember that many protein foods are also high in fat—cut these down first—and also remember not to add too much fat to carbohydrate foods—e.g., butter to a baked potato, and so on.

The chart on the right shows an ideal breakdown of a day's calorie and fat intake for two different dieting levels. A diet of about 1,250 calories a day, such as that on page 200, is suitable for people with less than 14 lb (6.3 kg), to lose, for most women, for small men, and toward the end of a diet. A diet of about 1,500 calories a day, such as that on page 201, is suitable for people with a lot of weight to lose, as well as for many men, and at the start of most diets.

There is no need to stick rigidly to these amounts (it would be very hard to do so anyway), but they provide a blueprint on which to build. Calorie and fat content of many foods is listed in the Food Charts at the end of the book, and more information is contained in Section One. The recipes in Section Five are calorie- and fat-counted, too, and indicated suitable for dieters as appropriate, to help you incorporate them into a weight loss plan.

■ Salt

This week try to reduce salt in your diet further by cutting the amount you add while cooking to just a few grains. The addition of fresh herbs and spices may help you miss the salt less. Check the list of high-salt foods on page 33, and start cutting back on the amount of those that you eat. In general, processed food contains a lot of salt.

DIET INTAKE LEVELS

1,250 calories a day

	Calories	Fat (g) *
Breakfast	250	5
Lunch	350	8
Main meal	350	12
Snack	100	5
Snack/Treat	100	5
Milk allowance	100	trace
	1,250	35

1,500 calories a day

	Calories	Fat (g)
Breakfast	300	6
Lunch	400	10
Main Meal	400	14
Snack	150	6
Snack/treat	150	6
Milk allowance	100	trace
	1,500	42

* based on 25% of total calorie intake.

CALORIE-CUTTING MAIN MEAL—CHICKEN

Chicken in the traditional manner	Calorie-cutting chicken ★ ★ ★ ★ ★
Chicken-leg portion, lean and skin, total weight 10½ oz (300 g), edible portion 5 oz (150 g), broiled; 4½ oz (125 g) new potatoes; 2 teaspoons (10 g) butter; 4 oz (115 g) salad of lettuce, cucumber, and tomato (1½ oz/50 g lettuce, ½ oz/20 g cucumber, 1¼ oz/40 g) tomato; 2 teaspoons (10 g) mayonnaise.	1 portion of Lemon Chicken (page 230); 6 oz (175 g), cooked weight, egg-thread noodles; 5½ oz (165 g) mixed vegetables (1½ oz/50 g carrot, ¾ oz/25 g zucchini, ½ oz/20 g green beans, 1½ oz/50 g broccoli, ½ oz/20g beansprouts) stir-fried in 1 teaspoon of oil.
530 calories and 26 g fat. Total weight of meal 14½ oz (410 g).	385 calories and 13 g fat. Total weight of meal 1 lb 1 oz (470 g).
Chicken is a favorite with dieters, but a typical weight-watcher's chicken meal isn't always as low-calorie as it may seem. The meal described on the left looks innocent enough, with its small portion of potatoes and salad. In fact, it	contains nearly one-third more calories than the bigger-looking, and heavier, plateful on the right.

CALORIE-CUTTING MAIN MEAL—STEAK

High-calorie, high-fat steak meal	Reduced-calorie, reduced-fat steak meal ★ ★ ★ ★ ★
8 oz (225 g) sirloin steak (including part-trimmed fat); 7 oz (200 g) deep-fried frozen fries; 1¾ oz (50 g) fried mushrooms; 1¾ oz (50 g) peas. 1,152 calories and 62 g fat. Total weight of meal 1 lb 2½ oz (525 g).	200 g (7 oz) sirloin steak, trimmed of fat; 200 g (7 oz) potato wedges brushed with 1 tsp oil and baked; l medium tomato, broiled; 60 g (2 oz) peas. 625 calories and 18 g fat. Total weight of meal 1 lb 2 oz (510 g).
A generous and satisfying steak meal needn't be off the menu for most weight-watchers. The plateful on the right contains approximately half the number of calories and one-third the fat of the plateful on the left, simply	because the amount of fat has been quite drastically reduced. Remember, when you're cutting fat, add more vegetables, then you will still have plenty to eat.

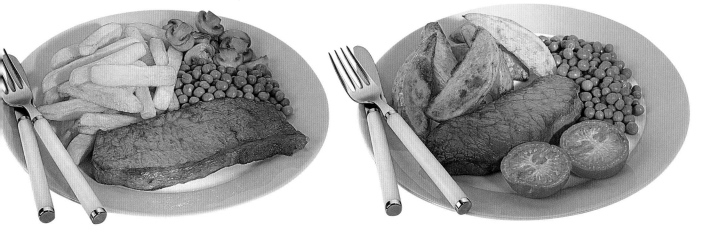

1,152 CALORIES AND 62 G FAT. TOTAL WEIGHT OF MEAL 1 LB 2 ½ OZ (525 G).   *625 CALORIES AND 18 G FAT. TOTAL WEIGHT OF MEAL 1 LB 2 OZ (510 G).*

Week four—getting back to nature

Goals for the Week:
* Treat your body with respect and give it high-quality fuel.
* Discover a taste for natural foods.
* Learn to manage "treat" foods within your diet.
* Lunch-time make-over.
* Consider long-term success.

It is hard to overeat on a diet high in natural wholesome foods, and that is why the two main keys to long-term success with weight-watching are:

1 To recognize that your body is important and that it deserves the best fuel you can give it.

2 For this reason to give it good-quality, nutritious and fresh food.

In this last week of the retraining course you should be fully appreciating the flavors, textures, and colors of your food. Instead of tasting just salt or sugar, you should be enjoying the subtleties of every type of food that you choose. This week try to:
* Eat as much unadulterated fresh food as possible. Eat fruits and vegetables raw or very lightly cooked.
* Try a variety of new foods, such as different breads, fish, fruits, salad leaves.
* Expand on the idea that "treating yourself" doesn't have to mean with something "naughty" (as in a pastry or chocolate), but can just as easily mean enjoying something nutrient-dense and light, such as a slice of perfect cantaloupe melon, or six fresh oysters on ice.
* Also consider the low-cost "top-quality" foods such as brown lentils, bulgur, wholegrain barley, and chickpeas, and enjoy them as much as you may enjoy that feast of shellfish.
* Get more quality, not quantity, into your diet. Think of having one glass of delicious wine rather than several glasses of *vin ordinaire*. Think of having a small organic filet mignon rather than a large steak of dubious origin.
* Think of yourself as a "foodie" rather than a gourmand.

* Long term, vow not to put any item of food or drink in your mouth that doesn't serve a useful purpose for your body or provide you with pure, unadulterated pleasure.

By following these tips and ideals, you will be able to control your weight, not by feeling deprived and miserable (as you will agree has been the case previously, which is why it didn't work), but by feeling in control, by enjoying your daily diet, and by feeling proud that you care enough about your body to provide for it well.

The diet plans that follow here are samples of how you may like to eat to lose weight now that the four-week course is over. (See page 196 for some guidelines on whether to try Diet 1250 or Diet 1500.)

■ Healthy low-calorie lunches
* Any of the soups from the recipe section (pages 216–19) with some slices of wholegrain bread and an average portion of fruit.
* Chickpea Salad with Peppers and Tomatoes (page 220); apple.
* Thai Salmon Salad (page 222).
* Panzanella (page 222); banana.
* Hummus; whole-wheat mini pita; orange.
* ½ avocado, sliced, with fresh crabmeat, and olive-oil dressing; slice

---

MANAGING "TREAT" FOODS

Most people who undertake a four-week course such as this find that, however much they enjoyed items such as confectionery, potato chips, cakes, and so on at the start, by the end of week 4 their tastes have changed and these foods no longer hold such appeal.

However, if you still want to include such items in your diet, you can do so even while dieting. The 1,250 calories-a-day plan overleaf allows 100 calories a day for a "treat," and the 1,500-a-day plan allows 150. Treats should be eaten or drunk with or after a meal, not on their own or when you are hungry (when you might easily eat more). Suggested options appear below:

100 calorie treats: 4 fl oz table wine; 3 (1-inch/2.5-cm squares) chocolate coated graham crackers; 1½ fl oz 80% spirits; 1 oatmeal cookie.

150 calories treats: 1 oz (30 g) tortilla chips; 1 small slice of angel food cake; 3 tablespoons (25 g) salted peanuts or cashew nuts.

of whole-wheat bread, green salad.
✱ Seafood and Tropical Fruit Salad (page 224); average portion of cooled cooked brown rice.

■ Long-term weight-watching

Once your desired body-weight is reached, maintain your weight by following all the ideas you have learned in the preceding weeks. You can eat more than you did while dieting—about 2,200 calories a day for women and 2,700 for men. As we have seen in the Question and Answer session, your metabolic rate is likely to be normal for a person of your size and age.

The Basic Healthy Diet given on page 53 is a good sample diet to follow; the food charts and recipes later in the book will help you build an enjoyable and satisfying diet for life.

Regular exercise is a vital key to long-term weight control. Try to ensure that you indulge in regular walking, cycling, or swimming, as well as generally building more activity into your daily life.

Try to combine aerobic exercise with muscle-toning exercise, such as window-cleaning or circuit-training. because the higher your muscle-to-fat ratio the more calories you will burn.

LUNCH MAKE–OVER

Within a busy life, lunch is often the one meal of the day that is eaten without any thought or planning. Most people believe that they "hardly eat a thing" at lunch and yet, when what they do actually eat is analyzed, it turns out to be much higher in calories and fat than they imagined.

The example below is typical. The cheese and crackers "snack" actually contains more calories and much more fat than the satisfying, healthy, and tasty (yet still quick) lunch on the right. Such a lunch will keep hunger pangs at bay and provide a better range of nutrients than the cheese snack.

High-calorie Snack	Low-calorie Meal	★ ★ ★ ★ ★
2½ oz (70 g) Cheddar cheese; 3 milk crackers; 1½ teaspoons (7.5 g) margarine.	3½ oz (100 g) tuna (canned in water, drained), flaked, with 1 medium chopped tomato, 2½ oz (70 g) cooked lima beans, 4 scallions, chopped, 2 teaspoons dressing made with olive oil and lemon juice, 1¼ oz (35 g) dark rye bread, 1 peach.	
446 calories and 30 g fat	390 calories and 7 g fat	

PROVING THAT YOU DON'T HAVE TO STARVE TO LOSE WEIGHT, THIS LUNCH WEIGHS MORE THAN THE SNACK BELOW AND IS MUCH MORE SATISFYING.

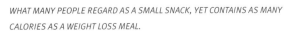

WHAT MANY PEOPLE REGARD AS A SMALL SNACK, YET CONTAINS AS MANY CALORIES AS A WEIGHT LOSS MEAL.

DIET 1250

Eat everything in the diet below plus:

* Daily 1¼ cups (275 ml) skim milk for use on its own or in tea and coffee.
* One extra snack/treat to the value of 100 calories to be eaten with or after a meal.
* Unlimited—fresh salad items, leafy green vegetables, lemon juice, fresh herbs and spices, water, mineral water.
* Tea and coffee—up to 4 cups a day altogether. No sugar or sweeteners.

Meals should be spaced out as evenly as possible. The daily snack should either be eaten mid-morning, mid- to late-afternoon, or shortly before bedtime. Calorie content works out at an approximate average of 1,250 per day, fat content averages 35 g a day maximum.

DAY ONE
Breakfast
½ cup (125 g) plain yogurt
¾ oz (25 g) All Bran
4½ oz (125 g) fresh fruit, chopped
Lunch
Lima Bean Soup
2 slices of Oat Bread, with a little 40% fat margarine
Evening
Chicken Cacciatore
6 oz (175 g), cooked weight, pasta shapes
large green salad
Snack
2 oz (60 g) ready-to-eat dried apricots

DAY TWO
Breakfast
¾ oz (25 g) Scotch oats, made into oatmeal using half water and half skim milk from allowance
1 orange
1 slice of Oat Bread with 1 teaspoon honey
Lunch
Feta and Pepper Spread
1 whole-wheat pita bread
1 apple
Evening
Rice and Beans
large mixed salad with fat-free dressing
Snack
1 large banana

DAY THREE
Breakfast
½ pink grapefruit
1 large boiled or poached egg
1½ thin slices of Oat Bread or wholegrain bread with a little 40% fat margarine
Lunch
Chickpea Salad with Peppers and Tomatoes
1 apple
Evening
Seared Tuna with Lemon Grass, large portion of green beans, 2¾ oz (75 g) new potatoes
Snack
One ¾-oz (25-g) slice of wholegrain bread OR Oat Bread, little 40% fat margarine and 1 teaspoon honey

DAY FOUR
Breakfast
1¼ oz (40 g) no-added-sugar muesli
½ cup (125 ml) skim milk extra to allowance, apple chopped in
Lunch
Sandwich of two 1¼-oz (40-g) slices of dark rye bread with a little 40% fat margarine, filled with plenty of salad items, plus 1 portion Canellini Bean and Basil Spread
Evening
Turkish Eggplant
large green salad with 2 teaspoons vinaigrette dressing
Summer Fruits Compote
Snack
Banana and Strawberry Smoothie

DAY FIVE
Breakfast
As Day 1
Lunch
medium slice of cantaloupe melon
1¾ oz (50 g) prosciutto
3½-oz (100-g) slice of Italian bread
green salad
Evening
Tabbouleh
Mushroom and Red Pepper Skewers
Snack
2 oz (60 g) ready-to-eat dried apricots

DAY SIX
Breakfast
As Day 2
Lunch
Baba Ganoush
1 whole-wheat pita bread
1 apple
Evening
1 small skinless, boneless, chicken breast, broiled or baked
Canellini Beans with Hot Tomato Vinaigrette
large green salad
Snack
1 large banana

DAY SEVEN
Breakfast
As Day 3
Lunch
Spinach, Parsley, and Garlic Soup
1¾ oz (50 g) French bread
1 apple
Evening
One 7 oz (200 g) shark steak, broiled or pan-fried without fat
Fresh Pepper Coulis
2¾ oz (75 g), cooked weight, bulgur wheat
broccoli
Snack
1 slice of Oat Bread with 1 teaspoon honey

Diet 1500

Eat everything in the diet below plus:

✱ Daily milk allowance of 1¼ cups (275 ml) on its own or in tea and coffee.

✱ One extra daily snack or treat to value of 150 calories, with or after a meal.

✱ Unlimiteds as diet 1250.

✱ Up to 4 cups of tea or coffee a day altogether.

Instructions as diet opposite. Provides an average 1,500 calories a day and 42 g fat.

DAY ONE
Breakfast
1¼ oz (40 g) Grapenuts with skim milk from allowance
1 orange
one 1 oz (30 g) slice of wholegrain bread with a little 40% fat margarine and 1 teaspoon honey
Lunch
Skordalia, selection of crudités
two 1-oz (30-g) slices of dark rye bread or Oat Bread
Evening
Parcels of Tilapia, Tomatoes, and Olives
4½ oz (125 g), cooked weight, pasta
large green salad
Snack
30 g (1 oz) ready-to-eat dried apricots
1 large banana

DAY TWO
Breakfast
1 large egg, boiled or poached
2 slices of Oat Bread or wholegrain bread with a little 40% fat margarine
1 peach or orange
Lunch
Carrot and Orange Soup
1 average wholegrain or rye roll
2 tablespoons cottage cheese
Evening
Potato and Mediterranean Vegetable Bake
green salad
Snack
1 medium banana; 1 graham cracker

DAY THREE
Breakfast
1 apple and date bar, ½ pink grapefruit,
3½ oz (100 g) low-fat ricotta cheese
Lunch
½ medium avocado, sliced, with tomato, onion, and iceberg lettuce, fat-free dressing,
1 medium wholegrain roll
1 kiwi fruit
Evening
Spiced Chicken and Greens
2¾ oz (75 g), cooked weight, brown rice
Snack
2 honey graham crackers

DAY FOUR
Breakfast
¾ oz (25 g) oatmeal, made with half water and half skim milk (extra to allowance),
1 medium banana
Lunch
Seafood and Tropical Fruit Salad
3½ oz (100 g) plain yogurt
Evening
Pasta with Milanese Sauce
large green salad
Snack
1 Oat-Apricot Bar

DAY FIVE
Breakfast
¼ oz (40 g) no-added-sugar muesli
½ cup (125 ml) skim milk extra to allowance,
1 apple chopped in
Lunch
Roast Tomato, Garlic, and Pepper Soup
3¼ oz (90 g) slice of Italian bread
1 orange
Evening
3½ oz (100 g) turkey cutlet or steak, peppered and broiled, Mango Salsa
4½ oz (125 g), cooked weight, brown rice
medium portion of green beans
Snack
½ cup (125 g) low-fat yogurt

DAY SIX
Breakfast
As Day 1
Lunch
Cucumber and Mint Soup
Sandwich of two 1-oz (30-g) slices of dark rye bread filled with a little 40% fat margarine and 1 tablespoon cottage cheese, plus plenty of salad
Evening
Chickpea and Vegetable Crumble, broccoli
Snack
Citrus Granita

DAY SEVEN
Breakfast
As Day 3
Lunch
6 oz (175 g), cooked weight, pasta, cooled and mixed with 6 oz (175 g) selection of raw, thinly sliced vegetables and tossed in 1 tablespoon tofu mayonnaise
1 apple
Evening
One 3¼ oz (90 g) fillet of salmon
Tomato and Bean Salsa
4½ oz (125 g) new potatoes
Snack
2 graham crackers, 1½ oz (45 g) grapes

Popular dieting methods evaluated

You may have been tempted to follow one or more of the popular diet methods that receive much publicity. Here we examine the theory behind each method, appraise its advantages and drawbacks, and rate each for various qualities (the more of the blank circles that are filled in, the better).

■ The Hay Diet (food combining)

Theory: If we mix "protein" and "carbohydrate" foods at the same meal, they are incompletely digested, leading to toxicity and weight problems; therefore, meals generally must not contain both. Vegetables and fruit form a large part of the diet, but fruit must be eaten in isolation. Only wholegrain or unprocessed starches should be eaten. Four hours should elapse between meals. Milk is restricted, and there are many other rules.

Typical lunch: Cheese with green salad; yogurt.

Appraisal: There is no scientific evidence or reason to believe the "protein fights carbohydrates" theory. Our digestive systems can happily cope with a meal containing both protein and starch. The theory falls down, anyway, because many foods contain both—e.g., the starchy foods like legumes, grains, and potatoes all contain protein too. For many people, the complicated rules may be hard to grasp and stick to, and don't fit in well with other people's eating habits. weight loss may be achieved simply because the system restricts calories.

Score: Ease ●○○○ Palatability ●○○○ Satiety level ●●○○ Safety ●●●○ Short-term effectiveness ●●●○ Long-term effectiveness ●●○○ Healthy eating basis ●●○○ Scientific basis ○○○○
Total score: 14/32

■ High-Protein Diet

Theory: Protein content of the diet is doubled, or more, to 30% or more of total calories. Carbohydrates and fats are restricted. There are various well-known diets based on the high-protein principle; each varies in its explanation of how they work. One, for instance, explains that a high-carbohydrate diet blocks utilization of calories and fat, because of various hormonal reactions; therefore, restricting carb intake will increase fat loss.

Typical lunch: Broiled skinless chicken, broccoli.

Appraisal: High-protein, low-carb flies in the face of all current nutritional knowledge. Restricting carbohydrates will also restrict fiber intake, which can cause constipation, bowel cancer, and other problems; and eating a diet high in protein can damage the liver, and increase excretion of calcium from the body (which could lead to increased chance of osteoporosis). High-protein diets work because they restrict overall calorie consumption rather than by hormonal reactions. On a high-protein, low-carb diet, ketosis may occur—characterized by acetone-smelling breath.

Score: Ease ●●○○ Palatability ●●○○ Satiety level ●●○○ Safety ●○○○ Short-term effectiveness ●●●○ Long-term effectiveness ●●○○ Healthy eating basis ○○○○ Scientific basis ●○○○
Total score: 13/32

■ Calorie Counting

Theory: All food contains calories (energy); weight loss is based on calorie restriction—by taking in less calories than the body needs to maintain its weight, stored body fat has to be used for energy, and weight loss results. With a guide to the calorie content of all foods, it is possible to include any food within a diet as long as it fits in with the overall chosen calorie level—usually between 1,200 and 1,500 calories a day.

Typical lunch: Shrimp sandwich with low-calorie mayonnaise; apple, small chocolate cookie.

Appraisal: Although the scope for including any food in a calorie-controlled diet may sound appealing to most people, the system doesn't necessarily teach healthy eating habits. Foods often need to be weighed or measured to ensure accuracy, which can be time-consuming and boring. With the right dietary advice, however, a calorie-controlled diet can be tailored to suit anyone and will work.

Score: Ease ●●○○ Palatability ●●●● Satiety level ●●○○ Safety ●●●○ Short-term effectiveness ●●●○ Long-term effectiveness ●●○○ Healthy eating basis ●●○○ Scientific basis ●●●●
Total score: 22/32

■ High-fiber, High-Carbohydrate

Theory: A diet high in fiber and carbohydrate helps the dieter to feel full for longer, while taking in fewer calories, because high-fiber foods take more chewing, swallowing, and digesting, and keep blood sugar levels more constant than many other types of diet. Calorie count will be restricted in such a diet, because fat levels are also controlled.

Typical lunch: Baked beans with whole-wheat toast; orange, a few prunes.

Appraisal: A sensible approach to dieting—the theory works well and is similar in approach to a basic healthy diet. It tends to have more long-term success than many other diets, but results may be slow. A high-fiber diet can also help to prevent certain ailments, and has even been linked with less risk of bowel cancer.

Score: Ease ●●●○ Palatability ●●○○ Satiety level ●●●● Safety ●●●● Short-term effectiveness ●●○○ Long-term effectiveness ●●●● Healthy eating basis ●●●● Scientific basis ●●●○

Total score: 26/32

■ Very-Low-Fat Diet

Theory: Fat is the nutrient highest in calories—at 9 calories per gram compared with 4 for protein and 3.75 for carbohydrate—therefore, more calories can be cut by avoiding fat than by any other method. Also, a high-fat diet is linked with some illnesses, so fat-cutting is healthy too, the theory goes.

Fat content of all foods is listed in various guides, and the theory is, if fat is avoided as far as possible but normal quantities of carbohydrate and low-fat protein foods are allowed, then weight loss must follow without the need to count calories.

Typical lunch: Vegetable soup made without added fat; skinless turkey breast sandwich (no margarine) with salad; fat-free fruit yogurt.

Appraisal: A reduced-fat diet can be healthy if it is mostly saturated fat that is reduced, but some very-low-fat diets also disallow the healthy fats found in items like nuts, plant oils, and oily fish.

Also, such diets may be short of essential fatty acids and of the fat-soluble vitamins A, D, E, and K. There is evidence that the EFAs can help weight loss rather than hinder it.

A very-low-fat diet can be quite unpalatable—less than around 25% of total calories is almost unworkable in most people's lives. There is also some evidence that people on a low-fat diet tend to eat more of the carbohydrate foods to make up the "lost" calories, so it isn't a guaranteed route to success. However, many people find fat cutting less bother than calorie counting, and it can fit in well with an overall healthy diet.

Score: Ease ●●●○ Palatability ●●○○ Satiety level ●●●○ Safety ●●○○ Short-term effectiveness ●●○○ Long-term effectiveness ●●●● Healthy eating basis ●●●○ Scientific basis ●●○○

Total score: 20/32

■ Meal Replacement

Theory: One, two, or three meals a day are replaced with a manufactured calorie-counted meal, such as a milk shake or a bar containing protein, vitamins, minerals, fiber, and so on. The idea is that this takes away the need to think about preparing reduced-calorie meals and provides all the nutrients the dieter needs while containing an exact stated low number of calories.

Typical lunch: One serving of meal-replacement chocolate milkshake, glass of water.

Appraisal: Many people do well on meal-replacement diets if used to replace one or two meals a day and the remaining meal(s) is/are healthy and balanced.

Long term, replacement diets can be boring. Critics say that the replacement meals don't provide phytochemicals, and that it is hardly possible to get the recommended five portions of fruit and vegetables or enough carbohydrate

every day on such a regime. Also, meal replacements do little to help re-educate people to long-term healthy eating and may encourage yo-yo dieting. Many are high in sugar—over 60% in some cases. Although guidelines for usage are given on packs, over-fast weight loss could result if used to replace too many meals.

Score: Ease ●●●● Palatability ●●○○ Satiety level ●○○○ Safety ●●○○ Short-term effectiveness ●●●○ Long-term effectiveness ●●○○ Healthy eating basis ●○○○ Scientific basis ●●●○

Total score: 18/32

■ Fasting

Theory: Existing on nothing but water (some "fasts" allow fruit and vegetable juices, too) for days or weeks at a time encourages rapid fat-loss; hunger pangs disappear within 2–3 days of the start of the fast, and the faster may feel highly energetic, clear-headed, and calm.

Typical lunch: Water.

Appraisal: On a fast, a high percentage of lean body tissue (muscle) can be lost, including that from the vital organs such as the heart, meaning that such a regime can be dangerous, especially if vigorous activity is undertaken while fasting. Headaches, dizziness, faintness, constipation, and bad breath (as a result of ketosis) are common side effects. Undertaken regularly, or for weeks at a time, deficiency in various vitamins and minerals will occur.

Score: Ease ●●○○ Palatability ○○○○ Satiety level ○○○○ Safety ○○○○ Short-term effectiveness ●●●● Long-term effectiveness ○○○○ (unsafe for long term) Healthy eating basis ○○○○ Scientific basis ●●○○

Total score: 8/32

Weight gain

Because of national preoccupation with obesity, it is not known how many in the US are underweight. However, there is evidence of a growing trend of young females worried about weight gain and about 1% of female adolescents have anorexia. According to most research, the greater the degree of underweight, the greater the risks of malnutrition, heart attacks, sexual and reproductive problems, osteoporosis, and reduced life span.

New research linking calorie restriction with increased life span contradicts much of these traditionally accepted statistics, so more research is needed, but it may be that BMIs at the lower end of "average" (i.e., 20–21) are healthy, while those under 20 are not.

Why do some people have trouble maintaining their body fat? Just like obese people, hereditary factors may be one reason for some. This could cause a predisposition to burning off the calories in food more quickly than average. Although not a great deal of research has been carried out on underweight people, it does seem that the main reason for underweight is the most obvious one—that low-weight people take more exercise and/or eat fewer calories.

In one recent study, people who thought they were naturally thin were fed a controlled high-calorie diet and, much to their surprise, every one of them put on the amount of weight that would be expected. They just hadn't been eating as much as they thought. It seems slim people prefer lower-calorie foods, such as fruits and vegetables, and are less tolerant of large, calorie-dense meals.

Some slim people also tend to be more active than normal-weight people, "fidgeting" more and perhaps even sleeping for fewer hours, perhaps with a natural inclination toward active hobbies.

Lastly, almost anyone can become too thin during or as a result of illness.

For everyone, a high-calorie diet can restore a suitable BMI. The trick is to offer a diet that the recipient will actually eat and doesn't find too daunting.

■ The Weight-Gain Diet

Nutritionists have found that an increment of 500 calories a day on average is about right in order to help most thin people put on weight. More than this may overwhelm most people; less means weight-gain would be slow. This amount is only a guide—it depends on starting weight and other factors. For instance, a very thin person who has been eating only a few hundred calories a day will probably gain weight on a diet that is lower in calories than a normal average diet (2,200 for women, 2,700 for men), but someone who is thin because they exercise a lot could need more than 500 calories a day above average.

The extra calories should be added to the diet so that the balance of nutrients is still healthy—with not too much fat, plenty of carbohydrate, and enough protein. Although fat is the most calorie-dense of the nutrients, at 9 calories a gram, it isn't suitable to offer the extra 500 calories in nothing but high-fat foods, as this would increase the fat content to unacceptably high levels. However, it is reasonable to offer a diet a little higher in fat than would be provided in the diet long term (especially if mostly in the form of the essential fatty acids). This is because thin people with a poor appetite often have difficulty in managing enough high-bulk foods, such as starchy carbohydrates, to provide enough extra calories, although sugars are easy to eat and digest.

SNACKS FOR WEIGHT GAIN

Healthy high-fat snacks: Fresh nuts, seeds, muesli, whole-milk yogurt.
Healthy high-carbohydrate snacks: Granola bars, bread, oatcakes.
Healthy high-calorie drinks: Whole or low-fat 2% milk, milky malted drinks, hot cocoa, fruit juice, 1–2 glasses wine or stout a day.

Examples of adding 500 calories' worth of snacks to the daily diet:
✳ 1 large slice of white bread with a little butter and jam; 1¼ cups (300 ml) low-fat 2% milk; 1 large banana.
✳ 2 small slices of nut and raisin bread with a little butter; ¾ cup (100 g) portion of vanilla ice cream; average portion of cornflakes with a little low-fat 2% milk.
✳ Ice cream milkshake; 2 cookies.

IDEAL CALORIES FOR GAIN

Daily milk and fruit juice allowance :	280 calories
Breakfast:	400 calories
Mid-morning snack:	200 calories
Lunch (or evening meal):	550 calories
Mid-afternoon snack:	150 calories
Evening meal (or lunch):	700 calories
Bedtime snack:	150 calories
Total:	2,430 calories

Sample weight gain diet for women

This sample diet gives an average of around 2,600 calories a day, divided up roughly as the blueprint opposite.
Daily allowance: 1¼ cups (275 ml) whole milk; 1¼ cups (275 ml) orange, or other fruit, juice.
Unlimited: Fresh or frozen vegetables; salad; fresh fruit.

DAY ONE
Breakfast
2 Shredded Wheat with 1 teaspoon brown sugar and 2 teaspoons sunflower seeds sprinkled over
⅔ cup (150 ml) low-fat 2% milk to cover (extra to allowance)
1 medium slice of white bread with butter and 1 teaspoon honey
1 apple or peach
Mid-morning
cheese and crackers
Lunch
tuna salad sandwich, ice cream
Mid-afternoon
1 Oat-Apricot Bar
Evening
Pasta with Basil and Ricotta
tomato salad
1 banana
Bedtime
mug of hot malted drink and 1 cookie

DAY TWO
Breakfast
poached egg on large slice of toast with a little butter
1 large slice of toast and butter with preserves
1 orange
Mid-morning
2 tablespoons shelled Brazil nuts and 5 halves of ready-to-eat dried apricots
Lunch
Squash, Potato, and Lima Bean Soup
medium whole-wheat roll with butter
Mid-afternoon
small slice of pound cake
Evening
Seafood Risotto with Ginger
fresh fruit salad with 2 teaspoons sour cream
Bedtime
mug of hot low-fat 2% milk
chocolate oatmeal cookies

DAY THREE
Breakfast
As Day 1
Mid-morning
As Day 1
Lunch
Brown Rice and Citrus Salad
Mid-afternoon
1 Oat-Apricot Bar
Evening
Avocado and Turkey Tortillas
Peach and Banana Fool
Bedtime
As Day 1

DAY FOUR
Breakfast
As Day 2
Mid-morning
As Day 2
Lunch
Quick Baked Beans
large slice of crusty bread with a little butter
Mid-afternoon
As Day 2
Evening
Steak and Spinach Stir-Fry
Raspberry Gratin
Bedtime
As Day 2

DAY FIVE
Breakfast
¾ cup muesli with 1 tablespoon chopped almonds added
4½ fl oz (125 ml) low-fat 2% milk to cover
1 pear or nectarine
Mid-morning
As Day 1
Lunch
Salad of Tuna, Avocado, and Tomato
1 large slice of whole-wheat bread
1 apple
Mid-afternoon
As Day 1
Evening
Almond, Chickpea, and Raisin Pilaf
green salad
Bedtime
mug of hot low-fat 2% milk
small slice of nut and raisin bread

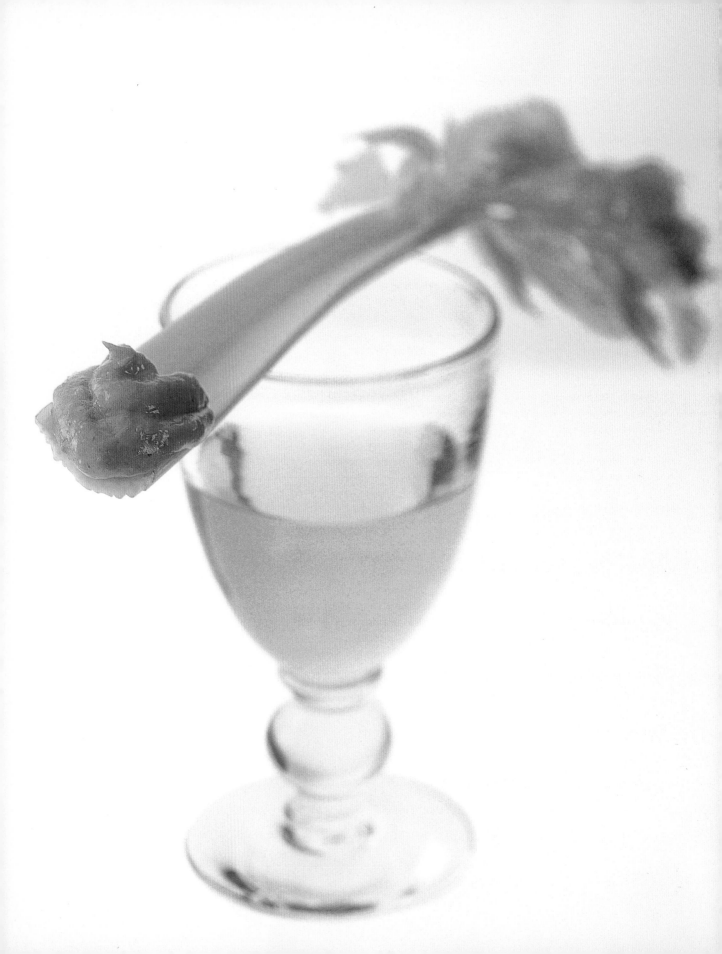

Food for health and pleasure

Knowing what foods to eat for your continuing good health is, of course, what this book is all about. Almost as important, however, is knowing how to put it all together. Apart from those occasions when you eat out, the kitchen is where you put all your knowledge into practice. Cooking well is important for two main reasons. Firstly, it is quite possible to turn healthy basic ingredients into less than healthy meals, and so a basic knowledge of healthy cooking is vital. Secondly, you need to provide meals that you and your family actually want to eat. No amount of diet theory will work unless you can convert it into tempting dishes that you really enjoy and which fit into your lifestyle and budget.

This section sets out to provide you with enough good ideas in the form of tips, healthy cooking charts, and carefully thought-out recipes to do just that.

Healthy Cooking Guidelines

The nutritional content of healthful ingredients and basic foods can be enhanced by careful cooking—or debased by poor cooking. For example, some cooking methods rob your food of vital vitamins, while others help to retain them. A classic example is the loss of vitamin C through boiling of vegetables —overboiling, in particular—whereas most other methods conserve almost all the vitamin C in your vegetables.

People catering for those with specific health problems need also to be aware that cooking methods may be important. If cooking for someone who needs to lose weight, say, shallow- and deep-frying are methods to restrict.

Another example is the case of people with digestive disorders or convalescents or long-term patients, who may find it hard to deal with raw and whole-grain foods, and who will get a more sustaining varied diet if offered plenty of foods puréed and turned into soups and casseroles.

Throughout the book, more detailed guidance is given on food and diets for specific ailments and conditions. The chart right shows the benefits and drawbacks of each common cooking method.

Cooking for pleasure—a guide to using the recipes that follow:

The 100 or so recipes that follow have been included to give you a wide selection of ideas on how to incorporate all the healthy foods into your regular diet and that of your family.

Most of the recipes are also featured within the various specialized diet plans throughout the book (for example, the recipe for Carrot and Orange Soup appears as a suggested lunch on Day One of the Anti-Cancer Diet, see page 140). They can also be used in the same way as you would the recipes in a general

COMMON COOKING METHODS COMPARED

✳ **Raw:** Retains maximum nutrients normally lost through cooking, with exception of carrots.
Not suitable for wide range of foods; may be indigestible.
Cut surfaces quickly lose vitamin C, so prepare at last minute.

✳ **Boiling:** No added fat.
Boiled vegetables lose up to 70% of their water-soluble vitamins B and C.
Retain more vitamins by using minimum water and cooking until crisp-tender.

✳ **Steaming:** Retains more nutrients than boiling.
Still 30% or more water-soluble vitamin losses.
Use cooking water in sauces, etc., to put back the vitamins.

✳ **Microwaving:** Retains most water-soluble nutrients if minimum water used.
Quite easy to overcook or undercook unless care taken. Food thermometer useful.
Reheated food should be stirred and served piping hot.

✳ **Baking/roasting:** No added fat necessary with meat—use foil; brush vegetables with olive oil.
Heat destroys vitamin C. Poultry needs thorough cooking.
Meat juices from roasting contain B vitamins—use in sauce.

✳ **Braising/casseroling/stewing:** Tenderizes low-cost meats; vitamins retained within dish.
Can be high in meat fats unless cooled and skimmed of surplus.
Ideal method for root vegetables and legumes.

✳ **Broiling/grilling:** Low-fat ways to cook meat; no added fats, plus fats melt and drip out of meat.
Overgrilled, charred meat linked with several types of cancer. Don't serve burned food.

✳ **Frying—deep- or shallow-:** High-fat—surface of foods absorbs fat; poor method for dieters. Retains water-soluble vitamins.
Frying in vegetable oils may be good idea on occasion for people needing to gain weight.
Use peanut oil—olive oil has too low a smoke-point.
(Change cooking oils frequently—much-used oils oxidize and may be carcinogenic.)

✳ **Stir-frying:** Retains water-soluble vitamins; little fat used.
Suitable method for 2–3 people at a time, as not much food can be stir-fried correctly in one batch. Cut surfaces of vegetables quickly lose vitamin C—prepare shortly before use.

healthy cook book. Each recipe has a panel of symbols above it, which will guide you to the recipe that is right for your purposes. For example, if you are looking for recipes suitable for someone with high blood-cholesterol, you look for the ♥ symbol, which appears on many of the recipes.

All the recipes are suitable for a general basic healthy diet (a sample of which appears in Section One on page 53) and also for childhood, pregnancy, menopause, and old age, although we give detailed advice in these areas and pick out recipes we consider especially suitable in the special features dealing with each of these times of life in Section Three.

The Nutrition Panels

Each recipe has a nutrition panel giving you information on the nutrient content of the recipe per serving. This information is mostly self-explanatory, but here are a few more notes for guidance:

* *Calories* per portion will vary according to size of raw ingredients (such as vegetables) used. I have tried to simplify your cooking life by not asking you to weigh or measure every last ingredient, so your idea of a "medium" onion might not be mine! Calories can also vary when using different manufactured products, for example, tuna in oil.

* *Total fat* is given in grams of fat. Section One gives all the information you need about how much fat you should be eating, and what types. Sometimes you may think that a recipe looks as if it is very high in fat, but serving suggestions are given where appropriate and, if followed, will bring the total meal into a good balance of the macronutrients— i.e. protein, fat, and carbohydrate.

For example, the recipe for Marinated Herbed Mushrooms looks quite high in fat (albeit mostly unsaturated fat), but if you team it with plenty of crusty bread or rice cakes, the total fat content of the meal by percentage goes down, and the total carbohydrate content of the meal by percentage goes up, creating a balance in accordance with the guidelines in Section One.

Also bear in mind that it is saturated fat that most people should be limiting in their diets and that the seemingly high-fat recipes, in fact, contain high levels of

---

the protective unsaturated fats and low levels of saturates.

* *Saturated* fat per portion is given in grams. For more information on how much saturated fat you should be eating in your diet, see Section One.

* *Protein content* per portion is given as "low," "medium," or "high." "Low" means less than 10% of the calories in the dish are in the form of protein; "medium" 10–15 %; and "high" over 15%.

* *Carbohydrate content* per portion is given as "low," "medium," or "high." "Low" means less than 35% of the total calories in the dish are in the form of carbohydrate; "medium" denotes 35–50 %; and "high" over 50%.

Section One gives you plenty of information on balancing your protein and carbohydrate intake, but, in brief, if you choose a meal high in protein at lunch you will know that your evening meal can be medium or low in protein; if you choose a meal that is low in carbohydrate, you should ensure that at the next meal you choose a high-carbohydrate one.

In practice, many of the recipes are designed to be part of a meal, not the sole item, and the rest of the items to be served with the recipe will balance the whole meal up very well. For example, a high-protein, low-carbohydrate sauce might be served with high-carbohydrate,

low-protein pasta, or a high-protein, low-carbohydrate fish dish might be served with low-protein, high-carbohydrate potatoes.

* *Fiber content* per portion is given in grams. Section One explains how much fiber intake you should be aiming for per day.

SYMBOLS

♥	Anti-heart-/-circulatory disease, high blood cholesterol
☺	Anti-cancer
✦	Immune system boost
◥	Anti-arthritis
⋈	Bone strength
!	Dairy-free
※	Gluten-/wheat-free
✖	Yeast-free
V	Vegetarian
◐	Low-calorie
●	Quick
⬧	Budget

All recipes serve 2 unless otherwise stated.

Assume that recipes are low in salt and dietary cholesterol, providing no more than one-third of the daily recommended maximum of either, unless otherwise stated.

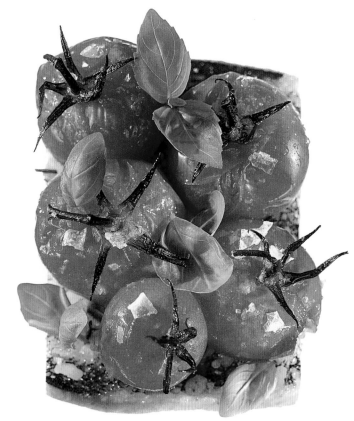

BAKED BABY TOMATOES WITH BASIL

Marinated shiitake mushrooms

Calories: 261	
Total fat: 22 g	
Saturated fat: 3.3 g	
Fiber: 1.6 g	
Protein: low	
Carbohydrate: low	
Vitamins: C	
Minerals: copper	

3 cups (225 g) shiitake mushrooms
4 tablespoons olive oil
2 garlic cloves, minced
*1 small hot red chili pepper, seeded
   and minced*
2 shallots, minced
1 tablespoon white wine vinegar
1 teaspoon balsamic vinegar
2 tablespoons chopped parsley
1 tablespoon chopped fresh tarragon
1 teaspoon chopped fresh thyme
1 teaspoon sea salt
black pepper

Tear the mushrooms into bite-sized pieces. Heat half the oil in a nonstick pan and stir-fry the garlic, chili pepper, and shallots for 1–2 minutes or until the shallots are softened. Add mushrooms and stir in remaining ingredients with rest of oil. Serve warm or cold.

Baked baby tomatoes with basil

Calories: 228	
Total fat: 13 g	
Saturated fat: 1 g	
Fiber: 1.6 g	
Protein: low	
Carbohydrate: medium	
Vitamins: C, E, carotenoids	

12 oz (325 g) baby tomatoes (about 12)
1 fresh, juicy garlic clove, chopped
2 tablespoons olive oil
1 teaspoon sea salt
black pepper
1 teaspoon fresh rosemary leaves
handful of fresh basil leaves, torn if large
two 1½-oz (40-g) slices of French bread

Preheat the oven to 400°F (200°C).
   Arrange the tomatoes in a small baking dish. Sprinkle with the garlic, half the olive oil, the salt, pepper, and rosemary. Bake for 25 minutes, or until the tomatoes are soft.
   Arrange on serving plates with the juices, topped with the remaining olive oil and basil leaves. Serve with the bread.

Smoked mackerel pâté salad

Calories: 571	
Total fat: 40 g	
Saturated fat: 8.5 g	
Fiber: 2.4 g	
Protein: high	
Carbohydrate: low	
Vitamins: B1, B2, niacin, B6, B12, D, E, folate	
Minerals: selenium, iodine, calcium, magnesium, potassium, iron, copper	

8 oz (225 g) hot-smoked mackerel fillets
⅔ cup (140 g) plain low-fat yogurt
2 tablespoons tomato paste
dash of Worcestershire sauce
*1 tablespoon chopped parsley, plus more
   parsley sprigs to serve*
black pepper
1 cup (50 g) mixed green salad leaves
hot whole-wheat toast

In a large bowl, flake the mackerel with a fork. Add the yogurt, tomato paste, Worcestershire sauce, chopped parsley, and black pepper to taste. Mix together well.
   Arrange the salad leaves and parsley sprigs on plates, spoon the pâté over, and serve with the toast.

Mushroom and red pepper skewers

🤍 ⏱ ✂ 🍷 🌿 V ⬇ 🗓

Calories: 111	
Total fat: 6.4 g	
Saturated fat: 1 g	
Fiber: 3.2 g	
Protein: medium	
Carbohydrate: medium	
Vitamins: A, niacin, B6, folate, C	
Minerals: copper	

2 medium red bell peppers, halved and seeded (about 7 oz / 200 g)
1 tablespoon olive oil
1 fresh, juicy garlic clove
1 teaspoon sea salt
½ small fresh hot red chili pepper, seeded and minced
2 teaspoons balsamic vinegar
8 small cremini mushrooms (about 4 oz / 115 g)

Preheat the broiler and place the pepper halves on the broiler pan, skin side up. Brush them with a little of the olive oil, and broil on both sides until softened but not charred.

Remove the pepper halves from the broiler and, when they have cooled a little, cut them into bite-sized squares.

Using a mortar and pestle, pound the garlic with the salt until well combined and creamy. Beat in the remaining olive oil, the chili pepper, and the vinegar.

Thread the pepper squares and mushrooms alternately on 2 skewers (soaked in water if wooden) and brush with the garlic-oil mixture.

Broil, about 5 inches from the heat, turning a few times and basting with remaining sauce, until the mushrooms are cooked through, about 5 minutes. Serve hot.

Turkish eggplant

🤍 ⏱ ✂ 🍷 🌀 V ⬇ 🗓

Calories: 186	
Total fat: 7.1 g	
Saturated fat: 1.1 g	
Fiber: 12 g	
Protein: medium	
Carbohydrate: high	
Vitamins: A, B1, niacin, B6, folate, C, E	
Minerals: potassium	

1 tablespoon olive oil, plus more for the baking sheet
1 large eggplant (about 9 oz / 250 g)
1 medium red bell pepper, seeded and finely diced
1 medium red onion, minced
1 teaspoon ground cumin
1 teaspoon sea salt
black pepper
2 medium tomatoes, halved
2 heaped tablespoons (25g) couscous
4 tablespoons boiling water

Preheat the oven to 350°F (180°C) and oil a baking sheet.

Halve the eggplant and scoop out all but the last ½ inch (1.5 cm) of flesh. Turn the shells upside down on the oiled baking sheet and bake for 25 minutes, or until the shells are just tender.

Meanwhile, heat the remaining olive oil in a nonstick frying pan. Chop the eggplant flesh and add it to the pan, along with the red bell pepper, onion, cumin, and seasoning. Stir-fry for a few minutes until soft.

Squeeze the tomato halves to remove the seeds, then chop them roughly and add to the eggplant mixture.

Soak the couscous in the boiling water until all water is absorbed, about 10–15 minutes. Stir the eggplant mixture into the couscous and adjust the seasoning.

Pile the mixture into the eggplant shells and return to the oven to warm through. Serve at once.

MUSHROOM AND RED PEPPER SKEWERS

All the following eight simple recipes are very versatile: they can be used as dips with crudités, bread, or crackers; they are good on toast or bruschetta; and some can be sandwich fillings. Some make excellent accompaniments to meat or fish or can be added by the spoonful to soups or casseroles to enrich them healthily. Individual usage notes appear below the recipes where appropriate.

Note regarding PORTIONS: It is hardly worth making these eight recipes in quantities to serve two, so each complete recipe will serve 4–6, depending on appetite.

They will all keep well, covered, in the refrigerator for several days. Filming the top with a little olive oil is a good way of preventing them from drying out and of prolonging their lives.

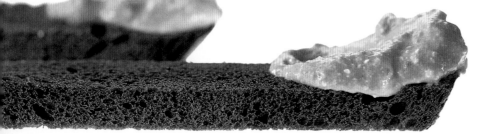

FETA AND PEPPER SPREAD

Feta and pepper spread

Calories: 179	
Total fat: 15 g	
Saturated fat: 7.5 g	
Fiber: 0.7 g	
Protein: high	
Carbohydrate: low	
Vitamins: niacin, B12, C, A, carotenoids	
Minerals: calcium	

1½ tablespoons olive oil
1 medium red bell pepper, seeded and chopped
½ fresh hot red chili pepper, seeded and chopped
dash of hot pepper sauce
2 cups (200 g) Greek feta cheese, roughly mashed

Heat the oil in a frying pan and stir-fry the bell pepper and chili pepper until soft but not browned. Add the hot sauce.

Place the cheese in a blender or food processor along with the contents of the pan and blend until you have a smooth spread. Serve at room temperature.

This is a lower-calorie, calcium-rich alternative to cheese, ideal for sandwiches.

Hummus

Calories: 186	
Total fat: 13 g	
Saturated fat: 1.8 g	
Fiber: 3.3 g	
Protein: medium	
Carbohydrate: low	

14-oz (400-g) can chickpeas, well drained and rinsed
juice of 1 lemon
3 tablespoons extra-virgin olive oil
1 tablespoon light tahini (sesame seed paste)
1 garlic clove, minced
1 teaspoon sea salt
black pepper or paprika to taste

Put all the ingredients in a blender or food processor and blend until you have a coarse-fine texture. Adjust the seasoning.

Canellini bean and basil spread

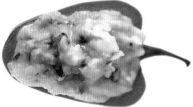

Calories: 86	
Total fat: 3 g	
Saturated fat: 0.5 g	
Fiber: 4.3 g	
Protein: high	
Carbohydrate: medium	

14-oz (400-g) can canellini beans, drained and rinsed
2 garlic cloves, minced
1 tablespoon olive oil
2 teaspoons lemon juice
1 teaspoon sea salt
black pepper
½ cup (25 g) fresh basil leaves

Place all the ingredients, except the basil, in a blender or food processor and blend until you have a texture that is still slightly rough—don't over-blend.

Add the basil leaves, fork them through, and blend for 2 more seconds. Check the seasoning.

You could use lima beans for a similar result.

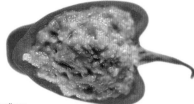

CANNELLINI BEAN AND BASIL SPREAD

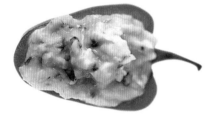

ANCHOÏADE

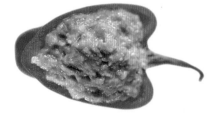

Anchoïade

Calories: 195	
Total fat: 20 g	
Saturated fat: 2.9 g	
Fiber: 0.4 g	
Protein: low	
Carbohydrate: low	
Vitamins: B12	

4 fresh, juicy garlic cloves, peeled
12 canned anchovy fillets in oil, drained
12 plump green olives, pitted
about 7 tablespoons (100 ml) extra-virgin olive oil
dash of white wine vinegar

Put the garlic, anchovies, and olives in a blender or food processor and blend until puréed. Pour in half the oil and the vinegar and blend again.

Add as much of the remaining oil as you need to make a paste or sauce, depending upon its intended use.

Good as a dip, as a quick sauce for a pasta first course, as a topping for crostini, or as a side sauce with eggs.

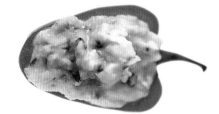

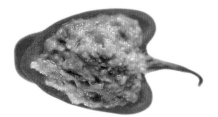

Rouille

Calories: 129	
Total fat: 8.5 g	
Saturated fat: 1.2 g	
Fiber: 0.3 g	
Protein: low	
Carbohydrate: low	

½ cup (50 g) slightly stale, rough white bread crumbs
7 tablespoons (100 ml) low-fat 2% milk
pinch of saffron
little hot water
2 fresh, juicy garlic cloves, minced
1–2 fresh hot red chili peppers, seeded and chopped
1 teaspoon sea salt
3 tablespoons olive oil

In a bowl, add the bread to the milk, stir, and let soak for a few minutes. In another small bowl, infuse the saffron in the hot water. Press out any surplus milk from the bread.

Using a mortar and pestle, pound together the garlic, chilies, and salt. Add the soaked bread and saffron infusion to the mortar and pound, gradually adding the olive oil to make a well blended purée.

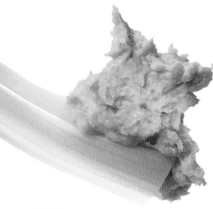

ROUILLE

Tzatziki

Calories: 96	
Total fat: 6.9 g	
Saturated fat: 3.9 g	
Fiber: 0.5 g	
Protein: high	
Carbohydrate: low	
Vitamins: B2	

½ English cucumber
4 fresh, juicy garlic cloves, minced
little sea salt
1¼ cups (300 g) Greek-style yogurt or thick, strained plain yogurt
2 teaspoons white wine vinegar

Peel the cucumber, then grate it on a medium-coarse grater. Wrap it in a clean dishtowel, and squeeze to remove as much moisture as you can.

Place the cucumber in a bowl, add the minced garlic and salt, and mix thoroughly. Add the yogurt and vinegar and mix well again. Serve chilled. **Ideal as a dip** or with grilled meats. More garlic can be added to taste.

Skordalia

Calories: 204	
Total fat: 18 g	
Saturated fat: 2.5 g	
Fiber: 3.3 g	
Protein: low	
Carbohydrate: low	
Vitamins: folate, C	

sea salt
2 cups (300 g) peeled and cubed celery root
1 cup (125 g) cubed boiling potatoes
3 fresh, juicy garlic cloves, minced
7 tablespoons (100 ml) skim or low-fat 2% milk
7 tablespoons (100 ml) olive oil

Bring a pan of lightly salted water to the boil. Add the celery root and potato and boil until tender, about 20 minutes. Drain until absolutely dry.

In a blender or food processor, blend the vegetables until smooth. Add the garlic and 1 teaspoon of salt and blend again.

Warm the milk and mix it with the olive oil, then pour this into the blender slowly, with the machine still running. The resulting purée should be smooth and silky. Adjust the seasoning.

Baba ganoush (eggplant purée)

Calories: 76	
Total fat: 5.7 g	
Saturated fat: 0.9 g	
Fiber: 4 g	
Protein: medium	
Carbohydrate: low	
Vitamins: folate	

2 large eggplants (about 1½ lb / 675 g in total)
1 teaspoon freshly ground cumin seed
1–2 garlic cloves, minced
1 tablespoon light tahini (sesame seed paste)
2 teaspoons olive oil
juice of ½ lemon
1 teaspoon sea salt
black pepper

Preheat the oven to 400°F (200°C). Prick the eggplants and bake them for 40 minutes or until soft right through.

Let them cool a little, then halve them and scoop their flesh into the bowl of a blender or food processor.

Add the remaining ingredients and blend until you have a purée. Check seasoning.

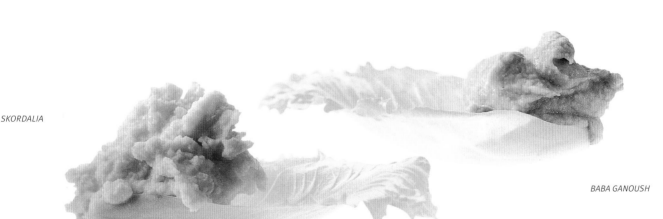

SKORDALIA

BABA GANOUSH

Cucumber and mint soup

❄ ⚔ V ⊙ ◐ ⬛

Calories: 131	
Total fat: 8.4 g	
Saturated fat: 1.8 g	
Fiber: 1.8 g	
Protein: medium	
Carbohydrate: low	
Vitamins: E	

½ English cucumber (about 9 oz / 250 g)
1 tablespoon sunflower oil
½ cup (125 g) minced onion
2 cups (450 ml) good-quality vegetable stock
handful of fresh mint
1 teaspoon sea salt
black pepper
2 tablespoons plain low-fat yogurt

Cut a ¾-inch (2-cm) chunk off the cucumber, chop it, and set this aside. Peel the remaining cucumber, halve it lengthwise, and scoop out the seeds. Chop the flesh.

Heat the oil in a saucepan and sauté the onion until soft. Stir in the cucumber. Add the stock, a couple of mint leaves, and seasoning. Simmer for 15 minutes.

Purée the soup in a blender or food processor, then leave to cool.

Chop the remaining mint leaves. Before serving, stir the chopped mint and yogurt into the soup and garnish with the reserved chopped cucumber.

Carrot and orange soup

♡ ⊙ ⚔ ❗ ❄ ⚔ V ⊙ ⬛

Calories: 109	
Total fat: 4.8 g	
Saturated fat: 0.7 g	
Fiber: 3.6 g	
Protein: low	
Carbohydrate: high	
Vitamins: B6, folate, A, C, E, carotenoids	

2 teaspoons corn or peanut oil
⅓ cup (75 g) minced onion
1 small garlic clove, minced
2 cups (225 g) peeled and chopped carrots
½ cup (125 g) good-quality canned crushed tomatoes (with their liquid)
juice of 1 large orange, freshly squeezed
½ teaspoon ground cumin
1 teaspoon sea salt
black pepper
1 cup (200 ml) good-quality vegetable stock
fresh green herbs, such as parsley, for garnish

Heat the oil in a saucepan and sauté the onion until soft, adding the garlic toward the end of cooking time.

Add the carrots and stir for a minute, then add the remaining ingredients except the herbs for garnish. Stir and bring to simmer (do not boil). Cook for 30 minutes or until the carrots and onions are tender.

Process the contents of the pan in a blender or food processor until smooth.

Adjust the seasoning, reheat, and serve garnished with the herbs.

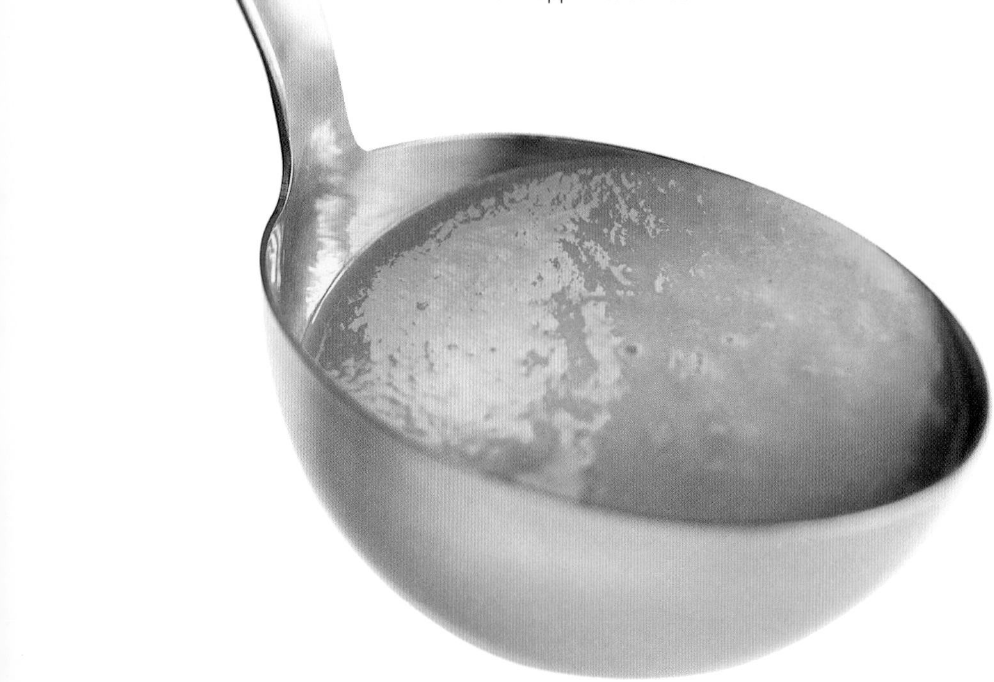

CARROT AND ORANGE SOUP

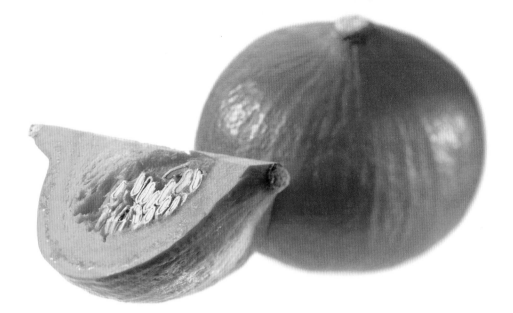

Squash, potato, and lima bean soup

🌿 ⊘ 🍴 ❤ ✂ ✕ ✅ ✚ ⚕

Calories: 252
Total fat: 6.5 g
Saturated fat: 0.8 g
Fiber: 7.3 g
Protein: medium
Carbohydrate: high
Vitamins: B1, niacin, B6, folate, A, carotenoids, C, E
Minerals: magnesium, potassium, iron, copper

1 tablespoon olive oil
⅓ cup (75 g) minced onion
3½ cups (400 g) orange-fleshed winter squash, such as onion squash or butternut, peeled and cut into cubes
1 medium potato, cubed
1 garlic clove, chopped
1 teaspoon fresh thyme leaves
1 teaspoon sea salt
black pepper
1¼ cups (300 ml) good vegetable or chicken stock
⅔ cup (100 g) frozen baby lima beans, thawed

Heat the oil in a nonstick frying pan and sauté the onion until soft.

Stir in the squash and potato. Add the rest of the ingredients except the lima beans, bring to a simmer, and cook for 30 minutes, adding the lima beans toward the end of cooking time.

When the vegetables are tender, purée the soup in a food processor. Adjust the seasoning. If the soup is too thick, add some water or stock and blend again. Reheat gently to serve.

Roasted tomato, garlic, and pepper soup

🌿 ⊘ 🍴 ❤ ✂ ✕ ✅ ✚ ⚕

Calories: 223
Total fat: 11 g
Saturated fat: 1.8 g
Fiber: 7.5 g
Protein: medium
Carbohydrate: medium
Vitamins: B1, niacin, B6, folate, A, carotenoids, C, E
Minerals: magnesium, potassium, iron

8 fresh, juicy garlic cloves, peeled
8 tasty ripe tomatoes (about 1 lb / 450 g) halved and seeded
1 medium red bell pepper, halved and seeded, then quartered
5 teaspoons olive oil
1 teaspoon sea salt
black pepper
1¾ cups (400 ml) good vegetable stock
⅔ cup (100 g) frozen baby lima beans, thawed
handful of fresh basil leaves

Preheat the oven to 400°F (200°C). Arrange the garlic, tomatoes, and red bell pepper quarters in a baking dish. Drizzle the oil over them, then sprinkle on the salt and pepper. Bake for 20–30 minutes, or until the vegetables are soft. (If the garlic looks like it is overcooking, remove it from the baking dish and set it aside.)

Transfer the contents of the baking dish to a blender or food processor. Add the stock and beans, and purée until smooth. Pour into a pan and reheat, adding the basil at the last minute. Adjust the seasoning.

Lentil and cilantro soup

Calories:	269
Total fat: 8.4 g
Saturated fat:
1.8 g
Fiber: 6.8 g
Protein: high
Carbohydrate:
medium
Vitamins:
B1, niacin, B6,
folate, A
Minerals:
magnesium,
potassium, iron,
copper,
selenium

1 tablespoon peanut oil
½ cup (125 g) minced red onion
1 garlic clove, minced
2¼ cups (500 ml) good-quality vegetable
*   stock*
½ cup (100 g) brown or
*   Puy lentils*
1 cup (100 g) peeled and chopped
*   carrot*
1 teaspoon sea salt
black pepper
2 tablespoons minced fresh cilantro
1 tablespoon plain low-fat yogurt

Heat the oil in a saucepan and sauté the onion until soft. Add the garlic and stir for a minute. Add the stock, lentils, and carrot and bring to a simmer.

Cook for 30 minutes or until the lentils are tender.

Add seasoning to taste, and stir in the cilantro and the yogurt.

Fava bean soup

Calories:	184
Total fat: 9.4 g
Saturated fat:
2.1 g
Fiber: 7.9 g
Protein: high
Carbohydrate:
low
Vitamins:
niacin, folate, C
Minerals: copper

1 tablespoon corn oil
½ cup (125 g) minced onion
1⅓ cups (225 g) shelled fresh (or
*   frozen), tender fava beans*
2¼ cup (500 ml) good-quality vegetable
*   stock*
1 tablespoon chopped fresh mint, plus
*   more leaves for garnish*
1 teaspoon sea salt
black pepper
2 tablespoons plain low-fat yogurt

Heat the oil in a pan and sauté the onion until soft and translucent.

Add the beans and stock and simmer for 20 minutes.

Add the chopped mint, salt, and pepper, and process in a blender or food processor until the soup is smooth. Adjust the seasoning, reheat, and stir in the yogurt before serving, garnished with mint leaves.

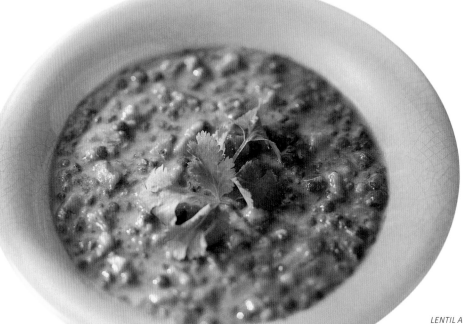

LENTIL AND CILANTRO SOUP

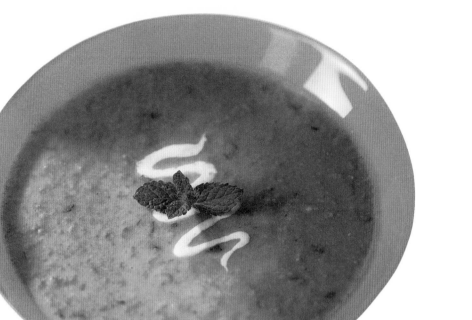

COUNTRY PEA SOUP

Country pea soup

🫀 ⏱ 🍃 🍷 ✳ 🏵 🅥 ➊ ◑ ⬧

Calories: 225	
Total fat: 7.4 g	
Saturated fat: 1 g	
Fiber: 8.8 g	
Protein: high	
Carbohydrate: high	
Vitamins: B1, niacin, B6, folate, C, E	
Minerals: magnesium, potassium, iron	

1 tablespoon sunflower oil
½ cup (125 g) minced onion
⅔ cup (100 g) chopped potato
2 cups (275 g) shelled fresh peas
1¼ cups (300 ml) good-quality chicken stock
1½ tablespoons chopped fresh mint
1 teaspoon sea salt
1 tablespoon plain yogurt

Heat the oil in a nonstick pan and sauté the onion until soft.

Add the potato, peas, stock, 1 tablespoon of the mint, and the salt, and simmer for 30 minutes.

Process the soup in a blender or food processor to a rough purée.

Reheat and serve with the remaining chopped mint and the yogurt stirred in at the last minute.

Spinach, parsley, and garlic soup

🫀 ⏱ 🍃 ✳ 🏵 🅥 ➊ ⬧

Calories: 150	
Total fat: 9 g	
Saturated fat: 2 g	
Fiber: 4.7 g	
Protein: high	
Carbohydrate: low	
Vitamins: B1, niacin, B6, folate, A, carotenoids, C, E	
Minerals: calcium, magnesium, potassium, iron	

1 tablespoon olive oil
½ cup (125 g) minced onion
3 garlic cloves, minced
1 cup (100 g) thinly sliced leek
6 tablespoons (50 g) chopped celery
2 cups (200 g) baby spinach leaves
large handful of chopped fresh flat-leaf parsley
1¾ cups (400 ml) vegetable stock
sea salt and black pepper
1 tablespoon freshly grated Parmesan cheese

Heat the oil in a saucepan and sauté the onion, garlic, leek, and celery until softened. Add the spinach, parsley, stock, and seasoning, then simmer for a few minutes.

Purée the soup using a blender or food processor. Adjust the seasoning.

Reheat and serve with the Parmesan sprinkled over.

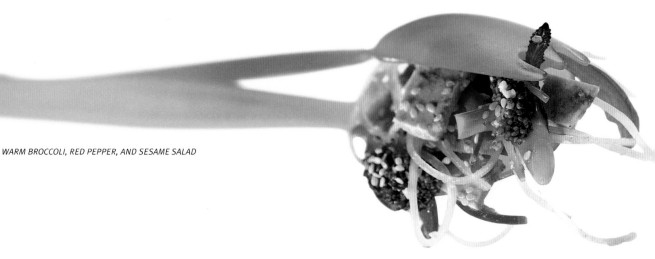

WARM BROCCOLI, RED PEPPER, AND SESAME SALAD

Warm broccoli, red pepper, and sesame salad

♥ ☺ ✤ ⧓ ♈ ✗✦ ⚒ Ⅴ ⊕ ◑ ⬙

Calories: 240	
Total fat: 18 g	
Saturated fat: 2.3 g	
Fiber: 4.5 g	
Protein: medium	
Carbohydrate: low	
Vitamins: niacin, B6, folate, A, carotenoids, C, E	
Minerals: potassium, iron	

2 tablespoons sesame oil
2 red bell peppers, seeded and thinly sliced (about 2 cups / 200 g)
1 cup (125 g) broccoli, cut into small florets
1 garlic clove, minced
½ cup (100 g) tofu, sliced
2 teaspoons light soy sauce
½ teaspoon Chinese chili sauce
1 teaspoon honey
½ teaspoon grated fresh ginger
1 teaspoon sesame seeds

Heat half the oil in a frying pan and stir-fry the bell peppers and broccoli for 5 minutes, until the peppers are tinged golden and slightly soft.

Add the rest of the ingredients, except the remaining oil and the sesame seeds, and stir-fry for a minute.

Turn onto serving plates, and serve warm with the sesame oil drizzled over and the sesame seeds sprinkled on top.

Chickpea salad with peppers and tomatoes

♥ ☺ ✤ ♈ ✗✦ ⚒ Ⅴ ⊕ ◑ ⬙

Calories: 300	
Total fat: 15 g	
Saturated fat: 2.1 g	
Fiber: 7.8 g	
Protein: medium	
Carbohydrate: medium	
Vitamins: niacin, B6, folate, A, carotenoids, C, E	
Minerals: magnesium, potassium, iron	

1½ cups (250 g) well-drained canned chickpeas
2 medium, ripe tomatoes
2 canned or bottled pimientos, well drained and thinly sliced
1 tablespoon each minced fresh mint, cilantro, and parsley
2 tablespoons extra-virgin olive oil
2 tablespoons lemon juice
pinch of sugar
pinch of mustard powder
1 teaspoon sea salt
black pepper
pinch of ground chili

Put the chickpeas in a serving bowl.
Halve the tomatoes and squeeze out the seeds, then roughly chop the flesh. Add to the bowl along with the pimientos and fresh herbs.

Combine the olive oil with the remaining ingredients and pour over the chickpea salad. Toss and serve.

Spiced lentils with mixed green vegetables

Calories: 272	
Total fat: 7.8 g	
Saturated fat: 1.5 g	
Fiber: 8.5 g	
Protein: high	
Carbohydrate: medium	
Vitamins: B1, B2, niacin, B6, folate, A, C, E	
Minerals: calcium, magnesium, potassium, iron, zinc, copper, selenium, iodine	

1 tablespoon peanut oil
1 medium onion, thinly sliced
1 teaspoon each freshly ground cumin seeds and ground ginger
1 small hot red chili, ground
1 teaspoon sea salt
black pepper
14-oz (400-g) can green lentils, well drained and rinsed
2 cups (200 g) mixed young, dark green, leafy vegetables (such as spinach, chard, or collard greens), torn
juice of ½ lemon
2 tablespoons plain low-fat yogurt

Heat the oil in a nonstick pan and sauté the onion until soft. Add the spices, chili pepper, and seasoning and sauté for 1 more minute.

Add the lentils and stir for a minute or two, then add the leaves and stir for another minute until slightly wilted.

Add the lemon juice and drizzle over the yogurt before serving slightly warm or at room temperature.

Brown rice and citrus salad

Calories: 545	
Total fat: 14 g	
Saturated fat: 1.9 g	
Fiber: 4.4 g	
Protein: high	
Carbohydrate: medium	
Vitamins: B1, niacin, B6, folate, C	
Minerals: magnesium potassium, copper	

1 large orange
2 cups (300 g) instant brown rice
3 ready-to-eat dried apricots, chopped
1 tablespoon chopped walnuts or brazils
7 oz (200 g) cooked lean chicken, sliced
1 tablespoon chopped fresh mint
1 tablespoon golden raisins
1 tablespoon walnut or sesame oil
1 teaspoon sea salt
black pepper

Peel and section the orange above a plate, retaining all the juices.

Place the rice, orange sections, apricots, nuts, chicken, mint, and raisins in a serving bowl.

Pour the retained orange juice into a bowl and combine with the walnut or sesame oil, salt, and pepper. Mix into the rice salad.

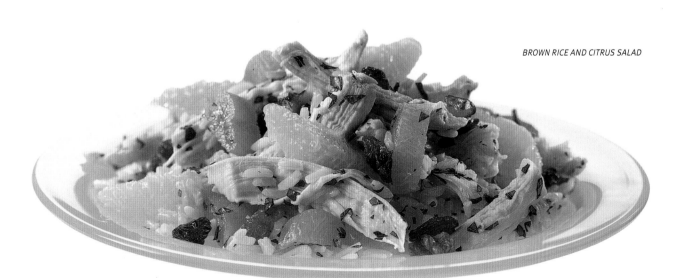

BROWN RICE AND CITRUS SALAD

Panzanella

♡ ⊙ ◐ ▼ V ↻ ⬗

Calories: 272	
Total fat: 15 g	
Saturated fat: 2.2 g	
Fiber: 4.6 g	
Protein: medium	
Carbohydrate: low	
Vitamins: B1, niacin, B6, folate, A, carotenoids, C, E	
Minerals: calcium, magnesium, iron, selenium	

2 slightly stale Italian crusty bread rolls
3 medium, ripe tomatoes
1½-inch (4-cm) piece of English cucumber, diced
1 small red onion (about 2¾ oz / 75 g), thinly sliced
6 black olives, pitted and halved
8 capers, well rinsed and drained
1 fresh, juicy garlic clove
1 teaspoon sea salt
5 teaspoons tomato juice or purée
2 tablespoons olive oil
1 tablespoon red wine vinegar
black pepper
1 tablespoon chopped fresh basil
1 tablespoon chopped fresh flat-leaf parsley

Tear the bread into small, bite-sized pieces and place these in a serving bowl.

Halve the tomatoes and gently squeeze out the seeds, retaining any juice that comes out. Roughly chop the tomatoes and add to the bread. Add the cucumber, onion, olives, and capers to the bowl.

Pound the garlic and salt with a pestle in a mortar until you have a paste. Gradually add the tomato juice or purée, olive oil, vinegar, and black pepper until you have a pourable dressing. Pour this over the salad. Add the chopped herbs and stir in lightly.

Leave for up to an hour for the bread to absorb the dressing.

A more substantial dish can be made with the addition of some diced mozzarella cheese or by grating some fresh Parmesan cheese over the top before serving.

This would add to the calcium, calorie, and increase fat content.

Thai salmon salad

♡ ⊙ ◐ ▦ ▼ ✕ ↻

Calories: 315	
Total fat: 17 g	
Saturated fat: 3 g	
Fiber: 2.9 g	
Protein: high	
Carbohydrate: low	
Vitamins: B1, B2, niacin, B6, B12, folate, A, C, D, E	
Minerals: magnesium, potassium, iron, copper, selenium, iodine	

2 medium salmon fillets (about 4 oz / 115 g each)
2 tablespoons teriyaki marinade
2-inch (5-cm) piece of English cucumber
1 medium zucchini
1 medium mango
1 cup (100 g) fresh beansprouts
2 teaspoons peanut oil
juice of 1 fresh, juicy lime
2 teaspoons fish sauce
1 garlic clove, minced
1 small hot green chili pepper, seeded and chopped
pinch of sugar
few fresh mint or cilantro leaves, chopped
2 lime wedges, to serve

Place the salmon fillets in a dish and pour the teriyaki marinade over them, coating well. Marinate, covered, in the refrigerator for at least 30 minutes, but no more than 1 hour.

Meanwhile, make the salad. Peel and stone the mango and slice into thin strips. Peel the cucumber and cut it into thin strips. Slice the zucchini similarly. Combine the cucumber, zucchini, mango, and beansprouts.

When the salmon is ready, preheat the broiler and put a heavy-duty baking sheet underneath it. Remove the salmon from the marinade and brush with a little of the oil. Put on the baking sheet under the broiler and cook for about 5 minutes, depending upon the thickness of the salmon. (If the baking sheet is good and hot, there's no need to turn the fish as the underside will cook nicely.)

While the salmon is cooking, mix together any remaining oil with the lime juice, fish sauce, garlic, chili, sugar, and herbs, and toss with the salad.

Arrange the salad on serving plates. Cut the cooked salmon into chunks and serve on the salad, with the lime wedges.

Seafood risotto with ginger

✳ 🔺 ◔ 🗓

Calories: 604	
Total fat: 22 g	
Saturated fat: 7.3 g	
Fiber: 2.5 g	
Protein: high	
Carbohydrate: high	
Vitamins: B1, B2, niacin, B6, folate, C	
Minerals: calcium, magnesium, potassium, iron, zinc, copper	

2¼ cups (500 ml) good-quality fish stock
1 teaspoon saffron threads
1 tablespoon (15 g) butter
1 tablespoon light olive oil
12 shallots, minced
½-inch (1.5-cm) piece of fresh ginger, grated
¾ cup (175 g) risotto rice
1 cup (150 g) crabmeat
2 tablespoons dry white wine or sherry
1 tablespoon chopped fresh cilantro
1 teaspoon sea salt
black pepper
1 tablespoon freshly grated Parmesan cheese

Heat the stock in a pan. Ladle a small amount into a small bowl when hot and infuse the saffron in this.

Heat the butter and oil in a nonstick frying pan and add the shallots. Sauté until soft, then add the ginger and stir for half a minute. Add the rice, stirring for a minute to coat all the grains.

Add one-quarter of the hot stock, stir, and bring to gentle simmer, stirring frequently. When all the stock is absorbed, add more and repeat, using the saffron stock toward the end of cooking.

When the rice is plump and cooked, but still with a moist and creamy texture, add the crabmeat, wine or sherry, cilantro, and seasoning. Serve at once, with the Parmesan cheese sprinkled over.

Salad of tuna, avocado, and tomato

🍃 ❢ ✳ 🔺 ◔ ◕

Calories: 409	
Total fat: 23 g	
Saturated fat: 4.3 g	
Fiber: 10 g	
Protein: high	
Carbohydrate: low	
Vitamins: B1, B2, niacin, B6, B12, folate, A, C, D, E	
Minerals: magnesium, potassium, iron, copper, selenium, iodine	

5 oz (150 g) fresh tuna steak
2 tablespoons extra-virgin olive oil
8 asparagus tips
2 beef tomatoes (about 9 oz / 250 g)
1 cup (170 g) cooked or canned canellini or lima beans, rinsed and drained
1 medium mild onion, thinly sliced
1 small ripe avocado (about 5 oz / 150 g)
1 tablespoon lemon juice
1 tablespoon chopped fresh oregano
1 teaspoon sea salt
black pepper

Brush the tuna steak with a little of the olive oil and broil or pan-fry for about 3 minutes on each side, until the outside is golden, but the inside is still pink.

Meanwhile, steam or microwave the asparagus tips until just tender. Halve the tomatoes and squeeze out the seeds, then chop roughly.

Arrange the beans on serving plates with the tomato, asparagus, and onion. Peel and slice the avocado and add to the plates.

Mix together the remaining oil, lemon juice, most of the oregano, and seasoning. Pour most of it over salad. Slice tuna and add. Drizzle remaining dressing over. Garnish with rest of oregano.

SALAD OF TUNA, AVOCADO, AND TOMATO

Shrimp, rice, and avocado

Calories: 619
Total fat: 28 g
Saturated fat: 8.3 g
Fiber: 6.4 g
Protein: high
Carbohydrate: medium
Vitamins: B1, B2, niacin, B6, B12, folate, A, C, E
Minerals: magnesium, potassium, iron, zinc, copper, selenium, iodine

⅔ cup (125 g) long-grain brown rice
1 tablespoon olive oil
½ cup (125 g) minced onion
1 garlic clove, minced
7 oz (200 g) large shrimp
1 red bell pepper, seeded and chopped
1 medium zucchini (about 3½ oz / 100 g), sliced across into rounds and then these halved
1 medium avocado
1 tablespoon lemon juice
2 tablespoons light sour cream
dash of hot pepper sauce
1 teaspoon sea salt
black pepper

Cook the rice in lightly salted boiling water until tender. Drain and reserve, keeping warm.

Heat the oil in a nonstick frying pan and sauté the onion until soft. Add the garlic, shrimp, bell pepper, and zucchini and stir-fry for a further 2–3 minutes.

Peel, pit, and chop the avocado and place in a bowl. Add the lemon juice, sour cream, pepper sauce, and seasoning, and mix roughly together.

Pour this mixture into the frying pan and stir into the shrimp, etc. Finally, fork in the cooked rice and serve still warm.

Seafood and tropical fruit salad

Calories: 251
Total fat: 5.2 g
Saturated fat: 0.8 g
Fiber: 4.1 g
Protein: high
Carbohydrate: medium
Vitamins: niacin, B6, B12, folate, A, C, E
Minerals: calcium, magnesium, potassium, iron, copper, selenium, iodine

10 large shrimp in shell (about 9 oz / 250 g)
2 teaspoons lime juice
1 teaspoon balsamic vinegar
2 teaspoons corn oil
1 teaspoon hot pepper sauce
pinch of sugar
1 pink grapefruit
1 small ripe mango
1 small banana
2 passion fruit

Make a charcoal fire or preheat the broiler. Peel the shrimp, but leave their tails on.

In a small bowl, mix together the lime juice, vinegar, oil, pepper sauce, and sugar. Brush the shrimp with a little of the mixture, then thread them on skewers (soaked in water if wooden). Grill or broil for 5 minutes, turning once.

Peel and slice the grapefruit and mango, adding any juice that runs out to the dressing and mixing well.

Arrange the sliced fruit on serving plates. Peel the banana, cut in half, then into long slices, and add to the plates. Spoon the flesh out of the passion fruit and add to the salad. Top with the shrimp and remaining dressing.
If using cooked shrimp, flash under the broiler for only 2–3 minutes.

SEAFOOD AND TROPICAL FRUIT SALAD

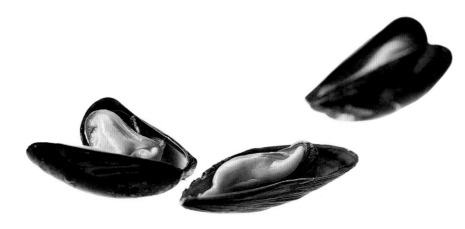

Tiger prawns with rice noodles

Calories: 413	
Total fat: 6.7 g	
Saturated fat: 1.3 g	
Fiber: 1.3 g	
Protein: high	
Carbohydrate: medium	
Vitamins: niacin, B6, B12, A, C, E	
Minerals: calcium, magnesium, potassium, iron, zinc, copper, selenium, iodine	

1 cup (about 100 g) chopped red bell pepper
1 fresh, juicy garlic clove, chopped
1 tablespoon chopped, flat-leaf parsley
juice of ½ lemon
1 tablespoon peanut oil
2 teaspoons Asian chili paste
1 teaspoon honey
12 raw tiger prawns (about 1 oz / 30 g each), tails left on
¾ cup (115 g) rice noodles
2 scallions, chopped
¾-inch (2-cm) piece of English cucumber, seeded and chopped
1 tablespoon coconut milk

In a shallow dish, mix the bell pepper, garlic, parsley, lemon juice, oil, chili paste, and honey. Place the prawns in the dish and toss to coat with the mixture. Marinate for up to 1 hour.

Cook the noodles and mix with the scallions and cucumber.

Preheat the broiler. Remove the prawns from the marinade, leaving some on each. Broil for 5 minutes or so, turning once or twice, until cooked.

While the prawns are cooking, heat the remaining marinade in a small pan with the coconut milk, stirring well. Serve the prawns with the sauce and noodles.

Scallops and mussels in the pan

Calories: 361	
Total fat: 9.5 g	
Saturated fat: 1.9 g	
Fiber: 3.3 g	
Protein: high	
Carbohydrate: medium	
Vitamins: B1, B2, niacin, B6, B12, folate, A, C, E	
Minerals: magnesium, potassium, iron, zinc, copper, selenium, iodine	

½ cup (125 g) minced red onion
1 small hot green chili pepper, seeded and chopped
1 medium yellow bell pepper, seeded and chopped
2 tomatoes, seeded and chopped
½-inch (1.5-cm) piece of fresh ginger, peeled and grated
large handful of fresh cilantro leaves
juice of 1 lime
1 teaspoon sea salt
black pepper
⅔ cup (150 ml) vegetable or fish stock
4½ tablespoons (50 g) couscous
1 tablespoon peanut oil
9 oz (250 g) sea scallops
1 garlic clove, chopped
7 oz (200 g) shelled mussels

In a bowl, combine the onion, chili pepper, bell pepper, tomatoes, ginger, cilantro, lime juice, salt and pepper. Leave for at least 30 minutes. Heat the stock and place in a bowl with the couscous. Set aside.

Heat the oil in a nonstick frying pan over a medium heat and cook the scallops (halved if very big) and garlic for a minute or two. Add the mussels and the onion mixture and stir for 2 minutes.

Fluff up the couscous and serve with the scallop and mussel dish.

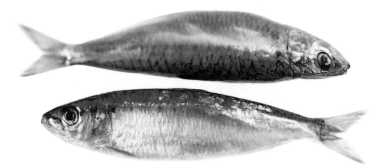

Speedy herbed swordfish

🐚 🐟 🦴 ❗ 🌿 ⚔ ⬇ ◕

Calories: 260	
Total fat: 13 g	
Saturated fat: 2.4 g	
Fiber: 0.4 g	
Protein: high	
Carbohydrate: low	
Vitamins: B1, B2, niacin, B6, B12	
Minerals: magnesium, potassium, selenium, iodine	

2 shallots, minced
1 tablespoon each chopped fresh flat-
    leaf parsley and dill
1 teaspoon fresh thyme leaves
juice of ½ lemon
1 tablespoon olive oil
2 medium swordfish steaks, each about
    6 oz (175g)
1 tablespoon fresh bread crumbs

In a blender or food processor, mix together the shallots, herbs, lemon juice, and olive oil. Place the fish steaks in a shallow dish and cover with the blended mixture. Marinate for 1–2 hours.

When you are ready to eat, preheat the broiler with a heavy-duty baking sheet underneath it. Remove the fish from the marinade (using a knife to return most of the marinade to the dish) and place on the hot baking sheet. Quickly mix the remaining marinade with the bread crumbs and use to coat the tops of the swordfish steaks. Broil for a few minutes until the steaks are cooked and the topping browned. (If the baking sheet is good and hot, the underside of the fish will cook nicely so there's no need to turn it.)

Sardines with red-currant glaze

🐚 🐟 🦴 ❗ 🌿 ⚔ ⬇ ◕ 🍶

Calories: 230	
Total fat: 11 g	
Saturated fat: 3.2 g	
Fiber: negligible	
Protein: high	
Carbohydrate: low	
Vitamins: B2, niacin, B6, B12, D	
Minerals: selenium, iodine	

8 fresh sardines (about 2¾ oz / 75 g
    each), cleaned and heads removed
1 teaspoon sea salt
black pepper
1 tablespoon chopped fresh parsley
lemon wedges, to serve
for the red-currant glaze:
1 tablespoon red-currant jelly
grated zest of 1 lemon
1 tablespoon medium-dry sherry

First make the red-currant glaze: in a small bowl, mix together the red-currant jelly, lemon zest, and sherry.

Make several diagonal cuts across the flesh of each sardine and season with the salt and pepper. Brush the red-currant glaze over the sardines and in the cavities.

Preheat the broiler, then broil the sardines for about 8 minutes, turning them once, until they are cooked through. Garnish with the parsley and serve immediately with the lemon wedges.

You could use cranberry jelly for the sauce, for a slightly more piquant change.

Spanish-style baked trout with chard

Calories: 471
Total fat: 19 g
Saturated fat: 3 g
Fiber: 5.4 g
Protein: high
Carbohydrate: low
Vitamins: B1, B2, niacin, B6, B12, folate, A, carotenoids, D, C, E
Minerals: magnesium, potassium, iron, copper, selenium, iodine

2 teaspoons olive oil
2 cups (225 g) potatoes, sliced and parboiled
1 beef tomato, sliced
1 large or 2 small trout, sea bass, or mackerel (total weight about 1 lb / 450 g), cleaned
4 black olives, pitted and halved
1 tablespoon pine nuts
1 tablespoon golden raisins
9 oz (250 g) tender Swiss chard leaves or spinach, cooked and thoroughly drained (about 1½ cups)
1 teaspoon sea salt
black pepper
3 tablespoons dry white wine
juice of ½ lemon

Preheat the oven to 400°F (200°C), and use the oil to brush a baking dish that will hold the fish snugly.

Cover the bottom of the dish with the sliced potatoes, then cover with the tomatoes. Lay the fish on top.

Scatter the olives, pine nuts, raisins, and Swiss chard around the fish, season with salt and pepper, and drizzle the white wine and lemon juice over.

Bake, uncovered, for 30 minutes, or until the fish is tender.

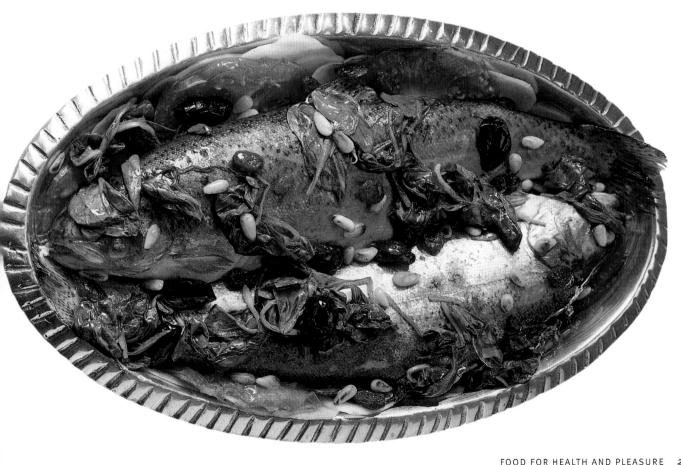

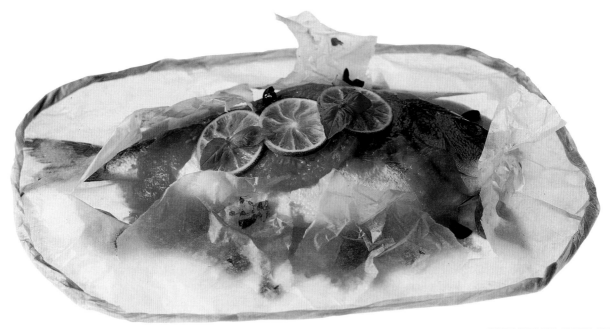

PARCEL OF TILAPIA, TOMATO, AND OLIVES

Parcels of tilapia, tomato, and olives

Calories: 225

Total fat: 8.3 g

Saturated fat: 1.3 g

Fiber: 2 g

Protein: high

Carbohydrate: low

Vitamins: niacin, B6, B12, C, E

Minerals: calcium, potassium, iron, copper, selenium, iodine

1 teaspoon olive oil

2 tilapia fish or small trout, cleaned

½ recipe-quantity of Tomato Sauce (see page 247)

1 medium tomato, sliced

1 fresh, juicy lime, sliced

6 pitted black olives, roughly chopped

2 tablespoons chopped fresh basil

Preheat the oven to 350°F (180°C). Brush two large sheets of foil with the oil and place the fish in the center of each. Spoon the sauce over each fish, then arrange the tomato and lime slices on top. Sprinkle the olives and basil over and seal up the foil tightly, though leaving plenty of air in the parcels.

Cook the parcels on a baking sheet in the oven for about 30 minutes.

Serve the fish parcels still closed so that when they are opened at the table their full aroma will hit!

Seared tuna with lemon grass

Calories: 216

Total fat: 6.8 g

Saturated fat: 1.7 g

Fiber: 0.3 g

Protein: high

Carbohydrate: low

Vitamins: B1, niacin, B6, B12, D

Minerals: magnesium, potassium, iron, copper, selenium, iodine

2 tuna steaks, each about 5 oz (150 g)

2 tablespoons teriyaki marinade

1 tablespoon black bean sauce

1 teaspoon Chinese chili sauce

1 stalk of lemon grass, crushed with a rolling pin to release aroma and chopped

1 tablespoon chopped fresh cilantro

Place the tuna steaks in a shallow dish. Mix together the remaining ingredients and spoon over the steaks. Marinate for 1 hour or so.

Remove the tuna from the marinade. Preheat the broiler and, when it is very hot, cook the steaks for about 4 minutes, turning once (depending upon the thickness of the steaks, which should be served rare).

If you can't get teriyaki marinade just use soy sauce.

Salmon and broccoli risotto

Calories: 634	
Total fat: 25 g	
Saturated fat: 5 g	
Fiber: 3.3 g	
Protein: high	
Carbohydrate: medium	
Vitamins: B1, B2, niacin, B12, folate, C, E	
Minerals: calcium, magnesium, potassium, iron, zinc, copper, selenium, iodine	

2 tablespoons light olive oil
1 medium onion, minced
1 garlic clove, minced
2/3 cup (140 g) risotto rice
3 cups (700 ml) good-quality fish stock, warmed
1½ cups (150 g) small broccoli florets
1¾ oz (50 g) smoked salmon, cut into small pieces
5 oz (150 g) salmon fillet, cubed
1 teaspoon sea salt
black pepper
1 tablespoon freshly grated Parmesan cheese

Heat the oil in a large nonstick frying pan and sauté the onion until soft. Add the garlic and rice, and stir for a minute or two to coat the rice well.

Add the fish stock, one-quarter of the volume at a time, stirring to absorb each quantity before adding more.

Meanwhile, blanch the broccoli for 1 minute in boiling water. About 5 minutes before the end of cooking time (when the rice is tender, moist, and creamy), add the smoked and fresh salmon, the broccoli, and seasoning.

Serve the risotto topped with the cheese.

Herring fillets with ginger and cilantro

Calories: 383	
Total fat: 26 g	
Saturated fat: 6.6 g	
Fiber: negligible	
Protein: high	
Carbohydrate: low	
Vitamins: B2, niacin, B6, B12, D	
Minerals: potassium, iron, copper, selenium, iodine	

4 herring fillets, each about 3½ oz (100 g)
2 teaspoons soy sauce
2 teaspoons lemon juice
1 teaspoon grated fresh ginger
little sea salt to taste
black pepper
2 teaspoons chopped fresh cilantro

Arrange the herring fillets on a plate and place this in a Chinese bamboo steamer (if you have one; otherwise use a conventional steamer). Sprinkle the fillets with the soy sauce, lemon juice, ginger, salt, and pepper. Steam for a few minutes over boiling water until cooked through.

Serve the fillets with the juices poured over, and garnished with the cilantro and a small amount of ground sea salt if you wish.

HERRING FILLETS WITH GINGER AND CILANTRO

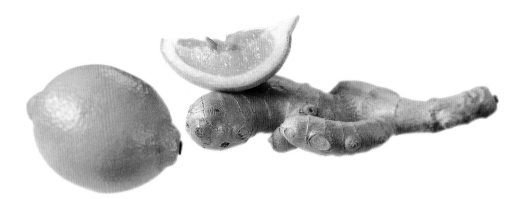

Chicken cacciatore

🫀 ☺ 🐟 🍷 🌿 🌾 ◐ 🍃 🍶

Calories: 214	
Total fat: 12 g	
Saturated fat: 2.4 g	
Fiber: 1 g	
Protein: high	
Carbohydrate: low	
Vitamins: niacin, B6, C, E	
Minerals: copper	

1 tablespoon olive oil
4 chicken thighs, part-boned and
   skinned
1 fresh, juicy garlic clove, crushed
few sprigs of fresh thyme, tarragon, and
   oregano, or 1 teaspoon each of the
   dried herb
7 tablespoons (100 ml) dry white wine
⅔ cup (200 g) canned crushed tomatoes
black pepper
6 pitted black olives, halved
6 capers, rinsed and drained

Heat the oil in a Dutch oven or heavy frying pan with a lid and brown the chicken on all sides.

Turn the heat down a little and add the garlic and herbs along with the wine. Stir for a minute or two. Add the tomatoes with their liquid and some pepper. Bring to a simmer and cook, covered, for 20 minutes or until the chicken is tender.

Add the olives and capers, stir well, and cook for a further 2–3 minutes, uncovered, until you have just a little thick sauce left. Adjust the seasoning and add a little sea salt if necessary.

Lemon chicken

🫀 ☺ 🐟 🍶 🍷 🌿 🥜 ◐ 🍃 🍶

Calories: 189	
Total fat: 6.9 g	
Saturated fat: 1.2 g	
Fiber: negligible	
Protein: high	
Carbohydrate: low	
Vitamins: niacin, B6	

2 medium skinless, boneless chicken
   breast halves
1 garlic clove
1 teaspoon sea salt
1 teaspoon grated lemon zest
juice of 1 juicy lemon
¾-inch (2-cm) piece of fresh ginger,
   peeled and grated
1 tablespoon toasted sesame or
   peanut oil

Put the chicken pieces in a shallow dish. Mash together the garlic and salt until you have a purée. Mix this with the lemon zest and juice, the ginger, and the oil and coat the chicken pieces. Marinate for 30 minutes, if possible.

Either bake the chicken in the dish in the oven preheated to 350°F (180°C) for 25 minutes, or, if you prefer, broil the pieces, about 5 inches (12.5 cm) from the heat. Alternatively, pan-fry them in a heavy nonstick skillet.

Spiced chicken and greens

Calories: 314	
Total fat: 13 g	
Saturated fat: 13 g	
Fiber: 3.9 g	
Protein: high	
Carbohydrate: low	
Vitamins: B1, B2, niacin, B6, folate, A, carotenoids, C, E	
Minerals: calcium, magnesium, potassium, iron, selenium	

1¼ cups (200 g) tender young green leaves of choice (bok choy, romaine, Napa cabbage, spinach, tender young chard, or a mixture)

2 medium skinless, boneless chicken breast halves

1 tablespoon peanut oil

½ cup (125 g) minced onion

2 garlic cloves, minced

1 fresh hot green chili pepper, seeded and minced

½ teaspoon each ground turmeric and cumin

2 large tomatoes (about 5 oz / 150 g in total), halved and seeded

7 tablespoons (100 g) plain whole-milk yogurt

about 3 tablespoons chicken stock

sea salt and black pepper

Chop the green leaves into thin slices. Slice each chicken breast across the grain into 4 pieces.

Heat the oil in a nonstick frying pan and sauté the onion until soft. Move the onion to one side and add the chicken pieces. Cook until they have turned slightly golden—if the onion is also slightly golden by now that is fine.

Reduce the heat and add the garlic, chili and spices, stirring everything in well for a minute or two. Chop the tomatoes and add to the pan, then cook for a further 2 minutes. Add the greens and stir for 2 more minutes, then spoon in the yogurt and bring to a simmer.

Using the chicken stock, thin the sauce down a little. Adjust the seasoning with a little sea salt and black pepper.

Avocado and turkey tortillas

Calories: 534	
Total fat: 13 g	
Saturated fat: 2.9 g	
Fiber: 5.9 g	
Protein: high	
Carbohydrate: medium	
Vitamins: B₁, B₂, niacin, B6, folate, E	
Minerals: magnesium, potassium, iron, copper, selenium	

4 wheat-flour tortillas
1 small avocado
2 teaspoons lime juice
sea salt and black pepper
7 oz (200 g) smoked turkey, sliced
for the salsa:
2 medium tomatoes, seeded and
   chopped
2 scallions, chopped
¾-inch (2-cm) piece of English
   cucumber, seeded and chopped
⅓ cup (50 g) cooked or canned black-
   eyed peas
1 tablespoon lime juice
1 tablespoon chopped fresh cilantro
1 teaspoon chili sauce

First make the salsa: In a bowl, combine all the ingredients and set aside for an hour or so, if you can.

When you are ready to serve, heat the tortillas in the oven preheated to 350°F (180°C), wrapped in foil or parchment paper.

Peel and pit the avocado and mash it with seasoning and lime juice. Fill each warm tortilla with some smoked turkey, salsa, and avocado.

You could use smoked chicken instead of the turkey.

Thai guinea fowl, cashew, and pineapple

Calories: 416	
Total fat: 28 g	
Saturated fat: 6.1 g	
Fiber: 2.2 g	
Protein: high	
Carbohydrate: low	
Vitamins: B₁, folate, C	
Minerals: magnesium, iron, copper	

2 guinea fowl breasts, skinned
1 tablespoon toasted sesame oil
1 heaped teaspoon each ground
   coriander, cumin, and fresh minced
   hot chili pepper
pinch of ground galangal or ginger
4 scallions, minced
juice of 1 lime
1 garlic clove, minced
1 tablespoon peanut oil
4 baby corn, blanched
1 tablespoon Thai fish sauce
2 tablespoons coconut milk
¾-inch (2-cm) piece of English
   cucumber, diced
3 rings of fresh pineapple, diced
⅓ cup (40 g) shelled roasted
   cashew nuts

Cut the guinea fowl breasts across the grain into bite-sized strips and place them in a shallow dish. Mix together the sesame oil, spices, scallions, lime juice, and garlic and coat the chicken with this. Set aside for 30 minutes if you can.

Heat the peanut oil in a nonstick frying pan and add the chicken and its marinade. Stir-fry for a few minutes.

Add the corn and Thai fish sauce and stir for a few more minutes. Add the coconut milk, cucumber, pineapple, and cashews and stir again for a minute or two. Serve immediately.

You can use skinless, boneless chicken or turkey breasts in this recipe, if you prefer. Thai fish sauce is now available from many supermarkets, healthfood stores, and Asian markets; if you can't find any, use good-quality soy sauce.

AVOCADO AND TURKEY TORTILLAS

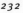

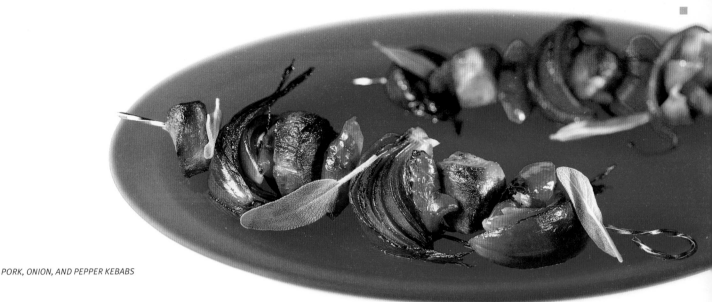

PORK, ONION, AND PEPPER KEBABS

Pork, onion, and pepper kebabs

Calories: 275
Total fat: 11 g
Saturated fat: 2.5 g
Fiber: 3.8 g
Protein: high
Carbohydrate: low
Vitamins: B1, B2, niacin, B6, B12, folate, A, carotenoids, C, E
Minerals: magnesium, potassium, zinc, copper, selenium

7 oz (200 g) pork tenderloin
1 garlic clove, minced
juice of 1 lemon
1 teaspoon sea salt
black pepper
1 red bell pepper, seeded and cut into squares
1 red onion, cut into wedges
2 teaspoons olive oil
½ recipe-quantity Tomato Sauce (see page 247)
1 teaspoon chopped fresh sage

Put the pork in a shallow dish. In a small bowl, roughly blend the garlic into the lemon juice along with the salt and pepper. Tip this mixture over the pork. Cover and set aside for an hour.

When ready to cook, preheat the broiler. Thread the pork pieces onto 2 kebab sticks, alternating them with pieces of red bell pepper and red onion. Brush with olive oil and broil for 8 minutes, turning occasionally.

Heat the tomato sauce and stir in the sage. Serve the kebabs with the sauce. **An alternative sauce** would be Tzatziki (see page 214).

Pork tenderloin in Chinese sauce

Calories: 237
Total fat: 12.4 g
Saturated fat: 2.6 g
Fiber: 0.6 g
Protein: high
Carbohydrate: low
Vitamins: B1, B2, niacin, B6, B12
Minerals: zinc

200 g (7 oz) pork tenderloin, cut into thin rounds
1 fresh, juicy garlic clove, crushed
¾-inch (2-cm) piece peeled fresh ginger
2 teaspoons clear honey
2 teaspoons light soy sauce
1 tablespoon dry sherry
1 tablespoon toasted sesame oil
2 teaspoons Chinese yellow bean sauce
2 teaspoons toasted sesame seeds

Preheat the oven to 400°F (200°C).

Place the slices of pork in a shallow baking dish that is just big enough to hold them in a single layer, overlapping them slightly.

Combine all the remaining ingredients, except the sesame seeds, in a small saucepan and heat through, stirring to mix well. Pour over the pork slices to coat evenly.

Cover the dish loosely with a piece of foil and bake for 20 minutes or until tender, basting two or three times.

Sprinkle with the toasted sesame seeds and serve.

Turkish lamb stew

Calories: 407

Total fat: 13 g

Saturated fat: 4.7 g

Fiber: 12 g

Protein: high

Carbohydrate: medium

Vitamins: B1, B2, niacin, B6, B12, folate, C, E

Minerals: magnesium, potassium, iron, zinc, copper

1 tablespoon olive oil

8 oz (225 g) lean boneless leg of lamb, cut into cubes

1 large onion, thinly sliced

1 garlic clove, minced

1¼ cups (175 g) peeled and cubed potato

4 canned tomatoes, drained

1 medium green bell pepper, seeded and sliced

⅔ cup (100 g) cooked or canned chickpeas

1 small eggplant, trimmed and cut into chunks

about 1 cup (200 ml) good-quality beef stock

black pepper

1 tablespoon red wine vinegar

1 teaspoon each chopped fresh thyme, rosemary, and oregano

4 black olives, pitted and halved

little sea salt

Heat the oil in a Dutch oven or heavy-based saucepan and brown the lamb over a fairly high heat.

Turn the heat down a little, add the onion and garlic, and sauté for a few minutes until soft.

Add the remaining ingredients, except the olives and sea salt. Stir well to mix, then bring to a simmer, and cook, covered, for 1–1½ hours, or until everything is tender.

Add the olives and sea salt and simmer, uncovered, for a further 15 minutes.

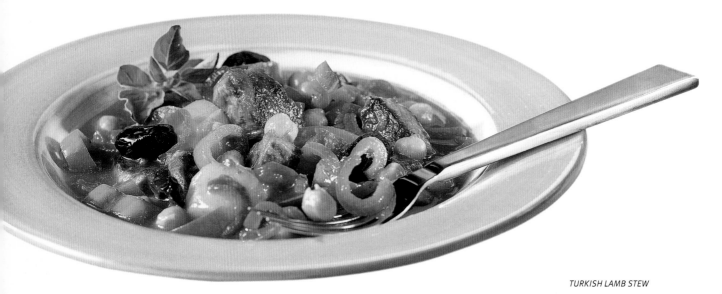

TURKISH LAMB STEW

Steak and spinach stir-fry

Calories: 482	
Total fat: 18 g	
Saturated fat: 5.3 g	
Fiber: 6.3 g	
Protein: high	
Carbohydrate: medium	
Vitamins: B1, B2, niacin, B6, B12, folate, A, carotenoids, C, E	
Minerals: calcium, magnesium, potassium, iron, zinc, copper	

7 oz (200 g) boneless sirloin steak
1 tablespoon Chinese black bean sauce
2 teaspoons red wine vinegar
2 teaspoons light soy sauce
2 teaspoons oyster sauce
1 teaspoon Chinese chili sauce
²⁄₃ cup (100 g) Chinese egg-thread noodles
1 tablespoon peanut oil
½ cup (40 g) small broccoli florets
1 red bell pepper, seeded and thinly sliced
4 scallions, halved lengthwise
1 cup (100 g) fresh beansprouts
1½ cups (150 g) fresh baby spinach leaves

Slice the beef across the grain into thin, bite-sized strips and place in a shallow dish. Mix together the black bean sauce, vinegar, soy sauce, oyster sauce, and chili sauce, and pour evenly over the beef. Set aside, covered, for an hour if you can.

Cook the noodles according to package directions, drain, and leave in their pan with a little of the cooking liquid to keep them warm and moist.

Heat the oil in a wok or large nonstick frying pan. Remove the beef from the marinade (some will cling to the pieces of beef, but that is fine) and add it to the wok. Stir-fry for 2 minutes.

Remove the beef from the wok and add the broccoli and red bell pepper. Stir-fry for 3 minutes.

Add the scallions, beansprouts, and spinach, and return the beef to the wok. Stir-fry again for 1 minute. Add the marinade and stir-fry some more.

If the mixture is too dry for you, add a little water or beef stock.

Toss the drained noodles into the wok to warm through and combine. Serve immediately.

Pasta with chicken livers

Calories: 477	
Total fat: 15 g	
Saturated fat: 5.6 g	
Fiber: 2.3 g	
Protein: high	
Carbohydrate: medium	
Vitamins: B1, B2, niacin, B6, B12, folate, A, C	
Minerals: magnesium, iron, zinc, copper	

5 oz (150 g) tagliatelle
little sea salt
1 tablespoon light olive oil
7 oz (200 g) chicken livers, trimmed and halved
2 garlic cloves, minced
7 tablespoons (100 ml) good-quality chicken stock
2 tablespoons light sour cream
juice of ½ lemon
black pepper
2 teaspoons chopped fresh parsley

Cook the tagliatelle in plenty of lightly salted boiling water until just tender. Drain well.

Meanwhile, heat the oil in a nonstick frying pan and, when very hot, add the chicken livers, stirring gently. When the outsides are browned but the insides still pink, remove with a slotted spoon and drain on some paper towels. Keep warm.

Add the garlic to the pan and stir for a minute or two, but don't let it burn.

Add the stock and bring to a simmer. Cook for a few minutes until the stock is reduced by about half, breaking the garlic up well with the back of a spoon to distribute.

Add the rest of the ingredients and return the livers to the pan. Stir to mix and cook gently for a minute or two. Adjust the seasoning if necessary. Serve the pasta with the chicken livers as soon as it is cooked and drained.

Pasta with olives and sardines

♡ ◷ ✦ ⬚ ⬚ ⬚ ✕ ◑ ⬚

Calories: 541	
Total fat: 23 g	
Saturated fat: 5.4 g	
Fiber: 2.7 g	
Protein: high	
Carbohydrate: medium	
Vitamins: niacin, B6, B12, D	
Minerals: calcium, magnesium, iron, copper, selenium, iodine	

about 1¼ cups (150 g) penne pasta
*1 teaspoon sea salt, plus more for
    cooking the pasta*
6 fresh sardines
2 tablespoons extra-virgin olive oil
6 black olives, pitted and chopped
juice of ½ lemon
*1 tablespoon chopped fresh flat-leaf
    parsley*
black pepper
*1 tablespoon freshly grated Parmesan
    cheese*

Cook the pasta in plenty of lightly salted boiling water until just tender.

Meanwhile, broil the sardines, turning once, until cooked (about 3 minutes per side). Carefully remove the central bone and any other bones you can see and chop the flesh into bite-sized pieces.

When the pasta is cooked, drain well and return to the pan. Add the sardines, olive oil, olives, lemon juice, parsley, and seasoning to the pasta. Stir well and heat through for 2 minutes over a low heat.

Serve with the Parmesan cheese sprinkled over.

Pasta with broccoli and anchovies

♡ ◷ ✦ ⬚ ⬚ ⵏ ✕ ◑ ⬚

Calories: 505	
Total fat: 20 g	
Saturated fat: 3 g	
Fiber: 6.6 g	
Protein: medium	
Carbohydrate: medium	
Vitamins: B1, niacin, B6, B12, folate, A, carotenoids, C, E	
Minerals: calcium, magnesium, potassium, iron, copper, selenium	

*about 1¼ cups (150 g) pasta shells or
    fusilli*
3 cups (300 g) small broccoli florets
1 fresh, juicy garlic clove
1 teaspoon sea salt
*1 small hot red chili pepper, seeded and
    chopped*
*4 large canned anchovies in oil, drained
    (reserving the oil) and chopped*
juice of ½ lemon
2 tablespoons extra-virgin olive oil
2 tablespoons slightly stale bread crumbs

Cook the pasta in plenty of lightly salted boiling water until just tender.

Meanwhile, blanch the broccoli for 1 minute, then drain.

Using a mortar and pestle, mash together the garlic, salt, and chili into a paste. Blend 2 teaspoons of the reserved oil from the anchovies and the lemon juice into this.

Heat 1 tablespoon of the olive oil in a nonstick frying pan and add the bread crumbs. Cook, stirring occasionally, until the crumbs are golden. Remove the crumbs and reserve.

Add the remaining oil to the pan and stir-fry the broccoli for a few minutes. Add the garlic mixture and stir for another minute, then add the anchovies. Lightly toss the broccoli mixture with the drained pasta and serve sprinkled with the bread crumbs.

PASTA WITH OLIVES AND SARDINES

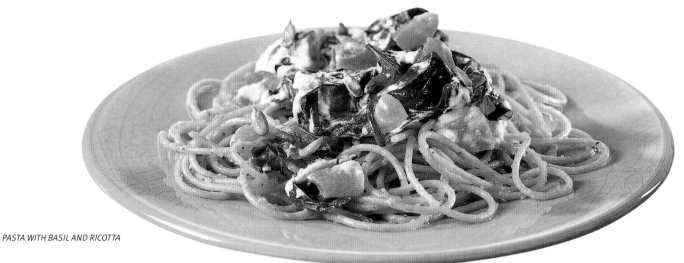

PASTA WITH BASIL AND RICOTTA

Pasta with milanese sauce

♥ ◐ ⬛ ❢ ⬥ ◉ ◕

Calories: 445

Total fat: 12 g

Saturated fat: 1.9 g

Fiber: 5.8 g

Protein: high

Carbohydrate: high

Vitamins: B1, B2, niacin, B6, folate, A, C, E

Minerals: magnesium, potassium, iron, zinc, copper

5 oz (150 g) spinach tagliatelle
salt
1 tablespoon olive oil
¾ cup (100 g) chopped tender celery
1 red bell pepper, seeded and chopped
1 garlic clove, minced
1½ cups (100 g) chopped fresh mixed
   mushrooms of choice (such as
   cremini, oyster, porcini)
½ cup (75 g) chopped extra-lean ham
½ recipe-quantity Tomato Sauce
   (see page 247)
1 tablespoon chopped flat-leaf parsley

Cook the pasta in plenty of lightly salted boiling water until just tender. Drain well.

Meanwhile, heat the oil in a nonstick frying pan and stir-fry the celery, bell pepper, and garlic for a few minutes until softened.

Add the mushrooms, ham, and tomato sauce. Stir well and leave to simmer for 20 minutes, adding a little chicken stock, water, or white wine if the sauce gets too thick.

Serve the sauce on top of the tagliatelle with parsley sprinkled over.

Pasta with basil and ricotta

♥ ◐ ⬛ ⬛ ⋈ V ◕ 🗋

Calories: 601

Total fat: 31 g

Saturated fat: 6.3 g

Fiber: 9.5 g

Protein: medium

Carbohydrate: medium

Vitamins: B1, B2, niacin, B6, folate, A, E

Minerals: calcium, magnesium, potassium, iron, zinc, copper

5 oz (150 g) whole-wheat spaghetti
1 teaspoon sea salt, plus more for
   cooking the pasta
1 fresh, juicy garlic clove
2 tablespoons pine nuts
⅓ cup (15 g) of fresh basil leaves
2 tablespoons extra-virgin olive oil
1 tablespoon sunflower seeds
5 tablespoons (40 g) chopped ready-to-
   eat dried apricots
1½ oz (40 g) young spinach or sorrel
   leaves (about ½ cup)
6½ tablespoons (100 g) ricotta cheese

Boil the pasta in a large pan of lightly salted water until just tender and then drain.

Meanwhile, using a mortar and pestle, crush the garlic with the sea salt until well combined. Add the pine nuts and pound again. Add most of the basil and crush, then add the olive oil to make a rich sauce.

Toss the warm, drained pasta with the basil sauce and all the remaining ingredients.

Serve garnished with the remaining basil leaves.

Potato and Mediterranean vegetable bake

Calories: 463	
Total fat: 18 g	
Saturated fat: 2.6 g	
Fiber: 13 g	
Protein: medium	
Carbohydrate: high	
Vitamins: B1, niacin, B6, folate, C	
Minerals: magnesium, potassium, iron, copper	

2 medium boiling potatoes (about 12 oz / 350 g in total)
1 teaspoon sea salt, plus more for cooking the potatoes
2 zucchini (about 7 oz / 200 g in total)
2 medium red bell peppers (about 9 oz / 250 g in total)
1 large eggplant (about 10 oz / 275 g)
5 teaspoons olive oil
1 recipe-quantity Tomato Sauce (see page 247)
black pepper
2 teaspoons chopped fresh oregano leaves

Preheat the oven to 400°F (200°C).

Peel the potatoes and cut them into ¼-inch (6-mm) slices, then parboil these in lightly salted water until almost tender. Drain and reserve.

Meanwhile, trim the zucchini and slice them thinly at an angle. Seed the pepper and cut it into quarters, then halve these. Trim the eggplant and slice it into ½-inch (1.5-cm) rounds. Place all the vegetables, except the potatoes, on a baking sheet, brush them with one-third of the olive oil, and sprinkle on the tablespoon of sea salt. Bake for 25 minutes, or until soft and turning golden.

Brush a suitable baking dish (small lasagne dish or similar) with a little of the remaining olive oil and put half the potato slices in the bottom. Arrange the baked vegetables over the potatoes, then pour on the tomato sauce to coat evenly.

Arrange the remaining potatoes evenly on top. Sprinkle with pepper and oregano and drizzle the last of the oil over.

Return to the oven to bake for 20 minutes before serving.

Potato gnocchi with cheese and cauliflower

Calories: 779	
Total fat: 23 g	
Saturated fat: 9.7 g	
Fiber: 6.7 g	
Protein: high	
Carbohydrate: high	
Vitamins: B1, B2, niacin, B6, B12, folate	
Minerals: calcium, magnesium, potassium, zinc, copper, iodine	

1 rounded tablespoon (¾ oz / 25 g) sunflower-oil margarine
about 3½ cups (500 g) ready-made potato gnocchi
1 small head cauliflower, broken into florets
1 heaped tablespoon (25 g) all-purpose flour
1¾ cups (400 ml) skim milk
6 tablespoons (40 g) grated reduced-fat Cheddar cheese
1 teaspoon sea salt
black pepper
1 medium tomato, sliced and halved
¼ cup (40 g) diced fontina cheese
1 tablespoon freshly grated Parmesan cheese

Brush a two-serving-size gratin dish with a little of the sunflower margarine. Cook the gnocchi in boiling water according to package directions, drain, and place in the gratin dish.

Cook the cauliflower florets in a very little boiling water (or steam or microwave) until tender, then carefully add them to the gnocchi, spreading them around the dish evenly.

Heat the remainder of the sunflower margarine in a saucepan and add the flour. Stir well for 1 minute, then add the milk. Bring to a simmer, stirring until you have a thickened sauce. Add the grated Cheddar, salt, and pepper, and stir for 1 minute.

Preheat the broiler.

Pour the sauce over the gnocchi and cauliflower and arrange the tomato pieces around the surface. Dot the fontina cheese over the top, then sprinkle on the Parmesan.

Broil until the top is bubbling and turning golden, then serve.

Winter squash with lentils and ginger

Calories: 388
Total fat: 7.8 g
Saturated fat: 1.3 g
Fiber: 13 g
Protein: high
Carbohydrate: high
Vitamins: B1, niacin, B6, folate, A, carotenoids, C, E
Minerals: calcium, magnesium, potassium, iron, zinc, copper, selenium

about 3 cups (450 g) orange-fleshed
   squash (see note)
1 tablespoon peanut oil
1 medium onion, thinly sliced
1 garlic clove, chopped
¾-inch (2-cm) piece of fresh ginger,
   grated
1 tablespoon Chinese black bean sauce
14-oz (400-g) can of green or brown
   lentils, drained and rinsed
⅔ cup (150 ml) good-quality vegetable
   stock
1 tablespoon chopped fresh cilantro

Peel the squash, remove the seeds and fibers. Cut the flesh into medium chunks.

Heat the oil in a Dutch oven or heavy frying pan and sauté the onion until just turning golden.

Add the garlic and ginger and stir for 1 minute. Add the squash and sauté until the chunks are tinged golden, then add the black bean sauce and lentils and give everything a good stir. Pour in enough stock barely to cover the squash, bring to a simmer, and cook, covered, for 20 minutes or until the squash is tender.

Adjust the seasoning, adding a little sea salt if necessary, then serve garnished with the cilantro.

NOTE: Suitable squashes for this sort of treatment include butternut, onion squash, Sweet Mama or Crown Prince, or any with firm, deep orange flesh. Watery, pale pumpkins or squashes aren't suitable for this dish.

WINTER SQUASH WITH LENTILS AND GINGER

Rice and beans

♥ ❢ ✗ ⚒ Ⅴ ⊕ ◑ ⬚

Calories: 356
Total fat: 3.1 g
Saturated fat: 0.8 g
Fiber: 5.3 g
Protein: medium
Carbohydrate: high
Vitamins: B1, niacin, B6, folate, A, C
Minerals: magnesium, potassium, copper

⅔ cup (125 g) basmati rice
1 teaspoon sea salt, plus more for cooking the rice
¼ cup (60 ml) coconut milk
1 hot green chili pepper, seeded and chopped
½-inch (1.5-cm) piece of fresh ginger, chopped
1 red bell pepper, seeded and chopped
2 scallions, minced
1 cup (155 g) drained canned mixed beans, rinsed
black pepper
1 tablespoon chopped fresh cilantro

Cook the rice in 9 fl oz (250 ml) boiling, lightly salted water, in a pan covered with a tight-fitting lid, until tender.

Meanwhile, put the coconut milk, chili, ginger, bell pepper, and scallions in a small saucepan and simmer for a few minutes.

When the rice is cooked, toss the rice, coconut sauce, beans, seasoning, and cilantro together and serve.

Almond, chickpea, and raisin pilaf

♥ ◔ ✦ ❋ ❢ ✗ ⚒ Ⅴ ◑ ⬚

Calories: 714
Total fat: 30 g
Saturated fat: 4.6 g
Fiber: 7.3 g
Protein: medium
Carbohydrate: high
Vitamins: B1, B2, niacin, B6, folate, E
Minerals: magnesium, potassium, iron, zinc, copper

1¼ cups (275 ml) vegetable stock
1 teaspoon saffron threads
¾ cup (150 g) long-grain brown rice
1 tablespoon peanut oil
¼ cup (35 g) unsalted cashews
⅓ cup (35 g) sliced almonds
½ cup (125 g) minced onion
½ teaspoon each ground coriander and cumin
⅔ cup (100 g) cooked or canned chickpeas
¼ cup (40 g) raisins
1 tablespoon chopped fresh cilantro

Heat the vegetable stock in a saucepan and add the saffron. Add the rice, bring a to simmer, and cook, covered, for 30 minutes or until the rice is tender and all the stock absorbed (add more stock or water if rice dries out before it is tender).

Heat a nonstick frying pan and brush the bottom with a little of the peanut oil. Add the cashews and almonds and stir-fry until golden. Remove from the pan and reserve.

Add the rest of the oil to the pan and sauté the onion until soft and just turning golden.

Add the ground coriander and cumin and stir-fry for 1 minute, then add the chickpeas and raisins and stir-fry for another minute. Add the rice, toasted nuts, and chopped cilantro, and stir together gently to combine.

ALMOND, CHICKPEA, AND RAISIN PILAF

Rice and greens

Calories: 516	
Total fat: 21 g	
Saturated fat: 0.8 g	
Fiber: 5.3 g	
Protein: medium	
Carbohydrate: high	
Vitamins: B1, niacin, B6, B12, folate, A, carotenoids, C, E	
Minerals: calcium, magnesium, potassium, iron, zinc, copper	

1 cup (100 g) sliced leek
¾ cup (100 g) sliced zucchini
1 cup (100 g) small broccoli florets
handful of fresh basil leaves
2 tablespoons extra-virgin olive oil
1 teaspoon sea salt
1 tablespoon pine nuts
2 tablespoons freshly grated Parmesan cheese
black pepper
⅔ cup (150 g) risotto rice
1¾ cups (400 ml) good-quality vegetable stock
1 cup (100 g) young leaf spinach
handful of arugula leaves (about ⅓ oz / 10 g), finely sliced

Blanch the leek, zucchini, and broccoli in boiling water for 1 minute; drain well.

Using a blender or food processor, blend the basil, half the oil, the salt, pine nuts, Parmesan, and pepper into a paste.

Heat the remaining oil in a nonstick frying pan, add the rice, and stir to coat.

Heat the stock to a simmer. Add one-quarter of the stock to the rice with the blanched vegetables, stir, and bring to a simmer. Stir from time to time and, when the stock is all absorbed, add another similar quantity. Continue like this until all the stock is used up and the rice is tender and moist. (Add extra stock if you need to.)

When the rice is nearly cooked, add the spinach, arugula, and the basil sauce and stir gently for a minute or two so that the greens wilt. Adjust the seasoning and serve immediately.

Asparagus can be used instead of broccoli in this dish.

Chickpea and vegetable crumble

Calories: 374	
Total fat: 14 g	
Saturated fat: 3.4 g	
Fiber: 10 g	
Protein: high	
Carbohydrate: medium	
Vitamins: B1, niacin, B6, B12, folate, A, C, E	
Minerals: calcium, magnesium, potassium, iron, copper	

1 tablespoon olive oil
½ cup (125 g) minced onion
1 garlic clove, chopped
1 cup (100 g) spinach or Swiss chard leaves
1¾ cups (200 g) diced carrots, parboiled
2 medium tomatoes, seeded and chopped
juice of ½ lemon
1⅓ cups (200 g) cooked or canned chickpeas
1 tablespoon chopped fresh flat-leaf parsley
1 hot red chili pepper, seeded and chopped
1 teaspoon sea salt
black pepper
3 tablespoons tomato purée
1 medium slice of stale bread
1 tablespoon Irish oatmeal
2 tablespoons freshly grated Parmesan cheese

Preheat the oven to 350°F (180°C).

Heat the olive oil in a nonstick frying pan and sauté the onion until soft and slightly golden.

Add the garlic and stir for a minute. Add the spinach or chard and the carrots and stir for a few more minutes, then add the tomatoes, lemon juice, chickpeas, parsley, chili, seasoning, and tomato purée. Stir well, bring to a simmer, and transfer everything to a gratin dish.

Chop the bread into small pieces or coarsely grate it. Mix this with the oatmeal and Parmesan and sprinkle over the chickpea mixture.

Bake for 30 minutes or until the top is golden.

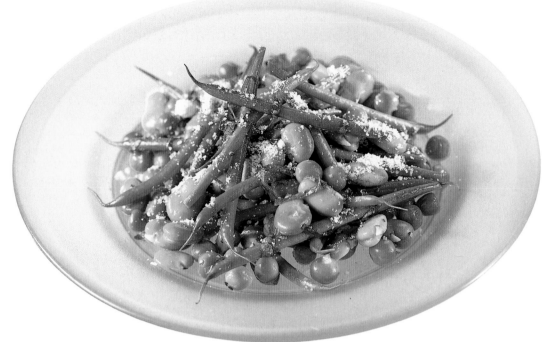

SUMMER VEGETABLES WITH MINT

Summer vegetables with mint

Calories: 136

Total fat: 7 g

Saturated fat: 1.8 g

Fiber: 6 g

Protein: high

Carbohydrate: low

Vitamins: B₁, niacin, folate, C

¾ cup (100 g) shelled fresh fava beans
⅔ cup (100 g) shelled fresh peas
½ cup (50 g) fine green beans (haricot verts), trimmed
sea salt
2 teaspoons extra-virgin olive oil
1 tablespoon chopped fresh mint
black pepper
2 teaspoons lemon juice
1 tablespoon freshly grated Parmesan cheese

Simmer the fava beans, peas, and green beans in a little lightly salted water until just tender.

Drain and add to a small frying pan with the oil, mint, seasoning, and lemon juice. Stir for a minute so that the flavors can combine. Serve with the grated cheese sprinkled over.

Stir-fried bok choy with almonds

Calories: 108

Total fat: 9.2 g

Saturated fat: 1.1 g

Fiber: 2.3 g

Protein: medium

Carbohydrate: low

Vitamins: folate, C

1 tablespoon toasted sesame oil
½-inch (1.5-cm) piece of peeled fresh ginger, grated
1 garlic clove, minced
3½ cups (300 g) bok choy leaves, any tough stalks discarded, thinly sliced
1 teaspoon soy sauce
2 teaspoons toasted chopped almonds

Heat the sesame oil in a wok or nonstick frying pan and add the grated ginger and chopped garlic, stirring for 30 seconds.

Add the sliced bok choy leaves and the soy sauce and stir-fry for 2 minutes.

Add the toasted chopped almonds, stir through, and serve immediately.

Eggplant and okra sauté

Calories: 137
Total fat: 6.9 g
Saturated fat: 1.1 g
Fiber: 7.1 g
Protein: high
Carbohydrate: medium
Vitamins: B1, B6, folate, C, E
Minerals: magnesium, potassium, copper

1 tablespoon olive oil
½ cup (125 g) minced red onion
1 fresh, juicy garlic clove, minced
1 cup (100 g) trimmed okra
½ cup (50 g) baby corn
1 medium eggplant
⅔ cup (200 g) canned crushed tomatoes
1 teaspoon chopped fresh thyme
1 teaspoon salt
black pepper
about 3 tablespoons vegetable stock
1 tablespoon chopped fresh cilantro

Heat the oil in a nonstick saucepan (which has a tight-fitting lid) and sauté the onion until soft.

Add the garlic and stir for a minute. Add the okra and corn and stir to combine.

Chop the eggplant into small cubes and add to the pan, with the tomatoes and their liquid, the thyme, seasoning, and stock. Mix well and bring to a simmer. Cook for 15 minutes, covered, then for a further 15 minutes uncovered, until you have a rich vegetable stew.

Serve sprinkled with the cilantro.

Peas and lettuce

Calories: 134
Total fat: 6 g
Saturated fat: 3.1 g
Fiber: 5.6 g
Protein: high
Carbohydrate: medium
Vitamins: B1, niacin, folate, C, A
Minerals: iron

1½ cups (200 g) shelled fresh small peas
1 head Little Gem lettuce or romaine heart, cut lengthwise into 8 pieces
4 scallions, chopped
2 teaspoons (10 g) butter
1 teaspoon balsamic vinegar
1 teaspoon chopped fresh parsley
1 teaspoon chopped fresh mint
1 teaspoon sea salt
black pepper

Put all the ingredients in a saucepan with 3 tablespoons of water and bring to a simmer.

Cook uncovered for a few minutes until the peas are tender.

EGGPLANT AND OKRA SAUTÉ

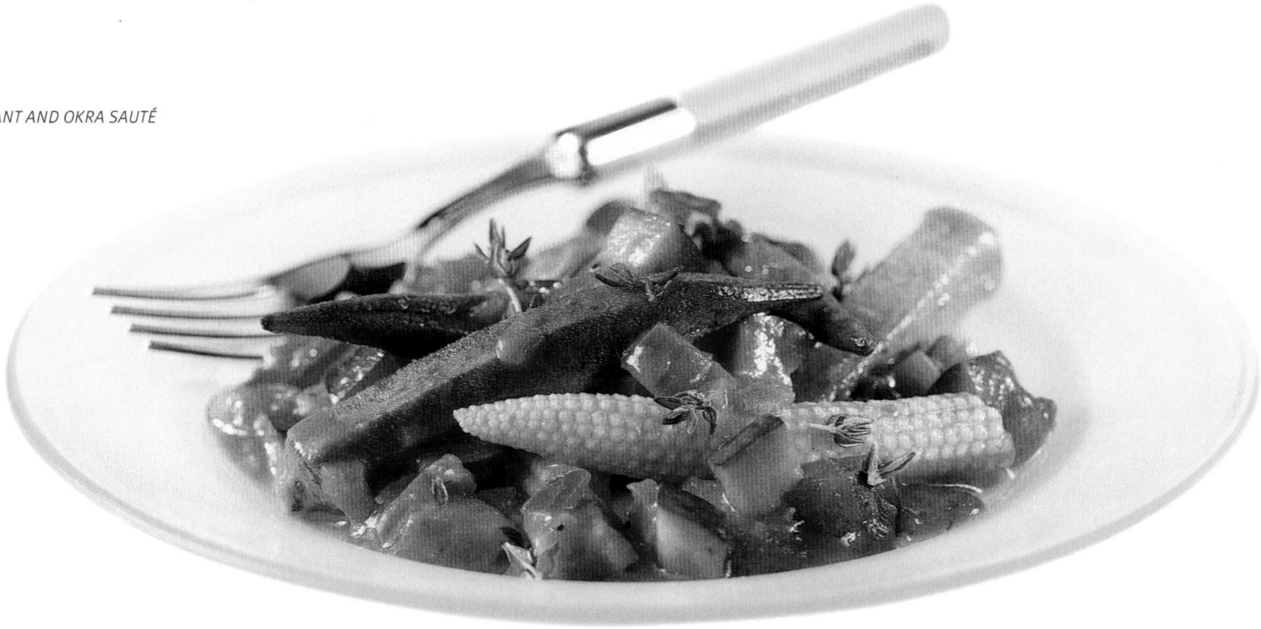

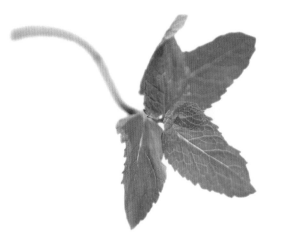

Green lentils with herbs

Calories: 220	
Total fat: 7.2 g	
Saturated fat: 0.9 g	
Fiber: 4.9 g	
Protein: high	
Carbohydrate: medium	
Vitamins: B1, niacin, B6, folate	
Minerals: magnesium, iron, copper, selenium	

½ cup (100 g) green lentils
1 small mild onion (about 2¾ oz / 75 g)
1¾ cups (400 ml) vegetable stock
1 tablespoon extra-virgin olive oil
juice of ½ lemon
2 tablespoons chopped fresh mixed
    herbs, such as oregano, mint,
    marjoram, thyme, sage, and parsley
1 teaspoon sea salt
black pepper

Put the lentils in a pan with the onion and stock. Bring to a simmer and cook for 45 minutes, or until lentils are tender.

Drain off any remaining stock and stir the olive oil, lemon juice, herbs, and seasoning into the lentils. Serve hot.

Spinach, broccoli, and walnut stir-fry

Calories: 107	
Total fat: 8.5 g	
Saturated fat: 0.8 g	
Fiber: 3.1 g	
Protein: high	
Carbohydrate: low	
Vitamins: folate, A, carotenoids, C, E	
Minerals: calcium, magnesium, iron	

1¼ cups (125 g) broccoli florets
2 teaspoons walnut oil
1¼ cups (125 g) baby spinach leaves
1 tablespoon chopped walnuts
1 teaspoon sea salt
black pepper
2 tablespoons vegetable stock

Blanch the broccoli in boiling water for 1 minute.

Drain and refresh in cold water. Dry on paper towels.

Heat the oil in a small nonstick frying pan and stir-fry the broccoli for 2 minutes.

Add the spinach, walnuts, and seasoning and stir-fry for 1 minute, adding the stock toward the end of the cooking time.

Tabbouleh

Calories: 299	
Total fat: 12 g	
Saturated fat: 1.7 g	
Fiber: 2.6 g	
Protein: low	
Carbohydrate: high	
Vitamins: B1, niacin, folate, A, C	
Minerals: magnesium, iron, copper	

⅔ cup (100 g) bulgur
1 large tomato, skinned, seeded, and
    chopped
2½-inch (6-cm) piece of English
    cucumber, chopped
handful of chopped fresh flat-leaf
    parsley
1 tablespoon chopped fresh mint
2 scallions, chopped
2 tablespoons olive oil
1 teaspoon sea salt
black pepper
juice of ½ lemon

Put the bulgur in a large bowl, pour over boiling water, and leave to soak for 30 minutes, or according to package directions, until plumped up. Drain.

Mix the bulgur with all the other ingredients in the bowl. Allow to stand, covered, for up to an hour before serving.

Quick baked beans

Calories: 361
Total fat: 13 g
Saturated fat: 1.6 g
Fiber: 12 g
Protein: medium
Carbohydrate: high
Vitamins: B1, niacin, B6, folate, E
Minerals: calcium, magnesium, potassium, iron, copper

14-oz (400-g) can canellini beans
1 tablespoon sunflower oil
½ cup (125 g) minced onion
1 teaspoon mustard powder
2 teaspoons brown sugar
1 teaspoon molasses
2 teaspoons lemon juice
1 teaspoon Worcestershire
    sauce
1 teaspoon sea salt
1 recipe-quantity Tomato Sauce
    (see page 247)

Preheat the oven to 300°F. Rinse the canellini beans well, drain them, and place them in a small casserole dish.

Heat the oil in a nonstick frying pan and sauté the onion until soft and just turning golden. Add the rest of the ingredients to the pan and stir well to heat through.

Pour the sauce over the beans, put the lid on the casserole, and bake for 1 hour, stirring once or twice.

If the mixture begins to look dry at any time, add a little water or tomato purée and stir.

Adjust the seasoning with salt, sugar, lemon juice, and Worcestershire sauce to taste and serve.

Canellini beans with hot tomato vinaigrette

Calories: 223
Total fat: 12 g
Saturated fat: 1.8 g
Fiber: 8 g
Protein: high
Carbohydrate: medium

1⅔ cup (250 g) drained canned canellini
    beans
1 juicy tomato (about 3½ oz / 100 g)
2 tablespoons olive oil
2 teaspoons red wine vinegar
pinch of mustard powder
pinch of sugar
1 teaspoon sea salt
black pepper
2 teaspoons chopped fresh basil

Rinse the beans well and drain them. Place them in a saucepan.

Blanch the tomato and skin it; halve it and remove seeds, then chop, retaining any juices that come out during this process.

In a bowl, mix together the oil, vinegar, tomato (with juices), mustard, sugar, and seasoning.

Pour this over the beans in the pan and heat gently, stirring, until all is warmed through.

Add the basil and serve warm.

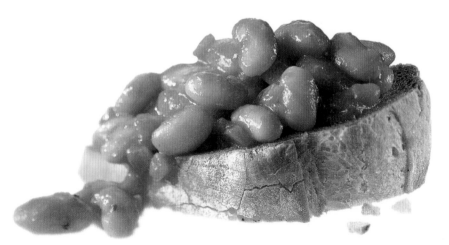

QUICK BAKED BEANS

Sauces serve 2–4, depending upon use. Nutrition details given are per portion, based upon each recipe serving 2. Halve these nutritional details if you are serving 4.

Mango salsa

Calories:	64
Total fat:	0.2 g
Saturated fat:	negligible
Fiber:	2.9 g
Protein:	low
Carbohydrate:	high
Vitamins:	A, carotenoids, C

1 ripe mango
1 small red onion
1 tablespoon lime juice
2 teaspoons chopped fresh mint
pinch of sea salt

Peel the mango and remove the pit, then chop the flesh, reserving any juice. In a bowl, combine this with all the remaining ingredients and leave in the refrigerator for 30 minutes.

Serve cold, with poultry, game, or fish.

Tofu mayonnaise

Calories:	33
Total fat:	1.6 g
Saturated fat:	0.2 g
Fiber:	negligible
Protein:	high
Carbohydrate:	low

½ cup (100 g) tofu, mashed
1 small garlic clove, minced
2 teaspoons white wine vinegar
1 teaspoon Dijon mustard
1 teaspoon sea salt
black pepper

Purée all ingredients together in a blender or food processor. Adjust the seasoning. Use to replace ordinary egg-based mayonnaise in your diet.

Vary the mayonnaise by adding chopped fresh herbs, such as dill, tarragon, or chives. Lemon juice can be used instead of the vinegar.

Fresh pepper coulis

Calories:	101
Total fat:	6.1 g
Saturated fat:	1 g
Fiber:	2.6 g
Protein:	low
Carbohydrate:	medium
Vitamins:	B6, folate, A, carotenoids, C

2 medium red bell peppers
1 tablespoon extra-virgin olive oil
1 teaspoon sea salt
black pepper

Simmer the peppers whole in water for 10 minutes, then drain, reserving the cooking water. When cool, peel off the skins. Remove seeds and chop the flesh.

Put the chopped peppers in a blender or food processor together with 2–3 tablespoons of the reserved cooking water, the oil, and seasoning. Process for a few seconds until you have a smooth sauce, adding a little more cooking liquid if the sauce is too thick. Adjust the seasoning. Serve hot or cold.

Hot pepper sauce to taste can be added for a sauce with more bite.

MANGO SALSA

AVOCADO SAUCE

FRESH PEPPER COULIS

Tomato and bean salsa

🫀 ⊙ 🥄 ❢ ☀ ☒ ✅ ⊕ ◔ ⬆

Calories: 194
Total fat: 6.5 g
Saturated fat: 1 g
Fiber: 6.9 g
Protein: high
Carbohydrate: high
Vitamins: A, B1, niacin, B6, folate, carotenoids, C, E
Minerals: magnesium, potassium, iron, copper

2 large tomatoes, halved, seeded, and chopped
1 medium red onion, chopped
1 small yellow bell pepper, seeded and chopped
2-inch (5-cm) piece of English cucumber, seeded and chopped
1½ cups (200 g) drained canned mixed beans, rinsed
1 green chili pepper, seeded and chopped
2 tablespoons chopped fresh cilantro
1 tablespoon olive oil
1 tablespoon lime juice
1 teaspoon sea salt
black pepper

Mix all ingredients in a bowl, and leave to marinate for 30 minutes. Serve cold.

Sauce verde

🫀 ⊙ 🥄 ❢ ☀ ☒ ✅ ⊕ ◔ ⬆

Calories: 108
Total fat: 11 g
Saturated fat: 1.6 g
Fiber: 0.3 g
Protein: low
Carbohydrate: low

1–2 garlic cloves, minced
1 teaspoon sea salt
1 teaspoon Dijon mustard
2 tablespoons chopped fresh flat-leaf parsley
2 tablespoons chopped fresh mint or basil
juice of ½ lemon
2 tablespoons extra-virgin olive oil
black pepper

Blend together the garlic and sea salt in a blender or food processor on low. Then, blend in the mustard, herbs, and lemon juice. With the machine still running, slowly add the olive oil, until you have a green sauce. Add black pepper to taste.

Tomato sauce

🫀 ⊙ 🥄 ❢ ☀ ☒ ✅ ⊕ ◔ ⬆

Calories: 126
Total fat: 5.9 g
Saturated fat: 0.8 g
Fiber: 2.7 g
Protein: medium
Carbohydrate: medium
Vitamins: B1, B6, folate, carotenoids, C, E
Minerals: potassium, copper

1 tablespoon olive oil
½ cup (125 g) minced onion
1 fresh, juicy garlic clove, chopped
16-oz (425-g) can crushed tomatoes
2 teaspoons tomato paste
1 heaped teaspoon brown sugar
2 teaspoons lemon juice
1 teaspoon salt
black pepper

Heat the oil in a nonstick frying pan and sauté the onion until soft. Add the garlic and stir for 1 minute.

Add the remaining ingredients, bring to a simmer, and cook, uncovered, for 30 minutes or more, until you have a rich sauce.

If too much liquid evaporates, add a little water or tomato juice.

Avocado sauce

🫀 ⊙ 🥄 🍴 ☀ ☒ ✅ ◔ ⬆

Calories: 257
Total fat: 25 g
Saturated fat: 7.3 g
Fiber: 3.3 g
Protein: low
Carbohydrate: low
Vitamins: B2, B6, E

1 large, ripe avocado
juice of 1 small lemon
½ cup (125 g) thick plain yogurt
black pepper
1 teaspoon sea salt

Peel and pit the avocado, and chop the flesh. Put it immediately in a blender or food processor with the lemon juice and process for a few seconds until smooth.

Stir in the yogurt (by hand) and the seasoning. Serve cold.
Good with fish and seafood, chicken, ham, and eggs, or as a pasta sauce or dip.

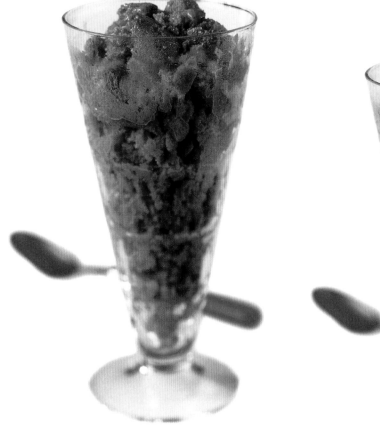
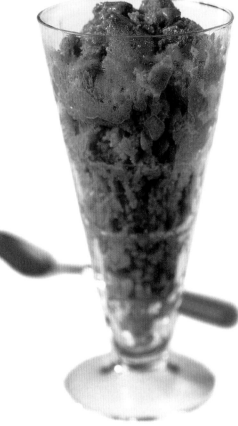

Blackberry ice sundaes

♥ ⊗ ☷ ❄ ✕ ∨ ◑ 🗂

Calories: 193	
Total fat: 1.2 g	
Saturated fat: 0.6 g	
Fiber: 6.3 g	
Protein: high	
Carbohydrate: high	
Vitamins: B2, folate, C, E	
Minerals: calcium, magnesium, potassium, iodine	

3 tablespoons (40 g) granulated fructose
   (fruit sugar)
1 teaspoon agar-agar (vegetable gelatin)
7 tablespoons (100 ml) skim milk
2 cups (275 g) blackberries
⅞ cup (200 g) thick plain low-fat yogurt
3 tablespoons orange juice

In a small pan, heat the fructose, agar-agar, and milk with 3 tablespoons water until the fructose and agar-agar are dissolved. Stir well.

Purée the berries in a blender or food processor and pass through a sieve to remove the seeds. Mix this well with the fructose syrup and the remaining ingredients and transfer to an ice cream machine. Freeze, following the manufacturer's instructions.

Other berries can be used in place of the blackberries; if using strawberries or raspberries you don't need to press the purée through a sieve. If using ripe fruit at the height of its season, you could reduce the amount of granulated fructose.

Summer fruit compote

🍶 ☺ ✎ 🍴 Y ✗ ✗ V ⊙ ◐ 🔥

Calories: 54	
Total fat: 0.3 g	
Saturated fat: negligible	
Fiber: 4.2 g	
Protein: medium	
Carbohydrate: high	
Vitamins: folate, C	
Minerals: copper	

1½ cups (200 g) strawberries
1 cup (100 g) raspberries
½ cup (100 g) black currants
3 tablespoons (40 g) granulated fructose
    (fruit sugar)
1 cinnamon stick
dash of lemon juice
thick plain yogurt or ice cream, to serve

Preheat the oven to 325°F (160°C).
Prepare the fruit if necessary, halving any
over-large strawberries, and removing
stems from the black currants.

Place the fruit, fructose, and
cinnamon in a shallow baking dish with
2–3 tablespoons water. Cover and bake
for 30 minutes, stirring gently once,
until the fruit is soft and there is a rich
juice.

Remove the cinnamon stick, and stir
in the lemon juice. Serve with yogurt or
ice cream.

Peach and banana fool

🍶 ☺ ✎ 🍴 ✗ ✗ V ⊙ ◐ 🔥

Calories: 174	
Total fat: negligible	
Saturated fat: 4 g	
Fiber: 1.4 g	
Protein: medium	
Carbohydrate: medium	
Vitamins: C	

1 ripe peach
1 medium, just-ripe banana
2 teaspoons confectioners' sugar
1 tablespoon orange juice
²/₃ cup (150 g) thick plain yogurt

Peel and chop the peach and banana
and place them in a blender or food
processor with the confectioners'
sugar and orange juice.

Blend until fairly smooth.

Fold the fruit mixture into the
yogurt, divide between 2 glass
dessert bowls or glasses and chill.

Citrus granita

🍶 ☺ ✎ Y ✗ ✗ V ⊙ ◐ 🔥

Calories: 142	
Total fat: negligible	
Saturated fat: negligible	
Fiber: 0.2 g	
Protein: low	
Carbohydrate: high	
Vitamins: C	

5 tablespoons (60 g) granulated fructose
    (fruit sugar)
²/₃ cup (150 ml) hot water
½ cup (125 ml) each fresh orange juice
    and lemon juice
3 tablespoons lime juice

Dissolve the fructose in the water. Stir in
the remaining ingredients and transfer to a
freezerproof tray. Freeze until the edges are
set, then fork these into the center. Repeat
the freezing and forking, to make a slushy,
granular texture. Serve frozen—it won't be
all that solid, even straight from freezer.

Raspberry gratin

☺ ✎ ⊟ ✗ V ◐

Calories: 218	
Total fat: 12 g	
Saturated fat: 7.7 g	
Fiber: 2.5 g	
Protein: medium	
Carbohydrate: low	
Vitamins: folate, C	
Minerals: calcium	

2 cups (200 g) fresh raspberries
2 teaspoons (7.5 g) granulated fructose
    (fruit sugar)
½ cup (100 g) thick plain yogurt
½ cup (100 g) light sour cream
1 teaspoon cornstarch
2 teaspoons brown sugar

Preheat the broiler. Divide the raspberries
between two individual soufflé dishes
and sprinkle the fructose on them.

Beat together the yogurt, sour cream,
and cornstarch, and spoon evenly over
the top of the r aspberries. Sprinkle the
brown sugar on top.

Put the soufflé dishes underneath the
broiler until the tops of the gratins begin
to bubble and
brown. Serve at once.

Stir-fried fruit salad

♡ ⊙ ⬦ ⬛ ⁂ ⚔ ✓ ⊙ ◑ ⬚

Calories: 214	
Total fat: 6.6 g	
Saturated fat: 3.1 g	
Fiber: 3.4 g	
Protein: low	
Carbohydrate: high	
Vitamins: A, C, E	
Minerals: magnesium, potassium	

1 large, barely ripe banana
1 teaspoon canola oil
½ tablespoon (7.5 g) unsalted butter
2 slices of fresh pineapple, each halved
1 small ripe mango, peeled, pitted, and quartered
2 teaspoons lime juice
1 tablespoon sweet wine
thick plain yogurt, light sour cream, or half-and-half, to serve

Peel the banana and cut it into wedges. Heat the oil and butter in a nonstick frying pan and, when very hot, add the fruit. When it starts to brown, stir gently.

Add the lime juice, stir again, and add the wine. When the wine has bubbled for a few seconds, serve, with some thick yogurt, sour cream, or half-and-half.

Mango phyllo tarts

♡ ⊙ ⬦ ⬛ Y ⚔ ✓ ⊙ ⬚

Calories: 232	
Total fat: 1.5 g	
Saturated fat: negligible	
Fiber: 4.5 g	
Protein: low	
Carbohydrate: high	
Vitamins: A, carotenoids, C	

3 rectangular sheets of phyllo pastry
butter-flavored nonstick spray coating
1 large, ripe mango
2 teaspoons granulated fructose (fruit sugar)
2 teaspoons lime juice
pinch each of ground cinnamon and ginger
1 tablespoon golden raisins
yogurt, ice cream, or raspberry coulis, to serve (optional)

Preheat the oven to 400°F (200°C). Cut the phyllo sheets in half to make six squares. Spraying each square with nonstick coating as you go, arrange three squares at angles to each other to produce a decorative edge in 2 muffin tins, or similar, to make 2 pastry shells. Bake for 10 minutes, or until just turning golden. Remove from the oven.

Meanwhile, peel, pit, and chop the mango. Mix this with the remaining ingredients. Heat through in a small saucepan or microwave to combine the flavors.

When the pastry cases are ready, fill them with the mango mixture and serve immediately with yogurt, ice cream, or a raspberry coulis, if you like.

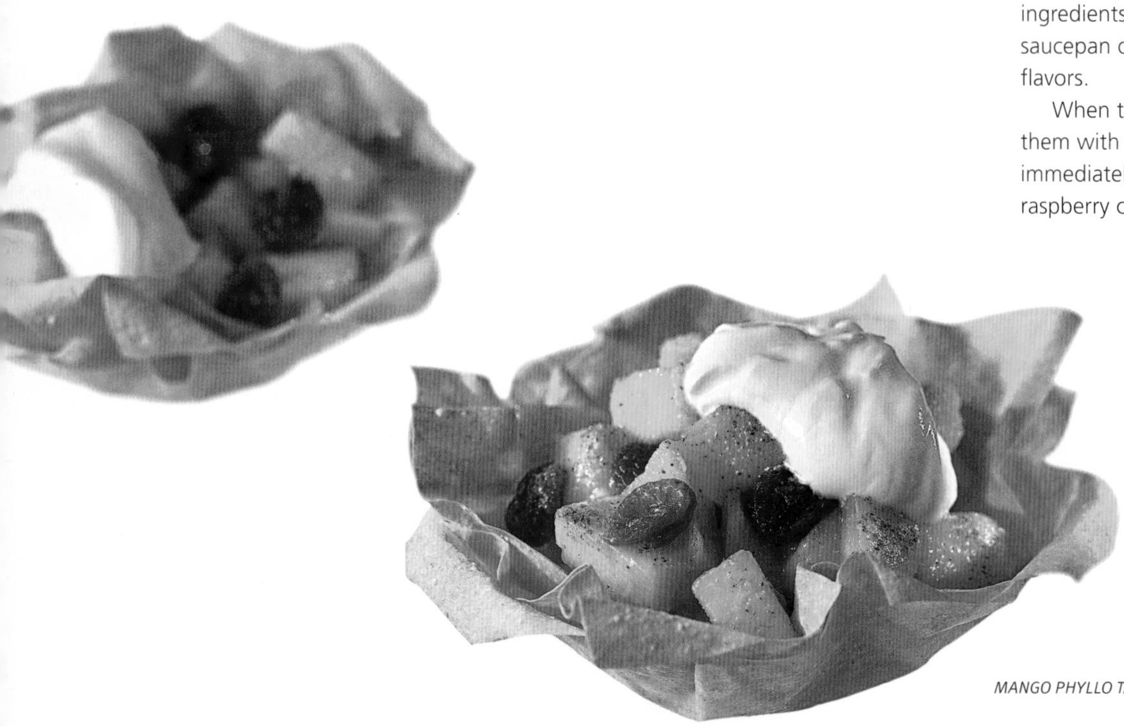

MANGO PHYLLO TARTS

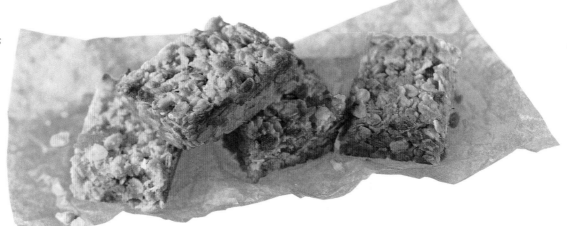

OAT-APRICOT BARS

Oat bread

🖤 ❢ ⩔ ◕ ⬧

Makes two 1-lb (450-g) loaves	
Calories: 78 per slice	
Total fat: 2 g	
Saturated fat: 0.4 g	
Fiber: 1.5 g	
Protein: medium	
Carbohydrate: high	
Vitamins: B, folate	
Minerals: magnesium, iron, zinc, copper	

3¾ cups (475 g) oat flour (see note)
⅓ cup (40 g) soy flour
1 packet (7.5 g) rapid-rise dry yeast
1 teaspoon sea salt
1 tablespoon brown sugar
1 tablespoon sunflower oil
1¾ cups (400 ml) water, slightly warm

Put the flours into a mixing bowl with the yeast, salt, and sugar. Add the oil and water and mix thoroughly. When a dough has begun to form, knead it thoroughly for 5–10 minutes.

Divide the dough between 2 lightly oiled 8½- x 4½- x 2½-inch (1-lb/450-g) loaf pans and leave in a warm place, covered with a dish towel, for 30 minutes until well risen. Preheat the oven to 350°F (180°C). Bake the loaves for 50 minutes, or until they sound hollow when tapped on the base. Turn out onto racks and leave to cool. The bread will keep for a day in an airtight container, or can be frozen.

NOTE: If your healthfood store cannot supply oat flour, simply process rolled oats in a blender or food processor until you have a flour, being careful not to over-process to dust. Soy flour can be found in most healthfood stores.

Oat-apricot bars

🖤 ❢ ✖ ⩔ ◕ ⬧

Makes 10	
Calories: 189 each	
Total fat: 8.7 g	
Saturated fat: 1.8 g	
Fiber: 2 g	
Protein: low	
Carbohydrate: high	
Vitamins: B, D, E	

⅔ cup (140 g) sunflower-oil margarine
⅔ cup (150 ml) apple cider concentrate
2¾ cup (225 g) rolled oats
pinch of sea salt
3 tablespoons (25 g) sunflower seeds
⅓ cup (50 g) chopped ready-to-eat dried apricots

Preheat the oven to 375°F (190°C).

In a saucepan, gently melt the margarine with the apple cider concentrate. Add the oats, salt, seeds, and apricots, and stir well to mix.

Spoon the mixture into a shallow 7-inch (17.5-cm) square cake pan. Press down well and smooth the top level. Bake for 20–25 minutes, until golden brown, then mark into 8 pieces before allowing to cool.

When cool, remove from the pan and cut through the marks to serve.

Vegetable cup

Calories:	48
Total fat:	0.6 g
Saturated fat:	
0.2 g	
Fibre:	12 g
Protein:	high
Carbohydrate:	
high	
Vitamins:	
niacin, folate, A,	
carotenoids, C, E	
Minerals:	
potassium	

8 oz (225 g) ripe tomatoes (about 2 medium-sized)
1 medium carrot
1 celery stalk
handful of watercress
1 teaspoon yeast extract dissolved in a little boiling water
½ cup (125 ml) tomato juice
pinch of celery salt
black pepper

Skin, halve, and seed the tomatoes. Peel and mince the carrot and chop the celery.

Put everything into a blender or food processor and process until smooth. Serve cold.

You can use a wide range of additional vegetables in this cup: Try adding some sorrel or spinach leaves, cauliflower and/or broccoli florets, and Swiss chard leaves.

CLOCKWISE FROM THE TOP: STRAWBERRY COOLER, MANGO AND PEACH BOOSTER, BANANA AND STRAWBERRY SMOOTHIE, VEGETABLE CUP

Strawberry cooler

Calories:	68
Total fat:	0.9 g
Saturated fat:	0.6 g
Fiber:	0.9 g
Protein:	high
Carbohydrate:	high
Vitamins:	C

1 heaped cup (150 g) strawberries
7 tablespoons (100 ml) skim milk
¾ cup (100 g) low-fat strawberry ice cream or frozen yogurt

Hull and halve the strawberries, then place in blender or a food processor.

Add the milk and ice cream and blend until smooth and frothy. Serve immediately.

Mango and peach booster

Calories:	150
Total fat:	0.8 g
Saturated fat:	0.4 g
Fiber:	3.3 g
Protein:	medium
Carbohydrate:	high
Vitamins:	B2, A, carotenoids, C
Minerals:	calcium, iodine

1 mango
1 peach
5 tablespoons orange juice
²/₃ cup (150 g) thick, plain low-fat yogurt
2 teaspoons clear honey

Peel, pit, and chop the mango and the peach. Place in a blender or food processor. Blend until smooth. Add the other ingredients and blend briefly to mix well. Serve chilled.

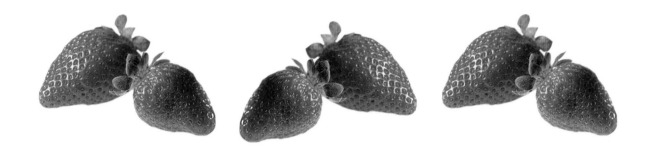

Banana and strawberry smoothie

Calories:	103
Total fat:	0.5 g
Saturated fat:	0.2 g
Fiber:	1.4 g
Protein:	high
Carbohydrate:	high
Vitamins:	B6, B12, C

1 medium banana
2 teaspoons lemon juice
²/₃ cup (75 g) fresh strawberries
1 teaspoon wheat germ
1 teaspoon granulated fructose (fruit sugar)
¾ cup (175 ml) skim milk

Peel and chop the banana, and put in a blender or food processor with the lemon juice. Add the chopped strawberries, wheat germ, fructose, and half the milk and blend until smooth.

Add the rest of the milk and blend again. Serve chilled.

Watermelon refresher

Calories:	50
Total fat:	0.4 g
Saturated fat:	negligible
Fiber:	0.2 g
Protein:	low
Carbohydrate:	high
Vitamins:	C

14-oz (400-g) piece of watermelon (about 2 cups chopped flesh)
1 teaspoon peeled and grated fresh ginger
2 teaspoons granulated fructose (fruit sugar)
3 tablespoons soda water or diet ginger ale

Peel the watermelon and remove seeds. Chop the flesh into pieces and put into a blender or food processor with the ginger and fructose. Blend.

Add the soda water or ginger ale and blend again. Serve chilled.

Summary punch

Calories: 39	
Total fat:	
negligible	
Saturated fat:	
negligible	
Fiber: 0.1 g	
Protein: low	
Carbohydrate:	
high	
Vitamins: C	

dash of Angostura bitters
dash of Grenadine
7 tablespoons (100 ml) pineapple juice
7 tablespoons (100 ml) orange juice
2 tablespoons lemon juice
7 tablespoons (100 ml) sparkling mineral
water

All the ingredients should be nice and cold. Mix together everything but the mineral water. Then stir in the mineral water and serve.

Orange and pineapple crush

Calories: 36	
Total fat:	
negligible	
Saturated fat:	
negligible	
Fiber: 0.6 g	
Protein: low	
Carbohydrate:	
high	
Vitamins: C	

2 rings of fresh pineapple
7 tablespoons (100 ml) orange juice
⅞ cup (200 ml) diet 7-Up

Chop the pineapple and process in a blender or food processor for a few seconds until it is well crushed.

Mix together the orange juice and 7-Up.

Divide the crushed pineapple between 2 glasses and top with the juice mixture. Serve chilled.

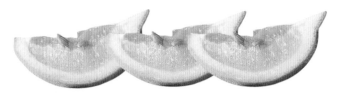

Apple and apricot shake

Calories: 169	
Total fat: 2.6 g	
Saturated fat:	
1.5 g	
Fiber: 3 g	
Protein: medium	
Carbohydrate:	
high	
Vitamins: B1, B12	
Minerals: calcium, potassium, iodine	

2 fresh and tasty apples
4 pieces ready-to-eat dried apricot
1½ cups (300 ml) low-fat 2% milk
2 teaspoons pouring honey
pinch of ground cinnamon

Peel, core, and chop the apples and put into a blender or food processor.

Chop the apricots and add to the blender with one-third of the milk, the honey, and the cinnamon. Blend to a purée, then gradually add the rest of the milk. Serve chilled.

Sangria

Calories: 132	
Total fat:	
negligible	
Saturated fat:	
negligible	
Fiber: 1.4 g	
Protein: low	
Carbohydrate:	
low	
Vitamins: C	

1 organic orange
1 organic lemon
1¼ cups (300 ml) light and fruity red
wine
7 tablespoons (100 ml) soda water

Wash the fruit and peel a few long strips of rind off each. Reserve. Peel the fruit, removing all the pith. Section the fruit over a suitable pitcher so that you retain all the juices, again removing all pith and seeds.

Halve the sections and add to the pitcher containing the retained juices, along with the rind. Pour the wine over, stir, and chill for at least 30 minutes.

When ready to serve, stir in the soda water.

Lemon balm tea

Calories:
negligible

Total fat:
negligible

Saturated fat:
negligible

Fiber: negligible

Protein:
negligible

¼ cup fresh lemon balm leaves, minced
5 cups (1.25 liters) boiling water
whole lemon balm leaves, for garnish
lemon slices, for garnish

Place the minced lemon balm in a warmed teapot and pour on the boiling water. Leave to infuse for 5 minutes, then strain into mugs.

Serve hot or cold garnished with lemon balm leaves and lemon.
Lemon balm tea is calming and also antiviral. Herbal infusions can also be made with various other fresh herbs such as mint (for indigestion), stinging nettle (diuretic and detoxifying), parsley (diuretic and stimulating), and rosemary (tonic and circulatory stimulant).

Dandelion and burdock tea

Calories:
negligible

Total fat:
negligible

Saturated fat:
negligible

Fiber: negligible

Protein:
negligible

1 oz (25 g) minced cleaned
    dandelion root
1 oz (25 g) minced cleaned
    burdock root

To make a tea out of plant roots, they must be simmered in boiling water for some time rather than simply steeped in boiling water—a decoction. Place the chopped roots in a pan, add 1 quart (1 liter) water, bring to a simmer, and simmer gently for 30 minutes until reduced by half. Strain and serve. The decoction can be kept in the refrigerator for a day or two.

Dandelion and burdock tea is a good detoxifier, aiding liver function. It is also diuretic and purifying, with a laxative effect.

CLOCKWISE FROM TOP: ORANGE AND PINEAPPLE CRUSH, SUMMER PUNCH, APRICOT AND APPLE SHAKE, SANGRIA

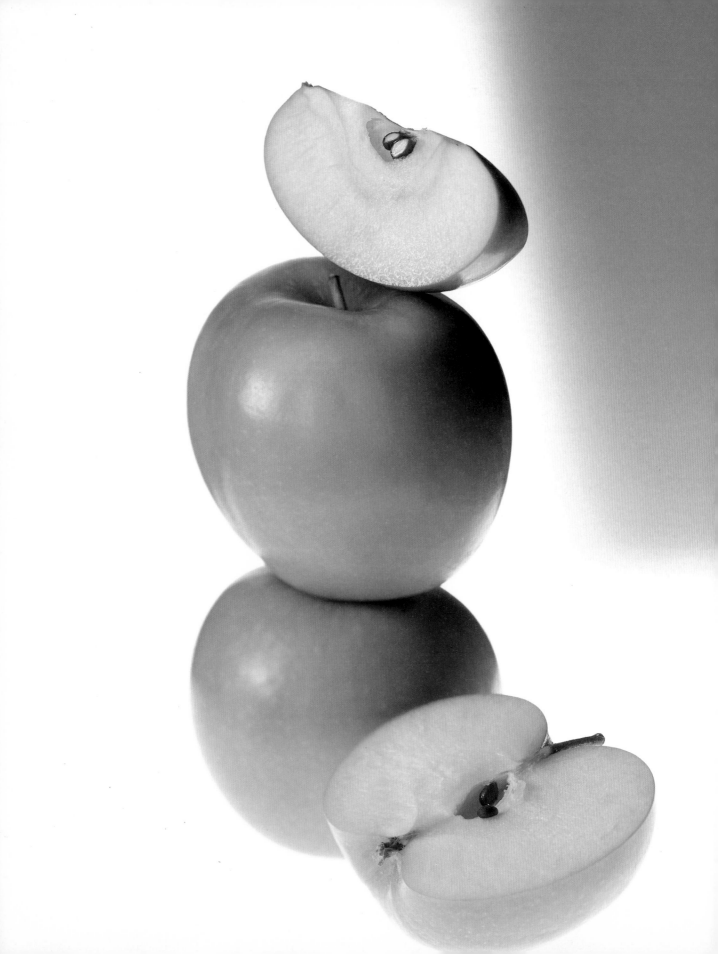

Food at a glance

The charts that follow list the nutrient breakdown of about 400 common and not-so-common foods. Whenever you want to know what is in the food you eat, this is the section to which you should refer. Where appropriate, there are also interesting health notes for individual foods and food groups, to give you extra information that the tables may not supply—for example, news about new micronutrients and their effect. The nutrient information is calculated from published analysis and manufacturers' data. However, individual foods vary in their precise nutrient content for various reasons—time of year (especially with fresh fruits and vegetables), method of storage (poor storage loses vitamins, for example), reformulation of manufactured products, and so on. There are also sometimes very significant variations in nutritional content of some branded foods made by different manufacturers—e.g., different brands of frozen hamburgers. However, the charts will still give you a very reasonable indication of nutrients.

The food charts

Name of food
Usually a general name (for staple foods) is given, but when a food is familiarly known under a manufacturer's name, (eg., Shredded Wheat), that is used.

Food state
This column tells you whether or not the food has been analyzed raw or cooked and, if the latter, how cooked.

Portion size (sometimes given at start of section)
We have tried as far as possible to give portion sizes that are quantities of the food that will normally be eaten, and portions as indicated by manufacturers. All other nutrient information refers to this portion size. The nutritional analysis of all the foods has been based on a portion weight in grams, but where appropriate we have given the nearest equivalent in cup or spoon meaures for ease of use.

We have tried to use our common sense when offering portion sizes—obviously, for a more accurate breakdown of what nutrients you are getting in your own diet, you may want to weigh your own portions and then raise or lower the nutrient content accordingly. Note that all data represent estimated values.

KiloCalorie content (calories) and KiloJoules (joules)
A KiloCalorie is a measurement of energy and is commonly known as a "calorie." Calorie content is given per portion stated.

A KiloJoule—commonly known as a "joule"—is another way of measuring energy, which is gradually overtaking the old KiloCalorie method in many countries. A KiloJoule is roughly 4.184 times each calorie, but as joules are measured in a slightly different way from calories, values can often be less or greater than this. For more information on typical energy (calorie/joule) content of various diets, see Section One.

Total fat (g) and percentages of types of fat
Total fat content of each portion of food is given in grams. The next three columns then offer a percentage breakdown of the types of fat within the total fat content. These are: percentage of polyunsaturated fats, percentage of monounsaturated fats, and percentage of saturated fat. This total fat column also includes trans (hydrogenated) fats, which have a similar effect within the body.

You will probably notice that, in all but a few cases, the three percentage columns don't actually add up to 100. This is because the total fat content of most foods also includes the non-fatty acid fats, such as glycerol and other fatty compounds, as well as polyunsaturated, monounsaturated, and saturated fatty acids, so that out of the total weight of fat in a particular food, the "missing" percentage will be these other fats.

If you are keeping a close eye on your fat intake, it is easy to work out what percentage of total calories in a particular food are fat calories. Check the total fat (g) column. Each gram of fat contains 9 calories, so multiply this column by 9. For example, Cheddar cheese contains 17 g fat, which equals 153 calories. Total calories in the cheese are 206. So the percentage of calories from fat in the cheese is (153 divided by 206 =) 74.27%. From this you can see Cheddar is a very high-fat food. You can also see that 63% of those fat calories are from saturated fat, making it also a food extremely high in saturated fat.

For more information on fat within your diet and how much we need of the different types, turn to Section One (pages 15–19).

Protein (g)
Protein content of the food is given in grams. In a similar way to fat, you can also work out the percentage of protein calories in any particular food.

Each gram of protein contains 4 calories. So, say, Cheddar cheese contains (13 g x 4 =) 52 protein calories. This is (52 ÷ 206 =) 25.24% protein, making cheese a high-protein food (because we need no more than 10–15% of our total daily calories as protein).

For more information on protein within your diet and how much we need for health, turn to Section One.

Total carbohydrate (g)

Total carbohydrate content of the food is given in grams and this total is then, in the next two columns, broken down into starches and sugars, both also given in grams. For an explanation of these different types of carbohydrate, turn to Section One.

If you would like to work out the percentage of calories from total carbohydrates, starch, or sugars, in any food, simply multiply the grams by 3.75, as each gram of carbohydrate contains 3.75 calories. For example, one scone contains 26 g of carbohydrate. That is (26 g x 3.75 =) 97.50 calories. The total calories in the scone are 151, so each scone contains (97.5 ÷151=) 64.56% of its calories as carbohydrate, making scones a high-carbohydrate food. For more information on carbohydrates and how much we need in our diets for health, turn to Section One.
NOTE: Due to US labeling regulations, a conversion factor of 4, not 3.75, is used for packaged foods; therefore, if calculating from package information, use 4 and not 3.75.

Fiber (NSP) (g) and soluble fiber (g)

The fiber columns give fiber content of each food, divided into the two different types of fiber—non-starch polysaccharides or insoluble fiber, and soluble fiber. These two different types of fiber have particular roles to play within a healthy diet. For more information about the types of fiber and how much we should get in our diets for good health, turn to Section One.

Cholesterol (mg)

Cholesterol content of foods is listed in milligrams (mg). This column will be useful for anyone who has been asked to follow a diet low in cholesterol by their physician, for instance, people with high blood cholesterol levels or a history of heart disease.

For more information on cholesterol within the foods we eat and its importance in a healthy diet, turn to Section One.

Vitamins (useful source of)

This column lists all the vitamins that appear in this portion size of food in useful quantities when available. A "useful quantity" in most instances is about 12% or more of the daily US RDI (Recommended Daily Intake). Where there is no US RDI for a nutrient, Recommended Dietary Allowances (RDAs) have been used.

The Health Notes will sometimes clarify this—for example, when content of a certain vitamin has come out at marginally below the 12%, if you eat a lot of that food it will still make a useful contribution to that vitamin content of your diet. This will usually be mentioned.

For more advice on vitamins and how much of them we need in our diets, turn to Section One, where you will also find charts listing the principal sources for all major vitamins and minerals.

Minerals (good source of)

Exactly the same criteria have been used for minerals as for vitamins (see above) and, again, for more information on minerals in your diet, and charts listing the best sources of each, see Section One.

Sodium content of foods has not been listed for each individual food, but if a food is particularly high in sodium this is mentioned in the Health Notes. For a list of the foods with high sodium content, see Section One, page 33.

In summary, chart headings are as follows:

name of food
food state
portion size
calories
k joules
total fat (g)
% poly
% mono
% sat
protein (g)
total carbohydrates (g)
starch (g)
sugars (g)
total fiber (NSP) (g)
soluble fiber (g)
cholesterol (mg)
useful source of vitamins
good source of minerals
special health notes (sometimes these are applicable to just one food in the group; at other times they run down several items as group notes)

VITAMIN ABBREVIATIONS

B1	also known as thiamine	pant ac	pantothenic acid
B2	also known as riboflavin	b-carotene	beta-carotene
niacin	also known as nicotinic acid		(pro-vitamin A)
B6	also known as pyridoxine	C	also known as ascorbic acid
folate	also known as folic acid		

MINERAL ABBREVIATIONS

cal	calcium	manga	manganese
cop	copper	phos	phosphorous
iod	iodine	potas	potassium
magnes	magnesium	sel	selenium

Breads and other baked goods

	food state	portion size	calories	k joules	total fat (g)	% poly	% mono	% sat	protein (g)	carbo (g)	starch (g)	sugars (g)
Ciabatta (Italian slipper bread)		4 slices (3½ oz/ 100 g)	143	605	2,6	12	73	15	9.7	20	18	1.9
Corn bread		1 lg. piece (3½ oz/ 100 g)	266	1,113	7.1	45	25	18	6.7	44	n/k	n/k
Croissant		2 (2½ oz/ 60 g each)	216	903	12.2	24	40	32	5	23	22	0.6
French		4 slices (3½ oz/ 100 g)	270	1,149	2.7	26	19	22	9.6	55	54	1.9
Mixed grain		4 slices (3½ oz/ 100 g)	235	999	2.7	26	22	19	9.3	46	44	2.2
Pita white		1 bread (3 oz/ 75 g)	195	827	0.8	46	n/k	46	7.1	40	37	1.7
Rye dark		3 slices (3½ oz/ 100 g)	219	931	1.7	n/k	n/k	n/k	8.3	45.8	n/k	n/k
Wheat germ		4 slices (3½ oz/ 100 g)	232	937	2.5	n/k	n/k	n/k	9.2	43	40	2.4
White		4 slices (3½ oz/ 100 g)	235	1,002	1.9	26	21	21	8.4	49	47	2.6
Whole-wheat		4 slices (3½ oz/ 100 g)	215	914	2.5	28	20	20	9.2	42	40	1.8
Oat cracker		2	115	482	4.8	29	44	21	2.6	16	16	0.8
Rice cake plain brown		2 lg. (1 oz/ 25 g)	90	376	0.7	36	40	20	2.1	20	n/k	n/k
Rye crispbreads		4 (1 oz/ 25 g)	81	338	0.45	50	17	17	2.7	16.5	14.4	2.1

total fiber (g)	soluble fiber (g)	chol (mg)	useful source of vitamins	good source of minerals	special health notes
2.6	n/k	0	niacin	cal, iron, sel, manga	Bread is a staple food and, for most people, a healthy one, as a source of carbohydrate and reasonable amounts of protein. Most breads are also low in fat, notable exceptions being croissants, breads made with milk, and some specialty breads, such as ciabatta.
0	0	40	B1, B2, niacin, folate	cal, iron, sel, potas, phos	Bread is usually made from wheat flour—whole-wheat contains the wheat germ (the central sprouting part), whereas white flour contains neither the germ nor the bran (the outer coating of the grain). Because many of the vitamins and minerals are contained in these parts of the
1.0	0.5	4.5	niacin, folate		grain, white bread is naturally much lower in vitamins and minerals than whole-wheat bread. In the US, however, most white bread flour is fortified with B1, niacin, iron, calcium, and folate, a vitamin especially important in pregnancy.
1.5	0.9	0	niacin	cal, iron, sel, manga	The salt content of bread can be high or fairly high, a point worth remembering if you eat a lot of bread and have been asked to follow a low-sodium diet.
4.3	2.1	0	B1, niacin, folate	magnes, phos	Bread is high on the list of foods that can produce allergic reactions in some people—the main allergens being gluten (the constituent that gives dough its elasticity), wheat, or yeast (see Gluten Intolerance, Allergies). Several manufacturers now make wheat-
1.5	n/k	0			and/or gluten-free loaves, and some flat breads are made without added yeast (check labels carefully as many flat breads, such as commercial pitas, DO contain yeast). Soda bread is a yeast-free alternative, though with a short shelf-life. Note that even breads that
4.4	n/k	0	B1, B2, niacin, E	cal, iron, phos	appear to contain no wheat—e.g., rye bread or oat bread—usually do, in fact, have a proportion of wheat in the recipe to give a lighter loaf. Check the ingredients list.
3.3	1.3	n/k	B1, niacin, folate	cal, magnes, iron, cop, iod, manga, potas, phos	Commercial, mass-produced budget loaves may contain several additives, such as bleach, soy flour, and caramel. Organic and traditionally made bread is now widely available.
1.5	0.9	0	B1, niacin	cal, manga	For people following a calorie-restricted diet, dark rye bread is a good choice as it has a medium glycemic index, unlike wheat loaves, which have a high glycemic index, and so keeps hunger at bay for longer.
5.8	1.6	0	B1, niacin, folate	magnes, potas, phos, iron, sel, manga	
1.5	0.9	2	manga		Most crackers tend to be high in salt and fat. Standard salted crackers are particularly high in saturated and trans fats and salt, and low in fiber. Oat crackers are higher in unsaturated fats and contain much more fiber; as regular eating of oat foods is linked with lowering of
2.1	n/k	0			blood cholesterol they could be a healthier alternative. Rye crisp-breads are a healthy wholefood, containing nothing but rye and a very little salt, and may be useful for people with wheat intolerance. Rice cakes are another low-fat, low-salt alternative to wheat crackers,
3.6	1.2	0		manga	though they are low in fiber.

	food state	portion size	calories	k joules	total fat (g)	% poly	% mono	% sat	protein (g)	carbo (g)	starch (g)	sugars (g)
Saltine cracker oyster, soda		9 (1 oz/ 25 g)	105	426	3.0	15	52	16	2.3	18	n/k	n/k
Tortilla		3½ oz (100 g)	325	1,360	7.1	45	40	13	8.7	55.6	n/k	n/k
Apple pie		1 average slice (3¾ oz/ 110 g)	293	1,227	15	7	35	49	3.2	39	24	15
Buttermilk biscuit		1	95	397	4	14	56	25	1.9	13	n/k	n/k
Chocolate cake rich	not frosted	1 slice (2 oz/ 50 g)	228	954	13	43	32	9	3.7	25	11	14
Chocolate chip cookie		2	100	418	4.5	11	53	36	1.1	13.6	n/k	n/k
Donut jelly		1	252	1,061	11	25	37	29	43	37	23	14
Eclair chocolate	frozen	1 (1½ oz/ 35 g)	139	576	11	6	33	52	2.0	9	6.8	2.3
Fruit cake rich		1 slice (2 oz/ 50 g)	171	719	5.5	25	40	31	1.9	30	5.6	24
Granola bar		1 bar (1½ oz/ 33 g)	138	583	5.4	46	42	12	2.4	21	8	11
Oatmeal cookie		1	80	334	3.2	15	57	18	1.1	12	n/k	n/k
Scone plain		1	174	731	7.0	24	37	34	3.5	26	23	2.8
Sponge cake		1 thin slice (2 oz/ 50 g)	151	640	2.5	12	36	32	2.1	32	8.3	24
Phyllo pastry	unbaked	1 oz (25 g)	79	332	0.9	n/k	n/k	8	2.2	15	15	0.3

total fiber (g)	soluble fiber (g)	chol (mg)	useful source of vitamins	good source of minerals	special health notes
0.5	0.3	n/k			
3.1	n/k	0	B1, B2, niacin	cal, phos, iron, cop, manga	
1.9	1	n/k	C		Calorie content of an apple pie can be reduced by using fructose to sweeten the apples and by making a top crust only.
n/k	n/k	n/k			Most bakery items are high in fat, particularly saturated fats. Mass-produced commercial baked goods are often high in trans fats, which are now thought to be equally as bad—or even worse—for health than the saturates.
n/k	n/k	76	A, D, E		A few baked goods are not high in fat—check labels. Most bakery products are also low in fiber, vitamins, and minerals, and high in sugars and (often) in cholesterol. Cake-lovers should consider all these factors before indulging too often. Most people view granola
0.5	n/k	0			bars as a healthier alternative to cakes and cookies, but they are higher in sugars than many other sweet foods and fat content can also be high.
n/k	n/k	11			Nutritional values given here are for guidance only, as recipes vary from manufacturer to manufacturer. Homemade cakes using unsaturated fats, natural ingredients, whole-wheat flours, and less sugar will produce a much healthier nutritional profile.
0.3	0.1	53			
0.9	0.3	32	A, D, E*		(* Dependent upon type of fat used in recipe.)
1.1	n/k	0		manga	
0.6	n/k	0			
0.9	0.4	14			
0.9	n/k	76			
0.8	n/k	n/k			Phyllo comes with hardly any fat, so the cook controls the amount and type of fat added. If lightly brushed with olive oil, this is the healthiest pastry you can get. Values here are for the pastry before adding oil.

	food state	portion size	calories	k joules	total fat (g)	% poly	% mono	% sat	protein (g)	carbo (g)	starch (g)	sugars (g)
Piecrust		1/7 pieshell (1 oz/ 25 g)	110	459	7.1	18	41	36	1.1	11	11	0.2
Puff pastry		1 oz (25 g)	93	390	5.9	16	42	49	3	7.7	7.3	0.5
Biscuit		1 average (3 oz/ 75 g)	276	1,154	13	4	26	66	4.3	34	n/k	n/k
Burrito with beef		1/4 lb (110 g)	261	1,092	11	4	33	47	13	29	n/k	n/k
Pizza cheese and tomato		1 slice (7 oz/ 200 g)	474	1,990	24	18	31	45	18	50	46	4

Breakfast cereals

	food state	portion size	calories	k joules	total fat (g)	% poly	% mono	% sat	protein (g)	carbo (g)	starch (g)	sugars (g)
All Bran		1/2 cup (1 oz/ 30 g)	78	333	1.0	40	10	20	4.2	14	8.3	5.7
Bran Flakes		1 cup (1 oz/ 30 g)	95	406	0.6	50	17	17	3.1	21	15	5.6
Cornflakes		1 cup (1 oz/ 30 g)	108	461	0.2	50	0	0	2.4	26	23	2.5
Fruit 'n Fiber		heaping 1/2 cup (1 oz/ 30 g)	105	444	1.4	21	29	57	2.7	22	14	7.3
★ Muesli no added sugar		scant 2/3 cup (2 oz/ 50 g)	183	776	3.9	31	46	21	5.3	34	26	7.8
★ Oatmeal (rolled oats)	raw	1/3 cup (1 oz/ 30 g)	113	476	2.8	39	36	18	3.4	20	20	0.3
Oatmeal	made with water	heaping 3/4 cup (7 oz/ 200 g)	98	418	2.2	36	36	18	3.0	18	18	tr
Pop Tart		1	210	870	6.0	n/k	n/k	17	2.5	36	19	17

total fiber (g)	soluble fiber (g)	chol (mg)	useful source of vitamins	good source of minerals	special health notes
0.5	0.2	9			The fat content of these traditional pastries is quite high and saturates are high unless a polyunsaturated margarine, which is low in hydrogenated fats, is used (check labels).
1.5	n/k	n/k			
n/k	n/k	5.1	B1	phos	A high-fat food, but homemade biscuits could be considerably lower in fat.
1.3	n/k	73	B1, niacin, B12	phos	A burrito with beef is high in calories and fat, but the meat content gives some B vitamins and minerals.
2.8	1.2	44	A, b-carotene, B1, B2, niacin, E	cal, potas, phos, iod, manga	The tomato sauce is high in lycopene, which helps to protect against heart disease and cancer. Cheese and tomato pizza is also a very good source of calcium. Fiber content can be boosted with extra veg.
7.3	1.2	0	B1, B2, niacin, B6, B12, folate, D	magnes, potas, phos, iod, iron, cal	Very high-fiber cereal, useful for helping regular bowel movement and good source of nutrients, but contains reasonably high amount of sugar.
3.9	0.9	0	B1, B2, niacin, B6, B12, folate, D	iron	Wheat-bran-based cereal; less fiber than All Bran but still higher than most commercial cereals; vitamin- and mineral-fortified.
0.3	0.1	0	B1, B2, niacin, B6, B12, folate, D	iron	Wheat-free cereal, low in fiber but fortified with vitamins and minerals. Fairly high in sugar, but a better choice for people trying to limit their sugar intake than "frosted" cereals such as Frosties.
2.1	0.8	0	B1, B2, niacin, B6, B12, folate, D	iron	Wheat-based cereal, higher in saturated fats than other cereals because of the coconut content; vitamin- and mineral-fortified.
3.8	n/k	tr	niacin, E	manga, cop	Muesli is a wholegrain oat-based cereal (sometimes also with wheat flakes—check label if avoiding wheat), dried fruit, nuts, and seeds, providing a good range of vitamins and minerals (though mostly not in sufficient quantities to appear on chart). Oats are rich in soluble fiber, which can help lower blood cholesterol, and with a low glycemic index providing lasting energy and keeping hunger at bay. Muesli is high in natural sugars from the fruit, but low in salt and high in monounsaturated fats. Oatmeal is also a wholegrain oat cereal, high in unsaturated fats and soluble fiber, and with a medium glycemic index.
2.1	1.2	0		manga	
1.6	1.0	0			
0.8	n/k	0	B1, B2, niacin, B6, B12, folate		Wheat-based breakfast snack fortified with vitamins and minerals; rather high in fats and low in fiber.

	food state	portion size	calories	k joules	total fat (g)	% poly	% mono	% sat	protein (g)	carbo (g)	starch (g)	sugars (g)
Puffed Wheat		2 cups (1 oz/ 30 g)	96	410	0.4	50	2.5	2.5	4.3	20	20	0.1
Rice Crispies		2 cups (1 oz/ 30 g)	111	472	0.3	33	33	33	1.8	27	24	3.2
Shredded Wheat		2	146	623	1.4	43	14	14	4.8	31	30	0.4
Special K		3/4 cup (1 oz/ 30 g)	113	481	0.3	33	33	33	4.6	25	19	5.2
Weetabix		2	127	540	1.0	46	18	18	4.4	25.2	28	1.8

Dairy products and eggs

	food state	portion size	calories	k joules	total fat (g)	% poly	% mono	% sat	protein (g)	carbo (g)	starch (g)	sugars (g)
Cows' milk whole		scant 1/2 cup (3 1/2 fl oz 100 ml)	66	275	3.5	3	28	62	3.2	4.8	0	4.8
Cows' milk 2%		scant 1/2 cup (3 1/2 fl oz 100 ml)	46	195	1.6	tr	31	63	3.3	5	0	5
Cows' milk skim or nonfat		scant 1/2 cup (3 1/2 fl oz 100 ml)	33	140	0.1	0	0	100	3.3	5	0	5
Goats' milk		scant 1/2 cup (3 1/2 fl oz 100 ml)	60	253	3.5	3	23	66	3.1	44	0	4.4
Soy milk		scant 1/2 cup (3 1/2 fl oz 100 ml)	32	132	1.9	58	21	16	2.9	0.8	0	0.8
Cream half-and-half		1/4 cup (2 fl oz/ 50 ml)	68	272	5.8	4	29	62	1.5	2.2	0	2.2
Cream light or coffee		1/4 cup (2 fl oz/ 50 ml)	99	409	9.8	4	29	62	1.4	2	0	2
Cream light-whipping		1/4 cup (2 fl oz/ 50 ml)	146	610	15	3	30	64	0.9	1.5	0	1.5

total fiber (g)	soluble fiber (g)	chol (mg)	useful source of vitamins	good source of minerals	special health notes
1.7	n/k	0	niacin	cop	Wholegrain wheat cereal, high in polyunsaturates and low in salt and sugar.
0.2	0	0	B1, B2, niacin, B6, B12, folate, D	iron	Rice-based cereal fortified with vitamins and minerals; low in fiber.
4.4	0.9	0	niacin	magnes, cop	Whole-wheat cereal high in polyunsaturates and fiber and low in sugar and salt.
0.6	0.2	0	B1, B2, niacin, B6, B12, folate, D	iron	Rice- and wheat-based cereal, fortified with vitamins and minerals; low in fiber and fairly high in sugars and salt.
2.9	1.2	0	B1, B2, niacin	iron, cop	Whole-wheat cereal fortified with vitamins and iron; fairly low in salt and added sugars.
0	0	14	A, B2, niacin, B12	cal, iod, potas, phos	Skim and low-fat milks are a good source of protein and one of the Western world's most common sources of calcium, a low intake of which has been linked with heart disease, colon cancer, and, of course, osteoporosis. It is frequently fortified with Vitamins A and D. Whole milk contains more than half of its calories as fat, two-thirds of which is saturated, so people following a diet low in saturates should use skim milk or soy milk.
0	0	7	A, B2, niacin, B12,	cal, iod, potas, phos	
0	0	2	A, B2, niacin, B12,	cal, iod, potas, phos	Some people are allergic to, or intolerant of, cows' milk, either because of lactose intolerance or an inability to digest the milk proteins, in which case goats' milk is often an acceptable alternative. See Allergies.
0	0	10	A, B2, niacin, B12,	cal, iod, potas, phos	Goat's milk is almost as high in fat and saturates as whole cows' milk, but may be tolerated by people allergic to cows'-milk products.
0	0	0	B2, E	cop	People who eat no dairy products should probably buy calcium-fortified soy milk. Soy milk is made from the soybean, one of few sources of complete plant protein. See Soybeans on page 316.
0	0	18			Whatever type of dairy cream you buy, most of the calories it contains will be from fat, two-thirds of which is saturated. Cream should be used sparingly within a healthy diet. Cream is occasionally fortified; check the label to see if it has any significant source of vitamins (though it is not likely).
0	0	33			
0	0	55	A		

	food state	portion size	calories	k joules	total fat (g)	% poly	% mono	% sat	protein (g)	carbo (g)	starch (g)	sugars (g)
Cream sour, full-fat		¹/₄ cup (2 fl oz/ 50 ml)	89	372	8.5	4	31	65	1.3	1.7	n/k	n/k
Cream sour, reduced-fat		¹/₄ cup (2 fl oz/ 50 ml)	40	167	6	4	29	61	1.5	2.1	0	2.1
Yogurt plain low-fat		scant ¹/₂ cup (3¹/₂ oz/ 100 g)	56	236	0.8	tr	25	63	5.1	7.5	0	7.5
Yogurt plain whole-milk		scant ¹/₂ cup (3¹/₂ oz/ 100 g)	79	333	3	7	30	30	5.7	7.8	0	7.8
Yogurt creamy Greek		scant ¹/₂ cup (3¹/₂ oz/ 100 g)	106	442	7.5	5	25	64	4.4	5.6	0	5.6
Yogurt low-fat fruit		¹/₂ cup (4 fl oz/ 115 g)	111	464	1.4	2	26	60	4.5	21	0	21
Yogurt skim		¹/₂ cup (4 fl oz/ 115 g)	63	264	0.2	5	27	60	6.4	7.5	0	7.5
Cottage cheese creamed		scant ¹/₂ cup (3¹/₂ oz/ 100 g)	79	333	4.5	3	29	63	12.5	2.7	0	5.7
Cottage cheese 1% fat		scant ¹/₂ cup (3¹/₂ oz/ 100 g)	72	300	1	tr	29	65	12.4	2.7	0	6.8
Cottage cheese fruit		scant ¹/₂ cup (3¹/₂ oz/ 100 g)	72	300	3.4	3	29	63	10	13	0	14
Ricotta part skim		¹/₄ cup (2 oz/ 50 g)	69	288	3.9	3	29	55	5.7	2.55	n/k	n/k
American cheese		2 oz (50 g)	165	690	12	3	29	64	9.9	4.1	n/k	n/k
Blue cheese		2 oz (50 g)	174	719	15	3	29	63	10	tr	0	tr
Brie		2 oz (50 g)	160	662	13	3	29	63	9.6	tr	0	tr

total fiber (g)	soluble fiber (g)	chol (mg)	useful source of vitamins	good source of minerals	special health notes
0	0	28			See entry under Cream, pages 266–7
0	0	19			
0	0	4	B2, B12	cal, potas, phos	Plain low-fat yogurt is a good low-fat source of calcium and protein.
0	0	11	B2, B12	cal, potas, phos	Over one-third of calories in plain whole-milk yogurt are fat, but it is still a good source of calcium.
0	0	14	B2, B12	cal, potas, phos	Over 50% of calories in creamy Greek yogurt are fat and much of this is saturated fat.
0	0	5.6	B2	cal, potas, phos	Fruit yogurts tend to contain a lot of sugar; check the label for additives.
0	n/k	2.2	B2	cal, potas, phos	Skim-milk products have only a trace of fat and are good for weight-loss diets.
0	0	15	B2	phos	Eaten in reasonable quantities, creamed cottage cheese can make a good contribution to calcium intake, at 86 mg/100 g, but saturated fat content is quite high.
0	0	4	B2	phos	Calcium content same as Creamed Cottage Cheese above, but fat content much lower.
tr	tr	11	B2	phos	
0	0	15			
0	0	32	B12	cal, phos	Cheese is perceived by many as a "protein" food, yet, weight for weight, many cheeses contain more fat than protein—and, as a percentage of total calories, fat is by far the dominant nutrient in cheese unless specifically labeled otherwise. Even "low-fat" cheeses may contain up to 50% of their calories as fat. For further guidance see Food Labeling, page 77.
0	0	38	A, B12	cal, phos	Cheeses are particularly high in saturated fats and many are high in sodium. Hard cheeses are, however, an excellent source of calcium, which is important in helping to prevent osteoporosis, and cheese is one of few good sources of vitamin B2, and a good source of B12 for people who don't eat meat. Hard cheeses also provide iodine in
0	0	50	B2, A, B12	phos	

	food state	portion size	calories	k joules	total fat (g)	% poly	% mono	% sat	protein (g)	carbo (g)	starch (g)	sugars (g)
Cheddar full-fat		2 oz (50 g)	206	854	17	4	27	63	13	0.1	0	0.1
Cheddar low-fat		2 oz (50 g)	131	546	7.5	3	29	63	16	tr	0	tr
Cheese spread full-fat		4 tbsp	138	572	11	3	29	63	6.8	22	0	2.2
Cheese spread half-fat		4 tbsp	94	392	5	3	24	66	8	3.2	0	3.2
Cream cheese full-fat		4 tbsp	220	904	24	3	29	63	1.5	tr	0	tr
Cream cheese light or low-fat		4 tbsp	98	405	7.5	3	24	66	6.0	1.5	0	1.5
Edam		2 oz (50 g)	167	691	13	2	29	62	13	tr	0	tr
Feta		2 oz (50 g)	125	519	10	3	20	67	7.8	0.8	0	0.8
Mascarpone		4 tbsp	225	926	23	3	24	66	1.4	2.4	0	2.4
Mozzarella		2 oz (50 g)	159	665	12.3	3	29	63	11	1.2	tr	1.2
Parmesan Italian	grated	1 tbsp	45	188	3.3	2	29	63	4	tr	0	tr
Processed cheese slice		1	66	273	5	4	28	61	4.2	0.2	0	0.2
Roquefort		2 oz (50 g)	184	770	15	4	29	62	11	1	0	tr
Swiss		2 oz (50 g)	188	787	14	4	27	63	14	1.7	n/k	n/k

special health notes

total fiber (g)	soluble fiber (g)	chol (mg)	useful source of vitamins	good source of minerals
0	0	50	B2, A, B12, niacin	phos
0	0	22	B2, B12, niacin	phos
0	0	33	A, B12	cal, phos
0	0	n/k	B12	cal, phos
0	0	48	A, B12	
0	0	n/k	B12	
0	0	40		cal, iod, phos
0	0	35	B12	cal, phos
0	0	n/k	A, B12	unknown
0	0	44	A, B12	cal, phos
0	0	10	B2, B12	cal
0	0	17	B12	phos
0	0	45	B2, B12	cal, phos
0	0	46	A, B12	cal, phos

reasonable amounts. Vegetarians who want to avoid eating animal products should buy rennet-free cheeses, which may be found in specialty stores.

People with a cows'-milk intolerance can choose all kinds of cheeses—including Cheddar-types and blue cheeses—made from goats' or sheep's milk. These are now widely available in supermarkets as well as at specialist cheese stores (see Allergies).

Cheese is said to be a trigger for migraine in some susceptible people. Migraine sufferers may find they can eat soft cheeses, but may have to avoid mature, hard cheeses, which contain an enzyme called tyramine that may be the key to an attack.

There is some research to show that eating cheese at the end of a meal may help to reduce the formation of plaque and therefore help prevent gum disease.

	food state	portion size	calories	k joules	total fat (g)	% poly	% mono	% sat	protein (g)	carbo (g)	starch (g)	sugars (g)	
Eggs medium		1	69	288	5	12	44	30	6	tr	0	tr	
Eggs large		1	84	349	6.1	12	43	30	7.2	tr	0	tr	
Eggs extra-large		1	98	410	7.2	11	43	29	8.5	tr	0	tr	
Egg large	fried in vegetable oil	1	102	447	7.9	11	43	29	7.8	tr	0	tr	

Condiments, sauces, and other pantry items

	food state	portion size	calories	k joules	total fat (g)	% poly	% mono	% sat	protein (g)	carbo (g)	starch (g)	sugars (g)	
Applesauce		1 tbsp (15 ml)	10	41	tr	0	0	0	0	2.5	0	2.5	
Barbecue sauce		1 tbsp (15 ml)	12	50	0.3	41	44	25	0.3	2	0.1	1.9	
Cranberry sauce		1 tbsp (15 ml)	26	155	0	0	0	0	tr	6.7	n/k	n/k	
Hamburger relish		1 tbsp (15 ml)	19	59	tr	0	0	0	0.1	5.1	n/k	n/k	
Italian salad dressing		1 tbsp (15 ml)	69	285	7.4	25	61	9	0	0.7	0	0.7	
Mayonnaise		1 tbsp (15 ml)	104	426	11	60	23	15	0.2	0.3	0.1	0.2	
Mayonnaise reduced-fat		1 tbsp (15 ml)	43	178	4.2	n/k	n/k	16	0.2	1.2	0.5	0.7	
Pesto		1 tbsp (15 ml)	78	321	7.1	21	47	27	3.1	0.3	0.1	0.2	
Soy sauce		1 tbsp (15 ml)	10	40	0	0	0	0	1.3	1.2	n/k	n/k	

total fiber (g)	soluble fiber (g)	chol (mg)	useful source of vitamins	good source of minerals	special health notes
0	0	179	B12, folate, A, D	iod	Eggs can also significantly contribute toward intake of B2, E, niacin. Iron is present but not well absorbed. Eggs are high in cholesterol, but most experts now agree that this should not pose a problem for anyone whose blood cholesterol levels are normal. The WHO suggests an upper limit of 10 eggs a week, including those eaten in cakes, dressings, desserts, etc. Raw and lightly cooked eggs should be avoided by infants, elderly, pregnant, and invalids, because of the risk of salmonella.
0	0	217	B12, folate, A, D	iod	
0	0	255	B12, folate, A, D	iod	
0	0	217	B12, folate, A, D	iod	Make fried eggs as healthy as possible by using a nonstick griddle or pan just brushed with a good-quality pure vegetable oil. If shallow-frying, drain the eggs thoroughly before serving.
0.2	n/k	0			Fruit- and vegetable-based sauces, such as applesauce, tomato sauce, and relishes, are normally eaten in fairly small quantities and therefore don't make a great contribution to the nutritional content of our diets. However, some contain reasonable amounts of sugar and salt, and if tomato ketchup and tomato sauces are eaten regularly they may make a useful contribution to carotenoid intake.
0.2	n/k	0			
0.2	n/k	0			Condiments based on oil, such as Italian salad dressing, mayonnaise, and pesto, are much higher in calories and fat. They can make a surprising contribution to the calorie and fat content of a meal and should be treated with caution if following a reduced-calorie diet. However, the fats they contain are mostly unsaturated.
0.4	n/k	0			
0	0	0	E		
0	0	11	E		
0	0	3	E		
n/k	n/k	6			
0	0	0			Some sauces, particularly soy, teriyaki, and Worcestershire, are high in salt (though reduced-salt soy sauce is now available) and should be limited for those following a low-sodium diet.

	food state	portion size	calories	k joules	total fat (g)	% poly	% mono	% sat	protein (g)	carbo (g)	starch (g)	sugars (g)
Sweet pickle relish		1 tbsp (15 ml)	21	91	0	0	0	0	0.1	5.4	0.3	5.1
Thousand Island salad dressing		1 tbsp (15 ml)	58	242	5.6	62	15	13	0.2	2.5	tr	2.5
Tomato ketchup		1 tbsp (15 ml)	17	73	0	0	0	0	0.2	4.3	0.2	4.1
Tomato sauce Italian (jar)		1 tbsp (15 ml)	7	30	0.2	50	0	0	0.3	1.0	0.2	0.9
Tomato paste		1 tbsp (20 g)	15	65	0.1	tr	tr	tr	1	2.8	0	2.8
Worcestershire sauce		1 tbsp (15 ml)	10	41	0	0	0	0	0.2	2.3	0.1	2.2
Coconut dried, unsweetened		2 tbsp (1 oz/ 25 g)	171	714	17	2	6	86	1.3	5	0	5
Coconut milk canned		scant ½ cup (3½ fl oz/ 100 ml)	22	95	0.3	tr	tr	67	0.3	4.9	0	4.9
Vinegar		1 tbsp (15 ml)	3	13	0	0	0	0	0.1	0.1	0	0.1

Drinks, alcoholic

	food state	portion size	calories	k joules	total fat (g)	% poly	% mono	% sat	protein (g)	carbo (g)	starch (g)	sugars (g)
Beer standard		1¼ cups (10 fl oz/ 275 ml)	112	469	0	0	0	0	0.8	10	n/k	n/k
Beer light		1¼ cups (10 fl oz/ 275 ml)	77	322	0	0	0	0	0.6	3.5	n/k	n/k
Bloody Mary		⅔ cup (5 fl oz/ 150 ml)	116	484	0	0	0	0	0	4.8	n/k	n/k
Cider hard		1¼ cups (10 fl oz/ 275 ml)	99	418	0	0	0	0	tr	7.1	0	7.1

total fiber (g)	soluble fiber (g)	chol (mg)	useful source of vitamins	good source of minerals	special health notes
0.2	n/k	0			See entry under Soy Sauce, pages 272–3.
0.3	0	4.1			
0.1	n/k	0			
n/k	n/k	0			
0.6	n/k	0	b-carotene, E	potas, cop	Tomato paste is high in lycopene, the pigment that helps prevent cancer and heart disease.
0	0	0			
n/k	n/k	0		manga	Coconut is one of the few plant foods to contain a large proportion of its fats as saturated fat. However, there is some evidence that the saturated fat in coconut doesn't act like the saturated fat in animal and dairy products, so it may be, therefore, that coconut fat isn't such a risk factor for heart disease.
tr	tr	0		manga	
0	0	0			Vinegar is often used as an anti-inflammatory by arthritis sufferers, though there is no real proof that this works. Should be avoided by people with a yeast allergy.
0	0	0			Beer contains phytochemicals, which have been shown to help protect against heart disease (see also Spirits and Wine overleaf). It aids digestion by encouraging acid production in the stomach.
0	0	0			Light beer may not have the same protective effect as alcoholic beers.
n/k	n/k	0			The tomato juice in a Bloody Mary could also add vitamin A and lycopenes to your diet.
0	0	0			Hard cider is found in some areas. It is produced by fermenting apples.

	food state	portion size	calories	k joules	total fat (g)	% poly	% mono	% sat	protein (g)	carbo (g)	starch (g)	sugars (g)
Liqueur coffee and cream		2 tbsp (1 fl oz/ 25 ml)	101	425	4.8	0.2	1.4	3	0.8	6.5	n/k	n/k
Liqueur mint		2 tbsp (1 fl oz/ 25 ml)	124	518	0	0	0	0	0	12	n/k	n/k
Port		1/4 cup (2 fl oz/ 50 ml)	79	328	0	0	0	0	0.1	6.0	0	6.0
Sherry medium		1/4 cup (2 fl oz/ 50 ml)	58	241	0	0	0	0	0.1	3.0	0	3.0
Spirits all kinds		2 tbsp (1 fl oz/ 25 ml)	48	197	0	0	0	0	tr	tr	0	tr
Stout Guinness		11/4 cups (10 fl oz/ 275 ml)	83	347	0	0	0	0	1.1	4.1	0	4.1
Wine white, dry		2/3 cup (5 fl oz/ 140 ml)	92	385	0	0	0	0	0.1	0.8	0	0.8
Wine white, sweet		2/3 cup (5 fl oz/ 140 ml)	132	552	0	0	0	0	0.3	8.3	0	8.3
Wine red		2/3 cup (5 fl oz/ 140 ml)	95	396	0	0	0	0	0.1	0.3	0	0.3
Wine cooler		11/4 cups (10 fl oz/ 275 ml)	164	683	0	0	0	0	0	23	0	23

Drinks, non-alcoholic

	food state	portion size	calories	k joules	total fat (g)	% poly	% mono	% sat	protein (g)	carbo (g)	starch (g)	sugars (g)
Coffee instant		1 tsp	2	6	tr	tr	tr	tr	0.3	0.1	0.1	0
Coffee freshly ground	black	scant 1 cup (63/4 fl oz 190 ml)	4	15	tr	tr	tr	tr	0.4	0.4	0	0
Cocoa	made with whole milk	scant 1 cup (63/4 fl oz 190 ml)	171	716	7.8	2.6	30	62	6.5	20	0.6	20

total fiber (g)	soluble fiber (g)	chol (mg)	useful source of vitamins	good source of minerals	special health notes
n/k	n/k	4.7			
tr	n/k	n/k			
0	0	0			High levels of congeners, so more likely to produce hangover than "pale" alcoholic drinks, such as vodka and white wine. Also more likely to trigger migraine. May contain same flavonoids as Red Wine (below).
0	0	0			
0	0	0			Spirits taken in moderate amounts offer protection against heart disease (see also Beer and Wine).
0	0	0	niacin		Stouts and dark beers contain more of the protective flavonoids than light-colored beers.
0	0	0			Red wines contain higher levels of flavonoids than any other alcoholic drink, offering protection against heart and arterial disease, probably because their antioxidant effect helps keep arteries free from "furring." Red wines also help prevent blood clotting and help increase "good" HDL blood cholesterol. Optimum level appears to be a minimum of 1 drink and a maximum of 4 for men, and a minimum of 1 drink and a maximum of 2 for women, on 5–6 days a week. Also appears to protect against Alzheimer's disease in older people, and may help protect against peptic ulcers. White wines contain slightly lower levels of flavonoids and polyphenols, providing moderate protection against heart disease.
0	0	0			
0	0	0		iron	
0	0	0			
0	0	0			Coffee is a mild laxative and diuretic. It contains caffeine, which is a stimulant, and can rob the body of calcium. It is also a common cause of indigestion. Coffee has been shown to speed recovery from colds. Both ordinary and decaffeinated coffee contain antioxidants, which protect against heart disease, cancer, and aging. But strong coffee made in a cafetière or percolator, or boiled without filtering, has been shown to raise blood cholesterol; filtered and instant coffees don't.
0	0	0			
tr	0	23	B2, B12		Cocoa powder contains antioxidant flavonoids; an average cup of cocoa will have almost the same antioxidant strength as a glass of red wine.

	food state	portion size	calories	k joules	total fat (g)	% poly	% mono	% sat	protein (g)	carbo (g)	starch (g)	sugars (g)	
Instant low-calorie cocoa mix		1 packet	47	161	0.5	3	31	54	3.7	8.5	n/k	2.5	
Tea	black	scant 1 cup (6³/₄ fl oz/ 190 ml)	1	5	tr	tr	tr	tr	0.2	tr	0	tr	
Cola		1¹/₂ cups (12 fl oz/ 330 ml)	142	574	0	0	0	0	tr	36	0	36	
Diet cola		1¹/₂ cups (12 fl oz/ 330 ml)	1.3	5	0	0	0	0	tr	tr	0	tr	
Lemon/lime soda		1¹/₂ cups (12 fl oz/ 330 ml)	137	319	0	0	0	0	tr	35	0	20	
Orange drink		1¹/₂ cups (12 fl oz/ 330 ml)	54	229	0	0	0	0	tr	14	0	14	
Apple juice/ sweet cider		scant (¹/₂ cup/ 100 ml)	38	164	0.1	100	0	0	0.1	10	0	10	
Cranberry juice		scant (¹/₂ cup/ 100 ml)	57	238	0	0	0	0	0	14	0	14	
Grape juice		scant (¹/₂ cup/ 100 ml)	46	196	0.1	tr	tr	tr	0.3	12	0	12	
Grapefruit juice		scant (¹/₂ cup/ 100 ml)	33	140	0.1	tr	tr	tr	0.4	8.3	0	8.3	
Orange juice		scant (¹/₂ cup/ 100 ml)	36	153	0.1	tr	tr	tr	0.5	8.8	0	8.8	
Pineapple juice		scant (¹/₂ cup/ 100 ml)	41	177	0.1	tr	tr	tr	0.3	11	0	11	
Tomato juice		scant (¹/₂ cup/ 100 ml)	14	62	tr	tr	tr	tr	0.8	3	tr	3	
Vegetable juice		scant (¹/₂ cup/ 100 ml)	21	88	0.5	n/k	n/k	n/k	0.8	3.3	0.4	2.9	

total fiber (g)	soluble fiber (g)	chol (mg)	useful source of vitamins	good source of minerals	special health notes
0.3	n/k	1.2		manga	See entry under Cocoa, pages 276–7.
0	0	0			Black and green tea contain powerful antioxidants, flavonols called quercetin, which may reduce risk of stroke, some cancers, and heart disease. Tea has less caffeine than coffee, but still is a mild stimulant.
0	0	0			Cola contains caffeine, a stimulant (see Coffee). Apart from that, it contains little except a lot of sugar and various flavorings.
0	0	0			Diet drinks are high in artificial sweeteners; it is wise to limit intake of these to 1 a day, particularly if following a weight-loss diet containing several other reduced-sugar products.
0	0	0			
0	0	0			Most commercial fruit drinks contain little real fruit juice, but consist mainly of sugar and/or sweeteners, flavorings, and colorings. Check label for juice content.
tr	tr	0	C		Some commercial brands contain added vitamin C, because apples are not one of the better fruit sources of C.
n/k	n/k	0	C		Compounds in cranberry juice are said to help prevent, and relieve, attacks of cystitis by preventing bacteria adhering to cells in bladder walls and urinary tract.
0	0	0	C		Red grape juice contains antioxidant compounds on a similar level to red wine, as well as vitamin C, another antioxidant.
tr	tr	0	C		Good source of vitamin C. If taken with some medicines, it can lead to toxicity from inhibition of liver mechanism—check with doctor if taking any medications for blood pressure, Aids, anxiety, or hay fever.
0.1	0.1	0	C		Rich in vitamin C. Freshly squeezed orange juice is preferable to commercial brands, as fresh juice contains bioflavonoids that act together with vitamin C as antioxidants.
tr	tr	0	C	manga	Pineapple juice contains the enzyme bromelain, which helps to break down protein in the diet.
0.6	n/k	0	C, E, carotenoids	potas	Tomato juice is rich in lycopene, shown to be a powerful protectant against some cancers. Research shows a 50% reduction in heart attacks in men who eat tomato-rich diet. Also rich in beta-carotene, an antioxidant thought to help combat heart disease. There is evidence that tomatoes exacerbate rheumatoid arthritis. For other vegetable juices, see individual vegetables, but remember juicing removes most of the fiber.
1	n/k	0	C, carotenoids	potas	

	food state	portion size	calories	k joules	total fat (g)	% poly	% mono	% sat	protein (g)	carbo (g)	starch (g)	sugars (g)	

Fats and oils

	food state	portion size	calories	k joules	total fat (g)	% poly	% mono	% sat	protein (g)	carbo (g)	starch (g)	sugars (g)	
Butter		2 tbsp (25 g)	184	758	20	3.4	25	67	0.1	tr	0	tr	
Lard		2 tbsp (25 g)	223	916	25	10	44	41	tr	0	0	0	
Margarine regular		2 tbsp (25 g)	185	760	20	11	41	44	0.1	0.3	0	0.3	
Margarine 60% fat		2 tbsp (25 g)	135	565	15	12	64	20	tr	0	0	0	
Margarine 40% fat		2 tbsp (25 g)	86	36	9.7	41	3.7	15	tr	tr	tr	tr	
Margarine corn or sunflower oil		2 tbsp (25 g)	180	767	20	44	32	21	tr	0.2	0	0.2	
Margarine olive oil blend		2 tbsp (25 g)	137	571	15	18	54	21	0.1	0.3	0	0.3	
Shortening vegetable		2 tbsp (25 g)	221	923	24	34	30	30	0		0	0	
Suet animal		2 tbsp (25 g)	224	936	25	1	37	56	0.2	0	0	0	
Canola oil		2 tbsp (25 g)	225	924	25	29	59	6	tr	0	0	0	
Corn oil		2 tbsp (25 g)	225	924	25	51	30	14	tr	0	0	0	
Peanut oil		2 tbsp (25 g)	225	924	25	31	44	20	tr	0	0	0	
Olive oil		2 tbsp (25 g)	225	924	25	10	73	14	tr	0	0	0	

total fiber (g)	soluble fiber (g)	chol (mg)	useful source of vitamins	good source of minerals	special health notes
o	o	58	A, D		Butter is high in saturated fat, which is linked with heart disease.
o	o	23			Lard is high in saturated fat.
o	o	4	A, D, E		Margarine is lower in calories and fat than butter. Usually made from water blended with vegetable fats or butter. May contain trans fats, now believed by some to be linked with heart disease even more than saturated fat, though some formulations have now reduced trans fats to a minimum and will therefore contain a lower percentage than the averages given. Many margarines are made up of different fats and percentage of fat types will vary. Low-fat margarines have a high percentage of water and some very-low-fat margarines can be more than half water.
o	o	o	A, D, E		
o	o	o	A, D, E		
o	o	1	A, D, E		High in polyunsaturated fats. Higher vitamin E content than butter or low-fat spreads.
o	o	tr	A, D, E		This spread is high in monounsaturates; many experts now believe that these are the healthiest of all the types of fat, as they can lower blood cholesterol levels. For more information see pages 16–19.
o	o	o			Vegetable shortening contains high levels of trans fats.
o	o	15			Animal suet high in saturated fat.
o	o	o	E		All plant oils are a good source of unsaturated fats and vitamin E, although all do still contain some saturated fat. Corn, safflower, sesame, sunflower, walnut, and blended vegetable oils are highest in polyunsaturated fats. Olive, canola, and peanut oils are highest in monounsaturated fats. All oils are extremely high in calories and intake should be moderate in people attempting to lose weight or keep weight off—but it should not be banned, as unsaturated oils are now known to have health benefits, including lowering of blood cholesterol, and are a good source of the antioxidant vitamin E. For more detail on oils and fats in the diet, see pages 15–19.
o	o	o	E		
o	o	o	E		
o	o	o	E		

	food state	portion size	calories	k joules	total fat (g)	% poly	% mono	% sat	protein (g)	carbo (g)	starch (g)	sugars (g)	
Safflower oil		2 tbsp (25 g)	225	924	25	74	12	10	tr	0	0	0	
Sesame oil		2 tbsp (25 g)	225	924	25	44	38	15	0.1	0	0	0	
Sunflower oil		2 tbsp (25 g)	225	924	25	63	20	12	tr	0	0	0	
Vegetable oil blended		2 tbsp (25 g)	225	924	25	48	36	10	tr	0	0	0	
Walnut oil		2 tbsp (25 g)	225	924	25	70	16	9	tr	0	0	0	

Fish and seafood

	food state	portion size	calories	k joules	total fat (g)	% poly	% mono	% sat	protein (g)	carbo (g)	starch (g)	sugars (g)	
Cod		3¹/₂ oz (100 g)	80	337	0.7	43	14	14	18	0	0	0	
Cod	deep-fried in batter	3¹/₂ oz (100 g)	247	1,031	15	24	45	27	16	12	12	tr	
Fish fillet breaded	baked	3¹/₂ oz (100 g)	188	786	11	15	15	50	11	13	13	0.1	
Fish sticks		4	200	838	8.9	26	38	32	14	17	17	tr	
Haddock smoked fillet		3¹/₂ oz (100 g)	81	345	0.6	33	17	17	19	0	0	0	
★ **Herring fillet**		3¹/₂ oz (100 g)	190	791	13	21	42	25	18	0	0	0	
Kipper fillet	broiled	3¹/₂ oz (100 g)	255	1,060	19	22	53	16	20	0	0	0	
★ **Mackerel fillet**	fresh	3¹/₂ oz (100 g)	220	914	16	21	49	21	19	0	0	0	

total fiber (g)	soluble fiber (g)	chol (mg)	useful source of vitamins	good source of minerals	special health notes
0	0	0	E		See entry under Canola Oil, pages 280–1.
0	0	0	E		
0	0	0	E		
0	0	0	E		
0	0	0	E		
0	0	46	niacin, B12	phos, iod, sel, potas	Plain-cooked white fish, such as cod, haddock, or sole, is a good low-fat, low-calorie source of protein, vitamins, and minerals, and ideal for dieters. (Any plain white fish not in the list has a similar nutrient value to cod.)
0.5	n/k	n/k	niacin, B12	phos, iod, sel, potas	Oily fish, such as herring, mackerel, salmon, and bluefish, are one of the few nutritional sources of the Omega-3 polyunsaturated fatty acids, which help to prevent heart disease and strokes and may help to prevent some cancers and help minimize the symptoms of arthritis.
0.1	0.5	n/k	niacin, B12	phos, iod, sel, potas	Latest research shows that just one portion of fish per week can help prevent heart attacks. Some research indicates a link between a lack of Omega-3 fatty acids and depression. Most fishes are also a good source of the antioxidant mineral, selenium. For more detail about
0.7	n/k	35	niacin, B12	phos, iod, sel, potas	Omega-3 fats and a chart showing the amount in each fish, turn to Section One, page 16.
0	0	36	niacin, B6, B12	phos, iod, sel, potas	Smoked fish, such as kippers, may be carcinogenic due to the smoking process.
0	0	50	niacin, B6, B12, D	phos, iod, sel, potas	
0	0	0	niacin, B6, B12, D	phos, iod, sel, potas	
0	0	54	niacin, B6, B12, D	phos, iod, sel, potas	

	food state	portion size	calories	k joules	total fat (g)	% poly	% mono	% sat	protein (g)	carbo (g)	starch (g)	sugars (g)
Pike		3 1/2 oz (100 g)	119	460	1.6	35	23	20	24.5	0	0	0
★ **Salmon** fresh fillet		3 1/2 oz (100 g)	180	750	11	28	40	9	20	0	0	0
Salmon canned		3 1/2 oz (100 g)	153	644	6.6	29	36	20	24	0	0	0
Salmon smoked		2 oz (50 g average serving)	71	299	2.3	26	39	17	13	0	0	0
★ **Sardines** fresh	whole	3	281	1,176	16	29	36	20	21	0	0	0
Sardines canned in oil	drained	3 1/2 oz (100 g)	220	918	14	36	34	21	23	0	0	0
Swordfish steak		3 1/2 oz (100 g)	109	458	4.1	27	39	22	18	0	0	0
Trout fresh		1 medium (8 oz/ 225 g)	281	1,184	12	33	34	9	44	0	0	0
Tuna fresh		3 1/2 oz (100 g)	136	573	4.6	35	22	22	24	0	0	0
Tuna canned in brine	drained	3 1/2 oz (100 g)	99	422	0.6	33	17	33	24	0	0	0
Tuna canned in oil	drained	3 1/2 oz (100 g)	189	794	9	53	26	17	27	0	0	0
Whitebait	deep-fried	3 1/2 oz (100 g)	525	2,174	48	n/k	n/k	n/k	20	5.3	5.2	0.1
Crabmeat		3 1/2 oz (100 g)	128	535	5.5	29	27	13	20	tr	tr	tr
Lobster		1/2 average (9 oz/ 250 g)	93	393	1.5	33	20	20	20	tr	tr	tr

total fiber (g)	soluble fiber (g)	chol (mg)	useful source of vitamins	good source of minerals	special health notes
0	0	110	B2, niacin, B6, B12	phos, sel, potas	See entry under Cod, pages 282–3.
0	0	50	B1, niacin, B6, B12, D, E	phos, potas, sel, iod	
0	0	20	niacin, B12, D, E	cal, phos, potas, sel, iod	
0	0	18	niacin, B6, B12	phos, sel, potas	
0	0	92	B2, niacin, B6, B12, D, pant ac	cal, phos, potas, sel, iod, iron, magnes	
0	0	65	B2, niacin, B12, D, pant ac	cal, phos, potas, iron, sel, iod, zinc	
0	0	41	niacin, B6, B12	phos, potas, sel	
0	0	151	B1, B2, niacin, B6, B12, D, E, pant	potas, phos, sel, iod	
0	0	28	niacin, B6, B12, D	potas, phos, cop, sel, iod	
0	0	51	niacin, B6, B12, D	phos, potas, sel	
0	0	50	niacin, B6, B12, D, E	phos, potas, sel	
0.2	n/k	n/k		cal, phos, cop, sel, iod	
0	0	72	B2, niacin	potas, phos, zinc, cop, magnes	Plainly cooked shellfish is a low-fat, low-calorie source of protein, many minerals including the antioxidant selenium, zinc (which is not easy to come by in the average diet), and magnesium, as well as some B group vitamins. The shrimp family is high in cholesterol and sodium. Only crabmeat and mussels contain significant amounts of Omega-3 fatty acids.
0	0	100	niacin, B12, E	phos, zinc, cop, sel, iod, potas	

	food state	portion size	calories	k joules	total fat (g)	% poly	% mono	% sat	protein (g)	carbo (g)	starch (g)	sugars (g)
⭐ Mussels	shelled	3¹/₂ oz (100 g)	104	440	2.7	3.7	15	19	17	3.5	tr	tr
Oysters	shelled	3¹/₂ oz (100 g)	65	275	1.3	31	15	15	11	2.7	tr	tr
Scallops	shelled	3¹/₂ oz (100 g)	118	501	1.4	29	7	29	23	3.4	tr	tr
Scampi	deep-fried in breadcrumbs	3¹/₂ oz (100 g)	237	991	14	47	38	10	9.4	21	21	tr
Shrimp	shelled	3¹/₂ oz (100 g)	99	418	0.9	22	22	22	23	0	0	0
Squid		3¹/₂ oz (100 g)	81	344	1.7	35	12	24	15	1.2	tr	tr

Fruit

	food state	portion size	calories	k joules	total fat (g)	% poly	% mono	% sat	protein (g)	carbo (g)	starch (g)	sugars (g)
⭐ Apple		1	47	199	0.1	100	0	0	0.4	12	tr	12
Apple cooking		1	60	257	0.2	100	0	0	0.5	15	tr	15
Apricot fresh		3¹/₂ oz (100 g)	29	123	0.1	tr	tr	tr	0.8	6.6	0	6.6
⭐ Apricot dried ready-to-eat		¹/₂ cup (2 oz/ 50 g)	79	337	0.3	n/k	n/k	n/k	2.0	18.2	0	18.2
Banana		1 medium	95	403	0.3	33	tr	33	1.2	23	2.3	21
⭐ Black currants		²/₃ cup (3¹/₂ oz/ 100 g)	28	121	tr	tr	tr	0.4	0.9	6.6	0	6.6
Blackberries		²/₃ cup (3¹/₂ oz/ 100 g)	25	104	0.2	50	50	tr	0.9	5.1	0	5.1

total fiber (g)	soluble fiber (g)	chol (mg)	useful source of vitamins	good source of minerals	special health notes
0	0	58	B2, niacin, B12, folate	iron, zinc, cop, sel, iod, phos, manga	See entry under Crabmeat, pages 284–5.
0	0	57	niacin, B12, D	cal, magnes, phos, potas, zinc, cop, sel, iod, manga	
0	0	47	niacin, B12,	potas, phos, zinc, sel, iod	
n/k	n/k	110	niacin, B12	cal, phos, cop, sel, iod, manga	
0	0	280	niacin, B12, E	potas, phos, magnes, zinc, sel, iod	
0	0	225	niacin, B6, B12, E	potas, phos, sel, iod	
1.8	0.7	0	C	potas	Vitamin C content varies considerably with variety of apple and its freshness. Some research shows that the flavonoid quercetin in apples can help lower blood cholesterol. Useful for dieters, as apples have a low glycemic index and keep hunger pangs at bay longer than many other fruits.
2.7	1	0	C	potas	
1.6	0.9	0	b-carotene		Apricots have a low glycemic index and are very high in the antioxidant beta-carotene.
3.1	2.0	0	b-carotene	potas, iron, manga	
1.1	0.7	0	B6, C	potas, manga	
3.6	1.6	0	C, b-carotene	potas	Black currants are one of the richest sources of vitamin C, containing around 200 mg per 3 1/2 oz (100 g) fruit—that is, more than three times the RDI for adults. Also contain the anticancer carotenoid lutein.
3.1	1	0	C, folate, E	manga	Blackberries are one of few fruits to contain significant amounts of the antioxidant vitamin E, and they contain the flavonoid ellagic acid, which may block cancer cells.

	food state	portion size	calories	k joules	total fat (g)	% poly	% mono	% sat	protein (g)	carbo (g)	starch (g)	sugars (g)
Blueberries		²/₃ cup (3¹/₂ oz/ 100 g)	30	128	0.2	50	50	tr	0.6	6.9	0	6.9
⭐ **Cherries**	pits and stems removed	²/₃ cup (3¹/₂ oz/ 100 g)	39	168	0.1	tr	tr	tr	0.7	9.5	0	9.5
Coconut shredded	packed	³/₄ cup (3¹/₂ oz/ 100 g)	351	1,446	36	2	6	86	3.2	3.7	0	3.7
Cranberries		1 cup (3¹/₂ oz/ 100 g)	15	65	0.1	tr	tr	tr	0.4	3.4	0	3.4
Currants dried		¹/₃ cup (2 oz/ 50 g)	134	570	0.2	n/k	n/k	n/k	1.1	34	0	3.4
Dates fresh		100 g	107	456	0.1	tr	tr	tr	1.3	27	0	27
Dates dried	pitted	6 (2 oz/ 50 g)		135	576	0.1	0	50	50	1.6	34	0
Figs fresh		2 medium (3¹/₂ oz/ 100 g)	43	185	0.3	33	33	33	1.3	9.5	0	9.5
Figs dried		¹/₂ cup (2 oz/ 50 g)	114	484	0.8	n/k	n/k	n/k	1.8	27	0	27
Grapefruit		¹/₂	24	101	0.1	tr	tr	tr	0.6	5.4	0	5.4
⭐ **Grapes**		²/₃ cup (3¹/₂ oz/ 100 g)	60	257	0.1	tr	tr	tr	0.4	15	0	15
⭐ **Kiwi fruit**		1 average	29	124	0.3	n/k	n/k	n/k	0.7	0.4	0.2	6.2
Lemon		juice of 1	1	6	tr	tr	tr	tr	0.1	0.3	0	0.3
Lime		juice of 1	1	4	tr	tr	tr	tr	0	0.2	0	0.2

total fiber (g)	soluble fiber (g)	chol (mg)	useful source of vitamins	good source of minerals	special health notes
1.8	0.5	0	C	manga	
0.7	0.4	0	C		Cherries contain ellagic acid, a phytochemical that may fight cancer.
7.3	1	0		potas	Coconuts are one of the few fruits that is high in saturated fats, though some research indicates that the saturated fat it contains is not the "harmful" type founds in animal and dairy fats.
3	1.1	0	C	manga	Cranberries are often used to prevent or treat cystitis and urinary tract infections (see Cranberry Juice).
0.9	0.5	0		potas, cop, manga	
1.5	0.4	0	C	potas	
2	0.6	0		potas	
1.5	0.9	0	b-carotene		
3.8	2	0		potas, iron, manga	
1	0.7	0	C		Pink grapefruit contains beta-carotene.
0.7	0.4	0		potas	Red grape varieties contain powerful polyphenols, the same as those in red wine. These are antioxidants and have a positive effect in reducing heart disease. Also contain ellagic acid (see Cherries).
1.1	0.5	0	C	potas	Kiwi fuit is richer in vitamin C than oranges, an average fruit containing about 40 mg which is two-thirds of a day's RDI for adults.
0	0	0	C		As with all citrus fruit, lemons are a good source of vitamin C.
0	0	0	C		

	food state	portion size	calories	k joules	total fat (g)	% poly	% mono	% sat	protein (g)	carbo (g)	starch (g)	sugars (g)
★ Mango		1	107	457	0.3	n/k	n/k	n/k	1.4	26	0.6	25
★ Melon cantaloupe		1 7 oz (200 g) slice	26	110	0.2	tr	tr	tr	0.8	5.6	0	5.6
Nectarine		1	60	257	0.2	tr	tr	tr	2.1	14	0	14
★ Orange		1	60	253	0.2	tr	tr	tr	1.8	14	0	14
★ Papaya		1	74	319	0.3	tr	tr	tr	1.1	18	0	18
Passion fruit		1	5	23	0.1	33	33	33	0.4	0.9	0	0.9
Peach		1	36	155	0.1	tr	tr	tr	1.1	8.2	0	8.2
Pear		1	64	270	0.2	tr	tr	tr	0.5	16	0	16
Pineapple	fresh	2 rings (3¹/₂ oz/ 100 g)	41	178	0.2	50	50	tr	0.4	10	0	10
Plums		2	34	145	0.1	tr	tr	tr	0.5	8.3	0	8.3
Prunes	pitted	5 (2 oz/ 50 g)	71	301	0.2	tr	50	50	1.3	17	0	17
Raisins		¹/₃ cup (2 oz/ 50 g)	136	580	0.2	n/k	n/k	n/k	1	35	0	35
Raisins golden		¹/₃ cup (2 oz/ 50 g)	138	586	0.2	tr	tr	tr	1.4	35	0	35
★ Raspberries red		generous ³/₄ cup (3¹/₂ oz/ 100 g)	25	109	0.3	33	33	33	1.4	4.6	0	4.6

total fiber (g)	soluble fiber (g)	chol (mg)	useful source of vitamins	good source of minerals	special health notes
4.9	3	0	b-carotene, niacin, C, E	manga, potas	Mangoes are best fruit source of antioxidant carotenoids. Extremely rich in fiber, particularly soluble fiber, important in keeping blood cholesterol low. Also one of the few good fruit sources of vitamin E.
1.4	0.4	0	b-carotene, C	potas	Orange- and red-fleshed melons, such as cantaloupe and watermelon, contain good amounts of beta-carotene, but pale-fleshed varieties do not.
1.8	0.9	0	C	potas	
2.7	1.8	0	folate, C	potas	One of the least expensive fruit sources of vitamin C, providing the RDI for adults in one average fruit (about 6 mg per orange). Rich in flavonoids such as rutin that have an antioxidant effect.
4.7	2.8	0	carotenoids, C	potas	A papaya is rich in beta-carotene and fibers. Particularly good source of soluble fiber (see Mango) and contains enzymes that aid digestion.
0.5	0.1	0	C, carotenoids		
1.6	0.8	0	C		
3.5	1.1	0	C	potas	
1.2	0.1	0	C	manga	A pineapple contains the enzyme bromelain, which helps the digestion by aiding the breakdown of protein.
1.5	1	0	b-carotene	potas	Plums are a good source of fibers, and red-skinned varieties contain useful amounts of beta-carotene.
2.8	2	0		potas, iron	Laxative effect due to compounds that stimulate the bowel. Regular intake has been shown to reduce LDL cholesterol in the blood. May also protect against colon cancer. Good source of fiber and iron.
1	0.5	0		potas, iron	
1	0.4	0		potas, iron	
2.5	0.7	0	folate, C	manga	Raspberries are one of the best fresh fruit sources of fiber.

	food state	portion size	calories	k joules	total fat (g)	% poly	% mono	% sat	protein (g)	carbo (g)	starch (g)	sugars (g)
Rhubarb	raw, chopped	generous ³/4 cup (3¹/2 oz/ 100 g)	7	32	0.1	tr	tr	tr	0.9	0.8	0	0.8
Strawberries		heaping ²/3 cup (3¹/2 oz/ 100 g)	27	113	0.1	tr	tr	tr	0.8	6	0	6
Tangerine		1	23	99	0.1	tr	tr	tr	0.5	5.4	0	5.4

Meat, poultry, and game

	food state	portion size	calories	k joules	total fat (g)	% poly	% mono	% sat	protein (g)	carbo (g)	starch (g)	sugars (g)
Bacon Canadian	raw	3¹/2 oz (100 g)	157	567	7	9	46	31	19	0	0	0
Bacon cured	raw	3¹/2 oz (100 g)	556	2,326	57.5	12	46	37	8.7	0	0	0
Bacon cured	fried	3¹/2 oz (100 g)	576	2,410	50	5	47	36	31	0	0	0
Beef lean ground chunk	raw	scant 1 cup (3¹/2 oz/ 100 g)	137	934	5	4	38	36	19	0	0	0
Beef regular, ground	raw	scant 1 cup (3¹/2 oz/ 100 g)	310	728	27	4	42	40	16	0	0	0
Beef	roasted, lean meat only	3¹/2 oz (100 g)	175	736	5.1	4	45	41	32	0	0	0
Beef sirloin steak	raw, lean only	3¹/2 oz (100 g)	125	526	4.1	7	42	42	22	0	0	0
Hamburger	broiled	¹/4 lb (115 g)	254	1,057	19	3	46	45	21	0.1	0	0.1
Beef pastrami		3¹/2 oz (100 g)	350	905	29	3	50	38	17.2	3.1	n/k	n/k
Crocodile fillet	cooked	3¹/2 oz (100 g)	160	674	4	23	48	30	31	0	0	0

total fiber (g)	soluble fiber (g)	chol (mg)	useful source of vitamins	good source of minerals	special health notes
1.4	0.5	0		cal, potas	Contains good amounts of calcium, but the oxalic acid content of rhubarb hinders its absorption, and also hinders absorption of iron. Excellent laxative.
1.1	0.5	0	C		Strawberries are excellent source of vitamin C, with more than the RDI for adults (77 mg) in 3^1/$_2$ oz (100 g) of fruit. Also contains ellagic acid (see Cherries).
0.8	0.5	0	C		As with all citrus fruits, tangerines are good source of vitamin C, containing approximately 20 mg per average fruit, or one-third the RDI for adults.
0	0	50	B1, niacin, B6, B12, pant ac	potas, phos	Bacon, like most meats, is a good source of B vitamins and an important source of zinc, which helps to boost the immune system. Surprisingly, bacon contains more monounsaturated fat than saturated. Bacon can be an extremely high-fat food, especially if fried, but if well trimmed and broiled or pan-fried, is a good source of protein. Don't cook bacon to the point where it is burned, as the burned bits are carcinogenic. All bacon (and deli meats) are high in sodium, even the kinds labeled "reduced-salt," and should be avoided by people with high blood pressure or who have been asked to follow a low-salt diet by their doctor.
0	0	67	B1, niacin, B6, B12, pant ac	potas, phos	
0	0	65	B1, niacin, B6, B12, pant ac	potas, phos	
0	0	60	niacin, B6, B12, B2	potas, phos, zinc, iron	Beef, like most meats, is a good source of B vitamins, zinc, and iron. Lean cuts are not all that high in fat—just over one-quarter of lean beef's calories are fat calories. Of that, less than half is saturated. The World Cancer Research Fund says that red meat intake should be limited to 80 g a day. A recent International consensus study has suggested a strong link between meat eating and heart disease. American studies link grilled red meat with stomach cancer, and UK studies have shown increased production of carcinogenic nitrosamines in the intestines of people who eat large amounts of meat. Ground beef, including burgers, should be well cooked so that no pink meat remains, to prevent food poisoning such as E-coli, but don't cook meat until charred as the charred portion is carcinogenic. For further detail on red meat and your health, see pages 71–72 and 80–81.
0	0	85	niacin, B6, B12, B2	potas, phos, zinc, iron	
0	0	68	B2, niacin, B6, B12	potas, phos, zinc, iron	
0	0	59	B2, niacin, B6, B12	potas, phos, zinc, iron	
0	0	59	niacin, B6, B12	potas, phos, zinc, iron	
0	0	93	niacin, B12	zinc, iron	Pastrami is high in sodium, so it should be limited by anyone following a low-sodium diet.
0	0	n/k	n/k	n/k	Crocodile meat is very low in fat and high in protein, and a good alternative to higher-fat meats.

	food state	portion size	calories	k joules	total fat (g)	% poly	% mono	% sat	protein (g)	carbo (g)	starch (g)	sugars (g)	
Ham steak fat removed	broiled	3¹/₂ oz (100 g)	172	726	5.2	10	42	37	31	0	0	0	
Ham, cooked extra-lean		3¹/₂ oz (100 g)	107	451	3.3	15	46	33	18	1	0	1	
Ham Parma ham		2 oz (50 g)	111	466	6.5	n/k	n/k	33	13.5	tr	0	tr	
Lamb loin chop, trimmed	broiled	1	150	624	7.5	6	37	46	29	0	0	0	
Lamb leg	roasted, lean only	3¹/₂ oz (100 g)	203	853	9.4	6	42	40	30	0	0	0	
Lamb shoulder	roasted	3¹/₂ oz (100 g)	235	982	14	4	39	46	28	0	0	0	
Kidney lamb's	fat removed	1	91	385	2.6	19	23	35	17	0	0	0	
Liver lamb's		3¹/₂ oz (100 g)	137	575	6.2	15	29	27	20	0	0	0	
Ostrich	cooked	3¹/₂ oz (100 g)	188	794	3.4	32	35	32	39	0	0	0	
Pork tenderloin	raw	3¹/₂ oz (100 g)	122	514	4	8	45	40	22	0	0	0	
Pork leg	roasted, lean only	3¹/₂ oz (100 g)	185	779	5.1	14	41	35	35	0	0	0	
Pork chitterlings	roasted	3¹/₂ oz (100 g)	303	2,280	29	55	33	35	10.3	0	0	0	
Pork chop, loin, lean	broiled	1	220	929	7.7	16	16	34	38	0	0	0	
Pork Bologna		3¹/₂ oz (100 g)	247	1,033	20	10	49	36	15	tr	tr	n/k	

total fiber (g)	soluble fiber (g)	chol (mg)	useful source of vitamins	good source of minerals	special health notes
0	0	19	B1, B2, niacin, B6	potas, phos, zinc, cop	See entry under Bacon, pages 292–3.
0	0	58	B1, niacin, B6, B12,	potas	Extra-lean ham is a good source of fairly low-fat protein. All ham contains reasonably high amounts of sodium, due to the curing process.
tr	n/k	n/k	n/k	n/k	
0	0	96	B2, niacin, B6, B12, pant ac	potas, phos, iron, zinc	Lamb contains similar levels of saturated fat to beef and pork, but contains around twice as much total fat as either. Even the lean cuts of lamb, such as leg, are comparatively high in fat. Like most meat, however, lamb is a good source of B vitamins and iron and zinc. See health notes for Beef for general notes on red meat, and see also Heart Disease and Cancer in Section Two.
0	0	100	B2, niacin, B6, B12, pant ac	potas, phos, iron, zinc	
0	0	100	B2, niacin, B6, B12, pant ac	potas, phos, iron, zinc	
0	0	315	B1, B2, niacin, B6, B12, pant ac, biotin	potas, phos, iron, zinc, cop, sel	All variety meats are very high in nutrients. Kidneys are a good low-fat, low-calorie source of protein. Liver is one of the best dietary sources of iron and complete protein. However, it is high in cholesterol and should be avoided or limited by those on a low-cholesterol diet. Its very high content of vitamin A (which can be toxic) means it should be avoided by women during the first few months of pregnancy.
0	0	430	A, B1, B2, niacin, B6, B12, folate, pant ac, biotin	potas, phos, iron, zinc, cop, sel	
0	0	n/k	n/k	n/k	Ostrich is a low-fat source of protein.
0	0	89	B1, B2, niacin, B6, B12, pant ac	potas, phos, zinc, el	Pork is one of the best sources of the range of B vitamins, and the lean meat contains only a little more total fat than beef. Good source of zinc and a useful source of selenium, which, many experts now believe, may be lacking in many of our diets. See health notes for Beef for general notes on red meat, and see also entries for Heart Disease and Cancer in Section One.
0	0	105	B1, B2, niacin, B6, B12, pant ac	potas, phos, zinc, el	
0	0	143			
0	0	90	B1, niacin, B6, B12, pant ac	potas, phos, zinc, el	
0	0	59	B1, niacin, B6, B12, pant ac	potas, phos	

	food state	portion size	calories	k joules	total fat (g)	% poly	% mono	% sat	protein (g)	carbo (g)	starch (g)	sugars (g)
Salami		1 oz (25 g)	109	453	10	11	45	37	5	0.5	0	0.5
Sausage Spanish chorizo		3$\frac{1}{2}$ oz (100 g)	291	1,208	23	10	48	42	18	3.2	0.4	2.8
Sausage pepperoni		3$\frac{1}{2}$ oz (100 g)	551	2,279	51	10	45	38	22	0.6	tr	0.6
Sausage links pork	broiled	2 large	254	1,056	20	11	45	39	11	9.2	7.8	1.4
Sausage links turkey	broiled	2	90	369	16	26	37	33	12	1.2	n/k	n/k
Veal tenderloin		3$\frac{1}{2}$ oz (100 g)	109	459	2.7	15	44	33	21	0	0	0
Venison tenderloin		3$\frac{1}{2}$ oz (100 g)	103	437	1.6	25	25	50	22	0	0	0
Chicken boneless breast	skinless	1 half breast (3$\frac{1}{2}$ oz/ 100 g)	106	449	1.1	18	46	27	24	0	0	0
Chicken breast half	broiled, skin removed	1	192	814	2.9	18	46	27	42	0	0	0
Chicken leg	casseroled	1	257	1,075	12	19	46	27	37	0	0	0
Chicken roasted	meat only	3$\frac{1}{2}$ oz (100 g)	177	742	7.5	20	45	28	27	0	0	0
Duck	roasted, meat plus skin	3$\frac{1}{2}$ oz (100 g)	423	1,750	38	14	51	30	20	0	0	0
Duck	roasted, meat only	3$\frac{1}{2}$ oz (100 g)	195	815	10	13	50	32	25	0	0	0
Guinea fowl	raw, meat only	3$\frac{1}{2}$ oz (100 g)	148	622	6.2	23	37	33	23	0	0	0

total fiber (g)	soluble fiber (g)	chol (mg)	useful source of vitamins	good source of minerals	special health notes
0.1	n/k	83	B1, niacin, B6, B12, pant ac	potas, phos	Salami and other cooked sausages are high in fat, saturated fat, and sodium. Because of the smoking process, smoked sausages have been linked with some cancers.
tr	n/k	n/k	n/k	n/k	
tr	n/k	n/k	n/k	n/k	
0.6	n/k	42	niacin, B12	cop	Over 70% of the calories in an average pork sausage link are fat calories. Even broiled, the proportion remains high. Poultry sausages are less fatty, but may still contain over half their calories as fat.
n/k	n/k	80	niacin, B12, B6	cop	
0	0	84	B2, niacin, B6, B12	potas, phos, zinc	Veal is a low-fat, high-protein meat.
0	0	50	B2, niacin, B6, B12	potas, phos, iron, zinc, cop	Venison is a low-fat, high-protein meat, rich in vitamins and minerals. Good source of iron. The iron in all meats is more easily absorbed by the body than that in plant foods.
0	0	70	niacin, B6, pant ac	potas, phos, sel	Chicken is only a low-fat source of protein if the skin is removed, preferably before cooking. If you eat the meat and skin, the fat content of chicken is much higher than beef and other red meats. Chicken is a good source of selenium, an antioxidant mineral that may be lacking in our diets. Chicken should be cooked right through to avoid food poisoning, and stored and reheated carefully.
0	0	122	niacin, B6, pant ac	potas, phos, sel	
0	0	168	niacin, B6, pant ac	potas, phos, zinc, sel	
0	0	105	niacin, B6, pant ac	potas, phos, zinc, sel	
0	0	99	B1, B2, niacin, B6, B12	potas, phos, iron, zinc, cop, sel	Lean duck meat isn't as high in fat as many people believe, containing no more fat than lamb. But duck eaten with the skin—even crispy skin—becomes very high in fat, although it is much higher in unsaturated fats than is red meat. The lean meat is a good source of B vitamins and the important minerals iron, zinc, and selenium.
0	0	115	B1, B2, niacin, B6, B12, pant ac	potas, phos, iron, zinc, cop, sel	
0	0	n/k	n/k	n/k	Guinea fowl is a low-fat source of protein.

	food state	portion size	calories	k joules	total fat (g)	% poly	% mono	% sat	protein (g)	carbo (g)	starch (g)	sugars (g)	
Pheasant	roasted, meat only	3¹/₂ oz (100 g)	220	918	12	13	47	34	28	0	0	0	
Rabbit	raw, meat only	3¹/₂ oz (100 g)	137	576	5.5	33	24	38	22	0	0	0	
Turkey light meat	raw, meat only	3¹/₂ oz (100 g)	105	444	0.8	25	38	38	24	0	0	0	
Turkey dark meat	raw, meat only	3¹/₂ oz (100 g)	104	439	2.5	24	40	32	20	0	0	0	
Turkey light meat	roasted	3¹/₂ oz (100 g)	153	648	2	25	35	35	34	0	0	0	

Nuts, seeds, and savory snacks

	food state	portion size	calories	k joules	total fat (g)	% poly	% mono	% sat	protein (g)	carbo (g)	starch (g)	sugars (g)	
⭐ **Almonds**	shelled	¹/₃ cup (2 oz/ 50 g)	306	1267	28	25	62	8	11	3.5	1.4	2.1	
⭐ **Brazil nuts**	shelled	12 large (2 oz/ 50 g)	341	1407	34	34	38	24	7.1	1.5	0.3	1.2	
⭐ **Cashew nuts**	shelled	¹/₃ cup	287	1187	24	18	58	20	8.9	9.1	6.8	2.3	
Chestnuts	shelled	5 nuts (2 oz/ 50 g)	85	360	1.4	41	37	19	1	18	15	3.5	
⭐ **Hazelnuts**	shelled	heaping (¹/₃ cup (2 oz/ 50 g)	325	1343	32	10	79	7.5	7.1	3	1	2	
Macadamia nuts	shelled	heaping ¹/₃ cup (2 oz/ 50 g)	374	1541	39	2	78	14	4	2.4	0.4	2	
Nuts mixed, chopped	shelled	¹/₃ cup (2 oz/ 50 g)	304	1258	27	27	52	16	11	4	2	2	
Peanuts raw	shelled	18 nuts (2 oz/ 50 g)	282	1171	23	31	46	18	13	6.3	3.2	3.1	

total fiber (g)	soluble fiber (g)	chol (mg)	useful source of vitamins	good source of minerals	special health notes
0	0	220	B2, niacin, B6, B12, potas	phos, iron	Pheasant is higher in fat than some other game birds.
0	0	53	niacin, B6, B12	potas, phos, sel	Rabbit is a very low-fat source of protein.
0	0	57	niacin, B6, B12	potas, phos	Turkey is an extremely low-fat meat and a good choice for dieters, being high in protein, B vitamins, and selenium. The dark leg meat contains twice as much iron as the light breast meat and three times as much zinc, which is important for a healthy immune system.
0	0	86	B2, niacin, B6, B12,	potas, phos, sel	
0	0	82	niacin, B6, B12	potas, phos, sel	
3.7	0.6	0	B2, niacin, E	cal, magnes, potas, phos, cop, manga	All nuts contribute significant amounts of iron, zinc, and magnesium as a regular part of the diet. Nuts are quite high in protein, but the reason that their calorie content is so high is their high fat content. The fat in nuts is, however, mostly unsaturated. Most nuts, especially hazelnuts and macadamias, have a high monounsaturated fat content, but pine nuts and walnuts are higher in polyunsaturates. Chestnuts are the only low-fat nuts.
2.2	0.6	0	B1, E	magnes, potas, phos, zinc, cop, sel, manga	Brazil nuts are exceptionally high in magnesium and selenium, the antioxidant mineral that helps to protect against heart disease, cancer, and aging. Pecans are a good source of zinc, which helps to strengthen the immune system.
1.6	0.8	0	B1, niacin, folate	magnes, potas, phos, iron, zinc, cop, sel, manga	Some people are allergic to peanuts and, to a lesser extent, other nuts. A peanut allergy can produce an extremely serious reaction if even a minute amount of peanut is eaten, and can even cause death.
2	0.6	0		potas	All fresh nuts should be eaten quickly, as stale nuts can build up dangerous levels of contaminants that can cause illness. Children under five should not have nuts as they can choke on them.
3.3	1.3	0	B1, niacin, B6, folate, E	potas, phos, cop, magnes, manga	
2.7	0.9	0		magnes, cop, manga	
3	0.9	0	niacin, E	magnes, potas, phos, cop, manga	
3.1	0.9	0	B1, niacin, B6, folate, E	magnes, potas, phos, cop, manga	

	food state	portion size	calories	k joules	total fat (g)	% poly	% mono	% sat	protein (g)	carbo (g)	starch (g)	sugars (g)
Pine nuts	shelled	1/3 cup (2 oz/ 50 g)	344	1420	34	60	20	7	7	2	0.1	2
Pistachios	shelled	1/3 cup (2 oz/ 50 g)	301	1243	28	32	50	13	8.9	4.1	1.3	2.8
Walnuts	shelled	scant 1/2 cup (2 oz/ 50 g)	344	1419	34	69	18	8	7.3	1.6	0.3	1.3
Pumpkin seeds		1 tbsp	91	378	7.3	40	25	15	3.9	2.4	2.3	0.2
★ **Sunflower seeds**		1 tbsp	93	386	7.6	65	21	10	3.2	3	2.6	0.3
Popcorn	plain	4 cups (1 1/4 oz/ 30 g)	148	617	11	46	34	10	1.5	12	12	0.3
Potato chips salted		15 chips (1 1/4 oz/ 30 g)	159	665	10	15	40	41	1.7	16	16	0.2
Potato chips salted, reduced fat		15 chips (1 1/4 oz/ 30 g)	137	577	6.4	12	41	43	2	19	19	0.4
Prawn crackers		12 lg. crackers (1 3/4 oz/ 40 g)	205	857	12	10	79	11	n/k	24	n/k	2.4
Tortilla chips		heaping 1 cup (1 1/4 oz/ 30 g)	138	578	6.9	30	47	18	2.3	18	17.7	0.3

Purchased desserts

	food state	portion size	calories	k joules	total fat (g)	% poly	% mono	% sat	protein (g)	carbo (g)	starch (g)	sugars (g)
Egg custard sauce		scant 1/2 cup (3 1/2 floz/ 100 ml)	95	401	3	3	30	57	2.6	15	3.1	12
Ice cream vanilla		3/4 cup (3 1/2 oz/ 100 g)	194	814	9.8	3	25	65	3.6	24	tr	22
Mousse chocolate		scant 1/2 cup (3 1/2 floz/ 100 ml)	139	586	5.4	3	30	61	4	20	2.4	18

total fiber (g)	soluble fiber (g)	chol (mg)	useful source of vitamins	good source of minerals	special health notes
0.9	n/k	0	niacin, E	magnes, potas, phos, iron, zinc, cop, manga	See entry under Almonds, pages 298–9.
3	1.4	0	B1, niacin, E	potas, magnes, potas, phos, cop, manga	
1.8	0.8	0	B1, B6, folate, E	magnes, potas, phos, cop, manga	
0.8	0.3	0		potas, phos, magnes, iron, zinc, cop	Edible seeds are almost all a good source of many minerals and poly-unsaturated fats. They are high in calories because of their high fat content, but they weigh very little so they can be sprinkled on cereals, breads, soups, and so on without too much damage to a diet.
1	0.3	0	B1, E	magnes, iron, cop, manga	
n/k	n/k	0	E		Most snack products are very high in fat and salt without offering much nutritional benefit, and are best kept for occasional use.
1.6	0.8	0	E	potas	
1.8	1	0	E	potas	
0.6	n/k	0			
1.8	n/k	0	E	potas, manga	
0.1	n/k	11	A, B2	cal, potas, phos, iod	Most commercial desserts are high in sugar and fat unless specifically labeled otherwise. Puddings based on milk, such as custard and rice pudding, are a fairly good choice, as they contain good amounts of calcium, but sugar and fat content can vary greatly.
tr	0	31	A	cal	Many ready-to-eat desserts, particularly those with a long shelf-life stored on supermarket shelves at room temperature, are high in preservatives and other additives.
n/k	tr	n/k		cal	

Rice, grains, and pasta

	food state	portion size	calories	k joules	total fat (g)	% poly	% mono	% sat	protein (g)	carbo (g)	starch (g)	sugars (g)
★ **Barley** whole-grain	dry weight	1/4 cup (2 oz/ 50 g)	151	641	1	n/k	n/k	n/k	5.3	32	31	0.9
Barley pearl	dry weight	1/4 cup (2 oz/ 50 g)	180	768	0.9	n/k	n/k	n/k	4	42	42	0
Bulgur (cracked wheat)	dry weight	heaping 1/3 cup (2 oz/ 50 g)	177	739	0.9	n/k	n/k	n/k	4.8	38	n/k	n/k
Couscous instant	dry weight	heaping 1/3 cup (2 oz/ 50 g)	175	745	0.9	n/k	n/k	n/k	5.3	39	39	0
Flour all-purpose	unsifted, spooned into cup	scant 1/2 cup (2 oz/ 50 g)	171	725	0.6	50	17	17	4.7	39	38	0.8
★ **Flour** whole-wheat	stirred, spooned into cup	scant 1/2 cup (2 oz/ 50 g)	155	659	1.1	45	14	14	6.3	32	31	1
Pasta white macaroni	dry weight	scant 1/2 cup (2 oz/ 50 g)	171	728	0.9	44	11	11	6	37	35	1.6
★ **Pasta** whole-wheat twists	dry weight	scant 3/4 cup (2 oz/ 50 g)	162	690	1.3	44	12	16	6.7	33	31	1.9
Polenta (yellow cornmeal)	dry weight	scant 1/2 cup (2 oz/ 50 g)	172	720	0.8	n/k	n/k	33	4.3	37	36	1
★ **Rice** brown short grain	dry weight	1/4 cup (2 oz/ 50 g)	179	759	1.4	36	25	25	3.3	41	40	0.6
Rice white short grain	dry weight	1/4 cup (2 oz/ 50 g)	192	815	1.8	36	25	25	3.7	43	43	tr
Spaghetti in tomato sauce		7 1/2-oz (215-g) can	171	725	1.2	50	25	25	5.1	35	21	14
Wheat germ		2 tbsp	36	150	0.9	46	12	14	0.1	4	2.9	1.6

total fiber (g)	soluble fiber (g)	chol (mg)	useful source of vitamins	good source of minerals	special health notes
7.4	2	0	niacin, B6	potas, iron, manga, phos	Whole-grain barley contains the complete barley grain, which is rich in insoluble fiber and therefore good for helping constipation, and a good source of soluble fiber, which lowers blood cholesterol. Rich in minerals, good source of iron, and a useful source of protein. Contains gluten. In pearl barley the outer husk of the barley, containing most of the nutrients, has been removed. A high-cereal diet helps to protect against bowel cancer and possibly diverticulitis and breast cancer.
n/k	n/k	0		manga	
n/k	n/k	0	B1, niacin	phos, iron, cop	A cracked-wheat grain unsuitable for people with wheat or gluten intolerance or allergy. Good source of complex carbohydrate.
1	0.5	0			Pre-cooked wheat semolina which, although a low-fat carbohydrate, contains few nutrients. Traditional couscous, available at healthfood stores, contains more fiber, B vitamins, and iron, but takes longer to cook.
1.5	0.8	0		cal	White flour has been milled until most of the outer wheat husk has been removed, therefore contains few nutrients in good quantities, except calcium.
4.5	1	0	B1, niacin, B6	magnes, phos, cop, sel, manga	Whole-wheat flour is a good source of complex carbohydrate, containing all the goodness of the complete wheat husk and wheat germ, plenty of fiber, and useful amounts of protein.
1.5	0.8	0	niacin	manga, cop	Whole-wheat pasta is rich in niacin and fiber, with a low glycemic index. With twice as much iron (2 mg per 2 oz/50 g raw) as white, it is a helpful source of iron for vegetarians (even though iron does not appear in the chart as it is just under 17%, see page 259). White pasta contains less fiber, vitamins, and minerals, but is still a good source of low-fat complex carbohydrates, with a medium glycemic index.
4.2	1	0	B2, niacin	manga, cop, magnes	
0.5	n/k	0		iron	Cornmeal is usually cooked with a lot of added butter and cheese, rendering the finished dish very high in fat and saturates. Suitable for those with a gluten or wheat intolerance.
0.9	tr	0	B1, niacin	magnes, phos, cop, manga	Good source of B vitamins, with some fiber and low in fat, making brown rice an ideal complex carbohydrate, particularly for those with a gluten or wheat intolerance, but also with a medium glycemic index.
0.2	tr	0		manga	White rice contains less vitamins, minerals, and fiber than brown rice but still a good low-fat carbohydrate food, suitable for those with a gluten or wheat intolerance.
1.5	n/k	0		potas	Canned spaghetti is a fairly useful low-fat food, but it is high in salt and sugar. Contains useful amounts of lycopene and beta-carotene in the tomato sauce.
1.6	0.3	0	B1, B6, folate, E		You need at least 2 tablespoons of wheat germ a day to make a significant contribution toward your daily intake of B vitamins, vitamin E, or fiber (see note on vitamins and minerals on pages 259).

	food state	portion size	calories	k joules	total fat (g)	% poly	% mono	% sat	protein (g)	carbo (g)	starch (g)	sugars (g)	

Spreads, dips, and pâtés

	food state	portion size	calories	k joules	total fat (g)	% poly	% mono	% sat	protein (g)	carbo (g)	starch (g)	sugars (g)
Fruit preserves		heaping 1 tbsp (1 oz/ 25 g)	65	279	0	0	0	0	0.2	17	0	17
Jam		heaping 1 tbsp (1 oz/ 25 g)	30	130	0	0	0	0	0.2	7.8	0.2	7.8
Peanut butter		1¹/₂ tbsp (1 oz/ 25 g)	156	645	13	34	40	22	5.7	3.3	1.6	1.7
Hummus		2 tbsp (1 oz/ 25 g)	83	347	7.3	25	63	12	1.9	2.3	0.1	2.2
Taramasalata		2 tbsp (1 oz/ 25 g)	126	519	13	32	55	8	0.8	1	1	0
Chicken liver pâté canned		1 thin slice (1 oz/ 25 g)	50	210	3.3	18	40	30	3.3	1.6	n/k	n/k
Liverwurst		2 thin slices (1 oz/ 25 g)	79	327	7.2	9	35	29	3.3	0.3	0.2	0.1

Sweeteners and confectionery

	food state	portion size	calories	k joules	total fat (g)	% poly	% mono	% sat	protein (g)	carbo (g)	starch (g)	sugars (g)
Honey		1 tbsp (1 oz/ 25 g)	72	307	0	0	0	0	0.1	19	0	19
Fructose	powder	2 tbsp (1 oz/ 25 g)	96	401	0	0	0	0	0	25	0	25
Sugar brown		2 tbsp (1 oz/ 25 g)	91	387	0	0	0	0	0	25	0	25
Sugar white granulated		2 tbsp (1 oz/ 25 g)	99	420	0	0	0	0	0	26	0	26
Maple syrup		4 tsp (1 oz/ 25 g)	68	317	0	0	0	0	0.1	17	0	17

total fiber (g)	soluble fiber (g)	chol (mg)	useful source of vitamins	good source of minerals	special health notes
n/k	n/k	0			Fruit preserves are high in sugar but with small amounts of vitamin C, depending upon variety.
n/k	n/k	0			
1.4	0.4	0	niacin, E	magnes	Peanuts are high in fat and calories, and so is peanut butter, but the fat is mostly unsaturated. Fairly good source of protein and useful for vegetarians. If eaten regularly, contributes valuable amounts of iron.
3	n/k	0			Ready-made chickpea purée doesn't contain enough chickpeas to make a significant contribution to nutrients unless you eat lots. Homemade provides more, particularly magnes, iron, cop, manga, and niacin.
tr	n/k	6	B12		
0	0	98			See Liverwurst.
tr	n/k	42			Liverwurst is quite high in fats and cholesteral, but if eaten in reasonable amounts will contribute good amounts of iron and some B vitamins.
0	0	0			Honey is an antiseptic and spread on wounds helps healing. Nutrients are present in honey, but in such small quantities that a normal serving doesn't contribute to the diet. High glycemic index food.
0	0	0			Fructose (fruit sugar) has roughly the same calories as ordinary sugar (sucrose), but is twice as sweet and so offers a means of cutting calories. It is absorbed more slowly into the blood than sugar, so is less likely to produce fluctuations in blood sugar. It has also been shown to help disperse LDL cholesterols from the blood. However, an excess of fructose (around 25 g plus per day) can cause diarrhea and may raise triglyceride levels. Ordinary white sugar is the highly refined by-product of the sugar cane, containing no nutrients, fats, fiber, or anything except simple carbohydrate. Brown sugar is similar, though the darkest contain very small amounts of vitamins and minerals. High sugar intake has been linked with increased risk of various ailments, such as heart disease, but scientific evidence is scant, and the World Health Organization's 1998 report on carbohydrates says that moderate amounts of sugar can be included in a healthy diet. See page 12.
0	0	0			
0	0	0			
0	0	0			

	food state	portion size	calories	k joules	total fat (g)	% poly	% mono	% sat	protein (g)	carbo (g)	starch (g)	sugars (g)	
Molasses dark		4 tsp (1 oz/ 25 g)	67	279	0	0	0	0	0	17	0	15	
Chocolate milk		1 square (1 oz/ 25 g)	130	544	7.7	4	32	60	1.9	14	0	14	
Chocolate syrup		1½ tbsp (1 oz/ 25 g)	54	226	0.2	5	35	65	.5	15	n/k	n/k	
Carob bar		1 small piece (1 oz/ 25 g)	139	581	9.3	n/k	n/k	n/k	2.5	12	n/k	n/k	
Licorice		1 piece (1 oz/ 25 g)	70	296	0.3	n/k	n/k	n/k	1.4	16	5.1	10	
Hard candies		2 small pieces (1 oz/ 25 g)	93	39	tr	0	0	0	tr	24.5	tr	24	
Caramels plain		2 pieces (1 oz/ 25 g)	95	448	2.1	5	10	84	1.2	19	n/k	n/k	

Vegetables and legumes

	food state	portion size	calories	k joules	total fat (g)	% poly	% mono	% sat	protein (g)	carbo (g)	starch (g)	sugars (g)	
Artichoke globe		1 whole	9	39	0.1	100	0	0	1.4	1.4	tr	0.6	
Artichoke Jerusalem	boiled	3½ oz (100 g)	41	207	0.1	tr	tr	tr	1.6	11	tr	1.6	
★ **Asparagus**	½ in thick, cooked	7 spears (3½ oz/ 25 g)	25	103	0.6	50	25	25	2.9	2	0.1	0.9	
★ **Avocado**		½ medium	145	588	15	11	62	21	1.4	1.4	tr	0.4	
Bamboo shoots canned, drained		⅔ cup (3½ oz/ 100 g)	11	45	0.2	50	0	50	1.5	0.7	tr	0.7	
★ **Beans** fava, fresh	shelled	⅔ cup (3½ oz/ 100 g)	59	247	1	50	10	10	5.7	7.2	5.4	1.3	

total fiber (g)	soluble fiber (g)	chol (mg)	useful source of vitamins	good source of minerals	special health notes
tr	n/k	0		potas, magnes, manga	Molasses provides more nutrients than any other type of sweetener. In larger quantities, supplies good amounts of iron and calcium.
0.2	n/k	6			Chocolate is made from antioxidant cocoa beans, but milk chocolate doesn't contain a great deal of chocolate liquor. Semisweet chocolate contains more chocolate liquor (15–35%) and therefore has a greater antioxidant potential. It also contains more caffeine and theobromine, two stimulants, and twice the magnesium of milk chocolate and more iron, but very little calcium.
0.4	n/k	0			
n/k	n/k	0			Often eaten as a "healthier" alternative to chocolate, carob still contains a lot of fat and sugars, and therefore calories, but it is free from caffeine and other stimulants.
0.5	n/k	0		potas, cal, magnes, iron, manga	A natural laxative, licorice also contains useful amounts of several minerals. Virtually fat-free. A good choice if you must eat candy, especially as evidence that a compound in licorice may inhibit tooth decay.
0	0	0			Basically just sugar and additives, usually artificial flavorings and colorings. Frequent sucking and chewing of hard candies can contribute to tooth decay.
0	0	n/k			High in sugar and fat, and very little else. Chewing caramels can contribute to tooth decay.
n/k	n/k	0	folate	potas	Compound in artichokes called cynarin said to boost liver function and help regulate blood cholesterol, but there is little scientific evidence to support this.
3.5	2.3	0		potas	
1.7	0.8	0	b-carotene, E, folate	potas	One of few good vegetable sources of vitamin E. A natural diuretic. Its glycosides may be anti-inflammatory and of use in rheumatoid arthritis. Asparagus contains purines, which may trigger gout.
2.6	1.2	0	B6, E	potas	Avocados are a very good source of vitamin E and monounsaturated fats, and contains many other vitamins and minerals.
1.7	0.4	0		potas, cop	
6.1	1.4	0	b-carotene, niacin, folate, pant ac, C	potas	Fava beans are excellent source of fiber, including soluble fiber, which can help lower blood cholesterol, and a range of vitamins and minerals. Also contains flavonoid quercetin to help prevent CHD.

	food state	portion size	calories	k joules	total fat (g)	% poly	% mono	% sat	protein (g)	carbo (g)	starch (g)	sugars (g)
Beans green (haricot vert)	raw, chopped	scant 1 cup (3½ oz/ 100 g)	24	99	0.5	60	tr	20	1.9	3.2	0.9	2.3
Beans pole or runner	raw, chopped	scant 1 cup (3½ oz/ 100 g)	22	93	0.4	50	tr	25	1.6	3.2	0.4	2.8
Bean sprouts mung		½ cup (2 oz/ 50 g)	16	66	0.3	40	20	20	1.5	2	0.9	1.1
Beets	raw, diced	scant ¾ cup (3½ oz/ 100 g)	36	154	0.1	50	tr	tr	1.7	7.6	0.6	7
Bell peppers green	raw, cut into strips	1 cup (3½ oz/ 100 g)	15	65	0.3	67	tr	33	0.8	2.6	0.1	2.4
★ **Bell peppers** red	raw, cut into strips	1 cup (3½ oz/ 100 g)	32	134	0.4	50	tr	25	1	6.4	0.1	6.1
Bell peppers yellow	raw, cut into strips	1 cup (3½ oz/ 100 g)	26	113	0.2	50	tr	tr	1.2	5.3	tr	5.1
★ **Broccoli** green	raw	⅔ cup (3½ oz/ 100 g)	33	138	0.9	56	20	22	4.4	1.8	0.1	1.5
★ **Brussels sprouts**		3½ oz (100 g)	42	177	1.4	50	7	21	3.5	4.1	0.8	3.1
Cabbage red	raw, chopped	heaping 1 cup (3½ oz/ 100 g)	21	89	9.3	67	tr	tr	1.1	3.7	0.1	3.3
★ **Cabbage** Savoy	raw, shredded	scant 1½ cups (3½ oz/ 100 g)	27	114	0.5	60	tr	20	2.1	3.9	0.1	3.8
Carrots old		1¼ av. carrots (3½ oz/ 100 g)	35	146	0.3	67	tr	33	0.6	7.9	0.3	7.4
Cauliflower	raw, flowerets	1 cup (3½ oz/ 100 g)	34	142	0.9	56	11	22	3.6	3	0.4	2.5
Celery	raw, chopped	heaping ¾ cup (3½ oz/ 100 g)	7	32	0.2	50	tr	tr	0.5	0.9	tr	0.9

total fiber (g)	soluble fiber (g)	chol (mg)	useful source of vitamins	good source of minerals	special health notes
2.2	0.9	0	b-carotene, folate, C	potas	Green beans are a reasonable source of the antioxidant vitamins beta-carotene and C, and a good source of fiber.
2	0.8	0	b-carotene, folate, C	potas	As Green Beans.
0.8	0.3	0	folate, C		
1.9	0.9	0	folate	potas, manga	In some people, beets turn urine pink. Juice is said to be an aid to kidney function, but there is no scientific proof. The leafy greens are an excellent vegetable, containing calcium, beta-carotene, and iron.
1.6	0.7	0	b-carotene, folate, C	potas	Green bell peppers are one of the best vegetable sources of vitamin C, the antioxidant action of which is thought improved by flavonoids found in peppers. Red bell peppers are much higher in beta-carotene than other colors and, again, very rich in vitamin C. They contain the natural pain-killer capsaicin, clinically proved to be effective when rubbed on joints as a cream; the same effect may be gained by eating bell peppers and may be useful against arthritis pain.
1.6	0.7	0	b-carotene, B6, C		
1.7	0.7	0	b-carotene, B6, C	potas	As for Green Bell Peppers.
2.6	1.1	0	b-carotene, folate, C	potas	High in fiber and antioxidant vitamins beta-carotene and C, which help against heart disease, and rich in folate. Broccoli's phytochemicals (glucosinolates) have important properties, especially against cancer.
4.1	2.2	0	b-carotene, folate, C	potas	Brussels sprouts are an excellent source of fiber, folate, and vitamin C, and second-best source of the anti-carcinogenic glucosinolates (see Broccoli).
2.5	1.2	0	folate, C	potas	Red cabbage may be useful in fighting skin infections, as thought to contain natural antiseptic properties.
3.1	1.7	0	b-carotene, folate, C	potas	The dark green leaves contain most of the vitamins and minerals, while the pale center leaves contain much less. Contains similar anti-carcinogenic phytochemicals to broccoli and Brussels sprouts.
2.4	1.4	0	b-carotene		Carrots are richest source of beta-carotene (more available when cooked), converting in body to vitamin A, lack of which is associated with poor night vision. Also an antioxidant, helping fight heart disease and cancer.
1.8	0.9	0	folate, C	potas	Cauliflower is another good source of the cancer-fighting glucosinolates (see Broccoli).
1.1	0.5	0		potas	A phytochemical in celery lowers blood pressure by 13% and blood cholesterol by 7%—in rats! This has yet to be tested on humans, but Asian medicine has long used celery to lower blood pressure.

	food state	portion size	calories	k joules	total fat (g)	% poly	% mono	% sat	protein (g)	carbo (g)	starch (g)	sugars (g)	
Celery root	raw, chopped	scant 3/4 cup (3 1/2 oz/ 100 g)	18	73	0.4	n/k	n/k	n/k	1.2	2.3	0.5	1.8	
⭐ **Chili peppers** fresh	raw, chopped	4 large (3 1/2 oz/ 100 g)	20	83	0.6	n/k	n/k	n/k	2.9	0.7	tr	0.7	
⭐ **Collard greens**		3 1/2 oz (100 g)	33	136	1	60	10	10	3	3.1	0.4	2.7	
Corn fresh baby corn		3 1/2 oz (100 g)	24	101	0.4	n/k	n/k	n/k	2.5	2.7	0.8	1.9	
Corn frozen kernels		2/3 cup (3 1/2 oz/ 100 g)	85	361	0.8	40	25	25	25	17	15	1.9	
Cucumber English	sliced	scant 1 cup (3 1/2 oz/ 100 g)	10	40	0.1	tr	tr	tr	0.7	1.5	0.1	1.4	
Eggplant	raw, chopped	heaping 1/2 cup (3 1/2 oz/ 100 g)	15	64	0.4	50	tr	25	0.9	2.2	0.2	2	
Fennel	raw, chopped	heaping 1/2 cup (3 1/2 oz/ 100 g)	12	50	0.2	tr	tr	tr	0.9	1.8	0.1	1.7	
⭐ **Garlic**		1 clove	3	12	0	0	0	0	0.2	0.5	0.4	0.1	
Ginger fresh		1 small piece	2	10	0	0	0	0	0.1	0.5	0.3	0.2	
⭐ **Kale**		3 1/2 oz (100 g)	33	140	1.6	56	6	13	3.4	1.4	0.1	1.3	
Leeks	raw, chopped	heaping 3/4 cup (3 1/2 oz/ 100 g)	22	93	0.5	60	tr	20	1.6	2.9	0.3	2.2	
Lettuce Iceberg	raw, chopped	heaping 1 3/4 cup (3 1/2 oz/ 100 g)	13	53	0.3	67	tr	tr	0.7	1.9	tr	1.9	
Lettuce Romaine	raw, chopped	heaping 1 3/4 cup (3 1/2 oz/ 100 g)	16	65	0.6	67	tr	17	1	1.7	tr	1.7	

total fiber (g)	soluble fiber (g)	chol (mg)	useful source of vitamins	good source of minerals	special health notes
3.7	2.4	0	folate, C	potas	
n/k	n/k	0	C		Chilies contain high levels of pain-killer and antioxidant capsaicin (see Bell Peppers). Also stimulate metabolic rate, seem to have a cholesterol-lowering effect, relieve congestion, and aid to digestion.
3.4	1.7	0	b-carotene, folate, C	potas	See Kale or Cabbage.
2	0.4	0	b-carotene, folate, C		Corn is high in fiber and vitamin C.
2.1	n/k	0	folate, C	potas	
0.6	0.2	0			Mildly diuretic. Some evidence that the phytochemicals in cucumber called sterols (mainly in the skin) can lower blood cholesterol.
2	1	0	K		Eggplant has a range of vitamins and minerals, but none in rich quantities.
2.4	1.1	0	b-carotene, folate	potas	
0.1	0.1	0			Garlich contains allicin, which is antibiotic, antifungal, and possibly antiviral; sulfides, which may help prevent cancers; and an antioxidant that lowers blood cholesterol and prevents clotting.
n/k	n/k	0			A well-known antinausea remedy—ideal for travel and "morning" sickness. Also stimulates circulation and aids digestion. An infusion of grated ginger is said to help cold and bronchial symptoms.
3.1	1.9	0	b-carotene, folate, C, E	potas, potas, cal, manga	Kale is a good source of all three of the vitamin antioxidants, beta-carotene, C, and E, and rich in glucosinolates (see Broccoli), which help to fight cancers.
2.2	1.1	0	b-carotene, folate, C	potas	Leeks are mildly diuretic. Member of same family as onions and garlic and, as such, if eaten regularly may help to keep cholesterol levels low and the blood healthy.
0.6	0.3	0	folate	potas	Dark lettuce leaves contain useful amounts of beta-carotene, but pale leaves don't. Most lettuce is rich in folates. All lettuce contains phytochemicals that act as a mild sedative.
1.2	0.6	0	b-carotene, folate	potas	Romaine lettuce is much richer source of fiber and potassium than pale lettuce, as well as a good source of beta-carotene.

	food state	portion size	calories	k joules	total fat (g)	% poly	% mono	% sat	protein (g)	carbo (g)	starch (g)	sugars (g)
Mushrooms	raw, chopped	scant 1/2 cup (3 1/2 oz/ 100 g)	13	55	0.5	60	tr	20	1.8	0.4	0.2	0.2
Mustard greens	raw, chopped	scant 2 cup (3 1/2 oz/ 100 g)	15	63	0.2	50	50	0	2.3	2.1	0.2	1.9
Napa cabbage	raw, shredded	scant 1 1/2 cups (3 1/2 oz/ 100 g)	12	49	0.2	50	tr	tr	1	1.4	tr	1.4
Okra	raw, chopped	1 cup (3 1/2 oz/ 100 g)	31	130	1	30	10	30	2.8	3	0.5	2.5
Onions green (scallion)	raw, chopped	1 cup (3 1/2 oz/ 100 g)	23	98	0.5	40	20	20	2	3	0.2	2.8
★ **Onions** Spanish or Bermuda	raw, chopped	heaping 1/2 cup (3 1/2 oz/ 100 g)	36	150	0.2	50	tr	tr	1.2	7.9	tr	5.6
Parsnips	raw	1 1/4 parsnips (3 1/2 oz/ 100 g)	64	271	1.1	18	45	18	1.8	13	6.2	5.7
Peas canned, drained		heaping 1/2 cup (3 1/2 oz/ 100 g)	80	339	0.9	44	11	22	5.3	14	6.3	3.9
★ **Peas** fresh	raw, shelled	scant 2/3 cup (3 1/2 oz/ 100 g)	83	344	1.5	47	13	20	6.9	11	7	2.3
Peas frozen	shelled	scant 2/3 cup (3 1/2 oz/ 100 g)	66	279	0.9	56	11	22	5.7	9.8	45	2.6
Peas, snow	raw	3 1/2 oz (100 g)	32	136	0.2	50	tr	tr	3.6	4.2	0.8	3.4
Potatoes boiled, chipped	boiled, chipped	2/3 cup (3 1/2 oz/ 100 g)	72	306	0.1	100	0	0	1.8	17	16	0.7
Potatoes oven fries		3 1/2 oz (100 g)	162	687	4.2	14	38	43	3.2	30	29	0.7
Potatoes French fries	frozen, thick-cut, fried in corn oil	3 1/2 oz (100 g)	273	1,145	14	52	25	19	4.1	36	35	0.7

total fiber (g)	soluble fiber (g)	chol (mg)	useful source of vitamins	good source of minerals	special health notes
1.1	0.2	0	B2, niacin, folate, pant ac	potas, cop	Contains very little carbohydrate, but high in protein and fiber. Evidence that the shiitake mushroom contains phytochemicals lentinan and canthaxanthin, which help fight cancer.
0.4	0.2	0	carotenoids, C		Mustard greens are a rich source of glucosinolates.
1.2	0.6	0	folate, C	potas	Napa cabbage is a source of glucosinolates (see Broccoli), but not as rich as darker greens.
4	2.4	0	b-carotene	magnes, potas	Okra is very high in soluble fiber, which can help to lower blood cholesterol.
1.5	n/k	0	C		Onions are from same family as garlic, with several probable medicinal benefits. Many experts believe they can help lower blood cholesterol and blood pressure and "thin" blood to minimize risk of clotting. Also contain flavonoids and sulfurs that may help fight cancers, and natural antibiotics for help with bronchitis, colds, and flu, as well as quercetin, an antioxidant. The green portions of scallions contain beta-carotene and folate.
0.4	0.8	0			
4.6	2.6	0	b-carotene, B1, niacin, folate, C	potas, phos, iron	
5.1	1.4	0	b-carotene niacin	potas	Canning diminishes the vitamin C in vegetables.
4.7	1.3	0	b-carotene, B1, niacin, folate, C	potas	Peas are a popular source of vitamin C, fiber, and many other vitamins and minerals.
5.1	1.6	0	b-carotene, B1, niacin, folate, C	potas	Freezing peas hardly alters their nutritional value at all. In fact, if frozen soon after picking, will probably contain more vitamin C than fresh peas.
2.3	1	0	b-carotene, C	potas	Snow peas are an excellent all-round vegetable, containing good amounts of many nutrients, including protein and soluble fiber.
1.2	0.7	0	B6, C	potas, cop	Potatoes are one of the cheapest sources of vitamin C, potassium, and fiber, and, eaten in quantity (as is usual), provide many other vitamins and minerals. Green bits on the skin are poisonous and should be removed. The skins contain the most fiber and the flesh just under the skin contains the most vitamin C. New potatoes contain much more vitamin C than old. Potatoes should be cooked in their skin or peeled just before cooking, and should never be left soaking in water, both of which lose vitamin C. Oven fries are healthiest when the oil they contain is sunflower oil; check labels.
2	1.1	0	niacin, B6, C	potas, cop	
2.4	1.3	0	niacin, B6, C	potas, cop	

	food state	portion size	calories	k joules	total fat (g)	% poly	% mono	% sat	protein (g)	carbo (g)	starch (g)	sugars (g)
Pumpkin	raw	3¹/₂ oz (100 g)	13	55	0.2	tr	tr	50	0.7	2.2	0.3	1.7
Rutabaga	raw, chopped	scant ³/₄ cup (3¹/₂ oz/ 100 g)	24	101	0.3	67	tr	tr	0.7	5	0.1	4.9
Spinach fresh	raw, chopped	scant 2 cups (3¹/₂ oz/ 100 g)	25	103	0.8	63	13	13	2.8	1.6	0.1	1.5
⭐ **Squash** butternut	raw, chopped	³/₄ cup (3¹/₂ oz/ 100 g)	36	155	0.1	tr	tr	tr	1.1	8.3	3.4	4.5
⭐ **Sweet potato** orange-fleshed		¹/₂ av. potato (3¹/₂ oz/ 100 g)	87	372	0.3	33	tr	33	1.2	21	16	5.7
⭐ **Tomatoes** fresh		¹/₂ lg. tomato (3¹/₂ oz/ 100 g)	17	73	0.3	50	25	25	0.7	3.1	tr	3.1
Tomatoes canned		generous ¹/₃ cup (3¹/₂ oz/ 100 g)	16	69	0.1	tr	tr	tr	1	3	0.2	2.8
Turnips	raw, chopped	³/₄ cup (3¹/₂ oz/ 100 g)	23	98	0.3	67	tr	tr	0.9	4.7	0.2	4.5
⭐ **Watercress**		scant 1 cup (3¹/₂ oz/ 100 g)	22	94	1	40	10	30	3	0.4	tr	0.4
Zucchini	raw, sliced	³/₄ cup (3¹/₂ oz/ 100 g)	18	74	0.4	50	tr	25	1.8	1.8	0.1	1.7
⭐ **Adzuki beans**		¹/₄ cup (2 oz/ 50 g)	136	579	0.3	n/k	n/k	n/k	10	25	22	0.5
Baked beans in tomato sauce		5 tbsp (3¹/₂ oz/ 100 g)	81	345	0.6	50	25	25	4.8	15	9.3	5.8
Baked beans in tomato sauce	low-salt low-sugar	5 tbsp (3¹/₂ oz/ 100 g)	73	311	0.6	50	25	25	5.4	12	9.7	2.8
Black-eyed peas	dry weight	¹/₄ cup (3¹/₂ oz/ 100 g)	156	662	0.8	44	6	31	12	27	24	1.5

total fiber (g)	soluble fiber (g)	chol (mg)	useful source of vitamins	good source of minerals	special health notes
1	0.4	0	b-carotene, C		Pumpkin flesh contains the carotenoid phytoene, which may help prevent some cancers.
1.9	0.9	0	b-carotene, C		Rutabaga contains glucosinolates, which are thought to help fight cancers. Also contains the antioxidant vitamins beta-carotene and C, and is a good source of fiber.
2.1	0.8	0	b-carotene, folate, C, E	potas, cal	Oxalic acid content of spinach hinders absorption of iron and calcium. Contains large amounts of antioxidant beta-carotene and carotenoid lutein, which may be important in eye health. High in folate.
1.6	0.7	0	b-carotene, C, E	potas	Orange-fleshed squashes are rich in carotenoids, as well as the other antioxidants, vitamins C, and E.
2.4	1.1	0	C, E	potas	Orange-fleshed sweet potatoes are rich in beta-carotene, but the white-fleshed kind contains very little. Both are good sources of the other antioxidant vitamins C and E.
1	0.4	0	b-carotene, C, E	potas	Tomatoes are rich in lycopene, the antioxidant phytochemical that is important in helping to prevent heart disease and cancers. They also contain the antioxidants beta-carotene, vitamin C, and vitamin E.
0.7	0.3	0	b-carotene, C, E	potas	Lycopene (see above) is more potent in cooked and canned tomatoes than in raw ones. Tomato purées, pastes, and juices are all rich in lycopene.
2.4	0.9	0	C		Turnips contain a certain amount of glucosinolates (see Broccoli).
1.5	0.7	0	b-carotene, C, E	potas, cal, iron	Although rich in antioxidants and minerals, watercress is usually eaten in small quantities. Contains phenethyl isothiocyanate, which, in large amounts, fights lung cancer caused by tobacco.
0.9	0.4	0			
5.6	1.3	0	niacin	magnes, potas, iron, zinc, cop, manga	Though the nutritional content of each legume varies slightly, as a group they are, perhaps, almost the perfect health food. They are low in fat (apart from soybeans, the fat of which is mostly unsaturated anyway) and cholesterol-free, high in protein, high in complex carbohydrate, and high in fiber, and most are particularly rich in soluble fiber, which helps to lower blood cholesterol levels. Most contribute valuable iron and B vitamins to the diet of people who don't eat meat, and valuable for people who eat little or no dairy products. Regular legume eaters will also get plenty of zinc and other vitamins and minerals present in smaller quantities than will show on this chart. They are also low on the glycemic index.
3.5	2.1	0	b-carotene, folate	magnes, potas, phos, iron, manga	
3.8	2.3	0	b-carotene, folate	cal, magnes, potas, phos, iron, manga	Soybeans are of particular medical interest. Not only are they among the few plant sources of complete protein, containing all eight essential amino acids that make up protein, but research across the world now reveals that soy has many other health
4.1	1.5	0	folate	potas, phos manga, cop	

	food state	portion size	calories	k joules	total fat (g)	% poly	% mono	% sat	protein (g)	carbo (g)	starch (g)	sugars (g)
★ **Chickpeas**		1/4 cup (2 oz/ 50 g)	160	678	2.7	50	20	9	11	25	22	1.3
Chickpeas canned, drained		heaping 1/3 cup (3 1/2 oz/ 100 g)	115	487	2.9	45	24	10	7.2	16.1	7.6	0.2
★ **Fava beans** dried	dry weight	1/4 cup (2 oz/ 50 g)	123	521	1	52	14	14	13	16	12	3
Lentils red	dry weight	1/4 cup (2 oz/ 50 g)	159	677	0.6	39	15	15	12	28	25	1.2
★ **Lentils** brown and green	dry weight	1/4 cup (2 oz/ 50 g)	149	632	0.9	42	16	11	12	24	22	0.6
Lima beans	dry weight	1/4 cup (2 oz/ 50 g)	145	617	0.9	47	6	24	10	27	23	1.8
Red kidney beans	dry weight	1/4 cup (2 oz/ 50 g)	133	567	0.7	57	7	14	11	22	19	1.3
Red kidney beans canned, drained		heaping 1/3 cup (3 1/2 oz/ 100 g)	100	424	0.6	50	17	17	3.5	8.9	6.4	1.8
Refried beans canned		1/2 cup (3 1/2 oz/ 100 g)	108	451	1.1	11	50	36	6.3	19	n/k	n/k
★ **Soybeans**	dry weight	scant 1/4 cup (2 oz/ 50 g)	185	776	9.3	49	19	12	18	7.9	2.4	2.8
Split peas	dry weight	1/4 cup (2 oz/ 50 g)	164	698	1.2	50	13	17	22	29	27	0.9
★ **White beans** navy, pea		1/4 cup (2 oz/ 50 g)	143	609	0.8	31	25	19	11	25	21	1.4
Tofu firm		1 piece (3 1/2 oz/ 100 g)	73	304	4.2	48	19	12	8.1	0.7	0.3	0.3
Vegetable burger		one (2 oz/ 50 g)	98	411	5.6	n/k	n/k	n/k	8.3	4	2.2	1.8

total fiber (g)	soluble fiber (g)	chol (mg)	useful source of vitamins	good source of minerals	special health notes
5.3	1.6	0	folate, E	potas, iron, cop. manga	benefits. Soybeans contain phytoestrogens, naturally occurring estrogens, which can help to reduce menopause symptoms in women and may help to prevent breast cancer and osteoporosis, by acting like a natural hormone replacement therapy. Soybean products, such as soy milk and tofu, can also help lower LDL blood cholesterol and thus help prevent heart disease. However, for babies a diet high in phytoestregens may not be a good idea.
2	0.7	0	E	manga	
16	3	0	b-carotene, folate	manga	Baked beans in tomato sauce contain lycopene and can contribute good quantities of calcium in quantities larger than the 3¹/₂ oz (100 g) portion stated.
2.5	0.6	0		potas, iron	Beans canned in water are nutritionally similar to dried beans, except their sodium content will be higher. Baked beans in tomato sauce are also high in salt and sugar, unless the reduced-salt and -sugar brand is chosen.
4.4	1	0	B6, folate	potas, iron, sel, manga	
8	3.2	0		potas, manga, cop	
7.8	3.5	0	folate	potas, iron, manga, cop	
3.1	1.5	0		potas, iron, manga	
n/k	n/k	n/k	folate	phos, zinc, cop, manga	Commercially made refried beans can be much higher in fat than homemade.
7.8	3.4	0	B6, niacin, folate, E	magnes, potas, phos, iron, cop, manga	
3.2	1.1	0	niacin	manga	
8.5	4	0		magnes, potas, iron, manga	
tr	n/k	0		cal	Made from soybeans, tofu contains all their health benefits (see Soy Milk and Soybeans). Suitable protein food for vegans and a good alternative to dairy products for vegetarians.
2.1	1	0	B1, niacin, folate	potas, iron, manga	These nutrient notes are given for a typical vegetarian burger. Different brands of vegetable burger vary in their nutrient composition, but all contain reasonably high amounts of fat.

Index

Appendix

Alcoholics Anonymous
PO Box 459, Grand Central Station
New York, NY 10163
(212) 870 3400
www.alcoholics.anonymous.org
Alzheimer's Association
919 N. Michigan Avenue, Suite 1000
Chicago, IL 60611-1676
1-800-272-3900
www.alz.org
American Association for Chronic Fatigue Syndrome (AACFS)
7 Van Buren Street
Albany, NY 12206
1-800-232-8710
American Diabetes Association
1600 Duke Street
Alexandria, VA 22314
1-800-232-3472
www.diabetes.org
American Dietetic Association
216 West Jackson Boulevard
Chicago, IL 60806
(312) 899-0040
www.eatright.org
American Health Foundation
320 E 43rd Street
New York, NY 10017
(212) 953-1900
American Heart Association
7272 Greenville Avenue
Dallas, TX 75231
1-800-AHA-USA-1
American Institute for Cancer Research
1759 R Street N.W.
Washington, DC 20009
1-800-843-8114
Arthritis Foundation
1330 W. Peachtree Street
Atlanta, GA 30309
1-800-283-7800
www.arthritis.org
Association for the Promotion of Herbal Healing
2000 Center Street, Suite 1475
Berkeley, CA 94704
Asthma & Allergy Foundation of America
1125 15th Street N.W., Suite 502
Washington, DC 20005
(202) 466-7643
www.housecall.com/sponsors/nho/

1996vha/aafa.html
Consumer Health Information Resource Institute
300E Pink Hill Road
Independence, MO 64111
(816) 228-4595
Green Mountain Herbs
1-800-525-2696
Herbal Pathways
1-800-631-3575
National AIDS Hotline
1-800-342-AIDS
National Eating Disorders Association (NEDO)
6655 South Yale Avenue
Tulsa, OK 74136
(918) 481-4044
National Headache Foundation
428 W St James Place
Chicago, IL 60614
1-800-843-2256
www.headaches.org
National Osteoporosis Foundation
1150 17th Street N.W., Suite 500
Washington, DC 20038
(202) 223-2226
www.nof.org
National Women's Health Network
514 10th Street, N.W., Suite 400
Washington, DC 20004
(202) 347-1140
Office of Alternative Medicine
EPS Room 450
9000 Rockville Pike
Bethesda, MD 20892
(301) 496-7498
Public Health Service
Office of Communications, Room 728-H
200 Independence Avenue S.W.
Washington, DC 20201
(202) 690-6867
US Food & Drug Administration
Office of Consumer Affairs Inquiry Information Line
(301) 827-4420
www.fda.gov
Vegetarian Information Service
1-800-243-4143
World Health Organization
2 UN Plaza, Suite DC2-0970
New York, NY 10017
(212) 963-3952

The author would like to thank Lewis Esson for a mammoth editing task completed in his usual unflappable and professional way, also to Mary Evans, Vanessa Courtier, and all the team at Quadrille; Jane Turnbull and Tony Allen. Thanks also to the following for help with information, facts and figures in many subject areas: British Heart Foundation, British Medical Journal, Child Growth Foundation, Department of Health, Dunn Clinical Nutritition Centre, The Food Commission, The Lancet, MAFF, The National Food Alliance, Rowett Research Institute, The Soil Association, US National Cancer Research Institute, World Cancer Research Fund.

All photographs by Gus Filgate except: pp8, 10, 38, 54, 68, 70, 73, 76, 80, 84, 158, 186, 206—Martin Brigdale; pp161, 164–5, 168–9, 171, 173–5, 179–181, 183, 185, 188, 193, 195–7, 199, 201–3, 205—Patrick McLeavey. The publisher thanks the following for their permission to reproduce the following pictures: 160 The Image Bank/Steve Niedorf; 167 The Image Bank/Nicolas Russell; 170 Getty Images/Ken Fisher; 172 The Stock Market/N. Schafer; 176 Getty Images/Christopher Bissell; 182 Getty Images/Peter Correz; 198 Getty Images/Dale Durfee.